Ruminant Metabolic Diseases

Editor

ROBERT J. VAN SAUN

VETERINARY CLINICS OF NORTH AMERICA: FOOD ANIMAL PRACTICE

www.vetfood.theclinics.com

Consulting Editor
ROBERT A. SMITH

July 2023 • Volume 39 • Number 2

ELSEVIER

1600 John F. Kennedy Boulevard • Suite 1800 • Philadelphia, Pennsylvania, 19103-2899

http://www.vetfood.theclinics.com

VETERINARY CLINICS OF NORTH AMERICA: FOOD ANIMAL PRACTICE Volume 39, Number 2
July 2023 ISSN 0749-0720, ISBN-13: 978-0-443-18226-6

Editor: Taylor Hayes
Developmental Editor: Axell Ivan Jade M. Purificacion

Veterinary Clinics of North America: Food Animal Practice (ISSN 0749-0720) is published in March, July, and November by Elsevier Inc., 360 Park Avenue South, New York, NY 10010-1710. Subscription prices are $267.00 per year (domestic individuals), $533.00 per year (domestic institutions), $100.00 per year (domestic students/residents), $289.00 per year (Canadian individuals), $702.00 per year (Canadian institutions), $342.00 per year (international individuals), $702.00 per year (international institutions), $100.00 per year (Canadian students), and $165.00 (international students). To receive student/resident rate, orders must be accompained by name of affiliated institution, date of term, and the signature of program/residency coordinator on institution letterhead. *Clinics* subscription prices. All prices are subject to change without notice. **POSTMASTER:** Send address changes to *Veterinary Clinics of North America: Food Animal Practice*, Elsevier Health Sciences Division, Subscription Customer Service, 3251 Riverport Lane, Maryland Heights, MO 63043. Customer Service (orders, claims, online, change of address): Elsevier Health Sciences Division, Subscription **Customer Service, 3251 Riverport Lane, Maryland Heights, MO 63043. Tel: 1-800-654-2452 (U.S. and Canada); 314-447-8871 (ouside U.S. and Canada). Fax: 314-447-8029. E-mail: journalscustomerservice-usa@elsevier.com (for print support); journalsonlinesupport-usa@elsevier.com (for online support).**

Reprints. For copies of 100 or more, of articles in this publication, please contact the Commercial Reprints Department, Elsevier Inc., 360 Park Avenue South, New York, NY 10010-1710. Tel.: 212-633-3874; Fax: 212-633-3820; E-mail: reprints@elsevier.com.

Veterinary Clinics of North America: Food Animal Practice is covered in *Current Contents/Agriculture, Biology and Environmental Sciences, MEDLINE/PubMed (Index Medicus), and Excerpta Medica.*

Contributors

CONSULTING EDITOR

ROBERT A. SMITH, DVM, MS
Diplomate, American Board of Veterinary Practitioners; Veterinary Research and Consulting Services, LLC, Greeley, Colorado; Veterinary Research and Consulting Services, LLC, Stillwater, Oklahoma, USA

EDITOR

ROBERT J. VAN SAUN, DVM, MS, PhD
Diplomate, American College of Theriogenologists; Diplomate, American College of Veterinary Internal Medicine (Nutrition); Professor of Veterinary Science and Extension Veterinarian, Department of Veterinary and Biomedical Sciences, College of Agricultural Sciences, Pennsylvania State University, University Park, Pennsylvania, USA

AUTHORS

ANGEL ABUELO, DVM, MRes, MS (Vet Educ), PhD, MRCVS
Diplomate, American Board of Veterinary Practitioners (Dairy Practice); Diplomate, European College of Bovine Health Management; Department of Large Animal Clinical Sciences, College of Veterinary Medicine, Michigan State University, East Lansing, Michigan, USA

JENNA E. BAYNE, DVM, PhD
Diplomate, American College of Veterinary Internal Medicine (Large Animal); Associate Clinical Professor, Department of Clinical Sciences, Auburn University College of Veterinary Medicine, Auburn, Alabama, USA

GENARO ANDRES CONTRERAS, DVM, MS, PhD
Department of Large Animal Clinical Sciences, College of Veterinary Medicine, Michigan State University, East Lansing, Michigan, USA

MEREDYTH JONES COOK, DVM, MS
Diplomate, American College of Veterinary Internal Medicine; Oklahoma State University and Large Animal Consulting and Education, Stillwater, Oklahoma, USA

JOSEF J. GROSS, PD. Dr
Veterinary Physiology, Vetsuisse Faculty, University of Bern, Bern, Switzerland

WALTER GRÜNBERG, Prof., Dr. med. vet, MS, PhD
Diplomate, European College for Animal Reproduction; Diplomate, European College of Bovine Health Management; Associate Diplomate, American College of Veterinary Internal Medicine (Large Animal); Chair of the Clinic for Ruminants and Herd Health of the Justus-Liebig University Giessen, Clinic for Ruminants and Herd Health, Justus-Liebig University, Giessen, Germany

MEGAN S. HINDMAN, MS, DVM
Veterinary Production Animal Medicine Department, Iowa State University, Ames, Iowa, USA

SABINE MANN, Dr. med. vet, PhD
Diplomate, European College of Bovine Health Management; Diplomate, American College of Veterinary Preventive Medicine (Epidemiology); Assistant Professor of Ambulatory and Production Medicine, Department of Population Medicine and Diagnostic Sciences, College of Veterinary Medicine, Cornell University, Ithaca, New York, USA

JESSICA A. A. MCART, DVM, PhD
Diplomate, American Board of Veterinary Practitioners (Dairy Practice); Associate Professor of Ambulatory and Production Medicine, Department of Population Medicine and Diagnostic Sciences, College of Veterinary Medicine, Cornell University, Ithaca, New York, USA

MATTEO MEZZETTI, PhD
Department of Animal Sciences, Food and Nutrition (DIANA), Facoltà di Scienze Agrarie, Alimentari e Ambientali, Università Cattolica del Sacro Cuore, Piacenza, Italy

ANDREA MONGINI, DVM, MS
M&M Veterinary Practice, Inc, Ewetopia Dairy, Inc, Denair, California, USA

GARRETT R. OETZEL, DVM, MS
Emeritus Professor of Food Animal Production Medicine, Department of Medical Sciences, School of Veterinary Medicine, University of Wisconsin-Madison, Madison, USA

JOHN ROCHE, PhD
School of Biological Sciences, University of Auckland, Auckland, New Zealand

ERMINIO TREVISI, PhD
Professor, Department of Animal Sciences, Food and Nutrition (DIANA), Facoltà di Scienze Agrarie, Alimentari e Ambientali, Università Cattolica del Sacro Cuore, Piacenza, Italy

ROBERT J. VAN SAUN, DVM, MS, PhD
Diplomate, American College of Theriogenologists; Diplomate, American College of Veterinary Internal Medicine (Nutrition); Professor of Veterinary Science and Extension Veterinarian, Department of Veterinary and Biomedical Sciences, College of Agricultural Sciences, Pennsylvania State University, University Park, Pennsylvania, USA

Contents

(eg, propylene glycol, glycerol), intravenous glucose solutions, insulin, and other supportive care measures. Induction of parturition or C-section is often carried out to minimize ongoing energy deficits, with variable survival rates. Prolonging gestation to maximize fetal viability often requires intensive care in a hospital setting and carries significant risk to both dam and offspring.

Hyperketonemia: A Marker of Disease, a Sign of a High-Producing Dairy Cow, or Both? **307**

Sabine Mann and Jessica A.A. McArt

This review covers the history and nomenclature of ketosis, the source and use of ketones in transition cows, and the controversial role of hyperketonemia's association with health and production outcomes in dairy cows. With the goal of assisting veterinarians with on-farm diagnostic and treatment methods, the authors present current and evolving means of direct and indirect hyperketonemia detection as well as a summary of treatment modalities and their efficacy. They encourage veterinarians to include hyperketonemia testing as part of their routine physical examinations and contemplate day in milk at hyperketonemia diagnosis when designing treatment and management strategies.

Transition Management in Grazing Systems: Pragmatism Before Precision **325**

John Roche

Grazing cows undergo a similar degree of metabolic stress and immune dysregulation to those reported in high-yielding housed cows consuming total mixed rations, but the ability to manage diet precisely is much less. Feed quality varies from day-to-day and weather can greatly influence amount consumed on any given day. Transition cow management, therefore, tends to revolve around pragmatism as opposed to precision. Mid- and late-gestation management of body condition score is essential to a smooth transition period.

Metabolic Diseases in Beef Cattle **337**

Megan S. Hindman

Beef cattle are less prone to metabolic diseases as compared with dairy cattle; however, there are disease entities of concern in feedlot and cow-calf beef cattle operations. In one study, a prevalence of 2% was found for ruminant acidosis in a feedlot; however, there is little prevalence information published with regard to metabolic diseases in beef cattle.1 Metabolic diseases covered in this article are hypomagnesemia, ruminal acidosis, and all of the common sequelae, polioencephalomalacia, manganese deficiency, and protein-energy malnutrition (PEM).

Urinary Calculi of Small Ruminants **355**

Meredyth Jones Cook

Urolithiasis is a multifactorial disease of male ruminants causing significant economic loss and compromise of animal welfare. Known risk factors include anatomic factors, urine pH, water intake, dietary composition,

and genetic factors. Clinical cases of obstructive urolithiasis may be treated using a variety of medical and surgical interventions, including tube cystostomy, perineal urethrostomy, urinary bladder marsupialization, and modifications of these procedures designed to optimize patient outcome.

Hepatic Lipidosis in Ruminants **371**

Josef J. Gross

Hepatic lipidosis (ie, fatty liver) occurs primarily during the first weeks of lactation in dairy cows because of excessive lipolysis overwhelming the concomitant capacity for beta-oxidation and hepatic export of triglycerides. Besides economic losses due to reduced lactational and reproductive performance, close associations with concomitantly occurring infectious and metabolic health disorders, in particular ketosis, exist. Hepatic lipidosis is not only a consequence from the postpartal negative energy balance but also acts as a disease component for further health disorders.

VETERINARY CLINICS OF NORTH AMERICA: FOOD ANIMAL PRACTICE

FORTHCOMING ISSUES

November 2023
Vitamins and Trace Minerals in Ruminants
Robert J. Van Saun and William S Swecker, Jr., *Editors*

March 2024
Management of Bulls
A Lee Jones and Joseph C. Dalton, *Editors*

July 2024
Foreign Animal Diseases
Elizabeth Parker, Charles Foster, and Carla Huston, *Editors*

RECENT ISSUES

March 2023
Ruminant Diagnostics and Interpretation
John Dustin Loy, Jessie D. Monday, David R. Smith, *Editors*

November 2022
Liver Abnormalities in Cattle
John T. Richeson and Ty E. Lawrence, *Editors*

July 2022
Systems Perspective in Beef Practice
T. Robin Falkner, Dale M. Grotelueschen, and John T. Groves, *Editors*

Preface
Ruminant Metabolic Diseases

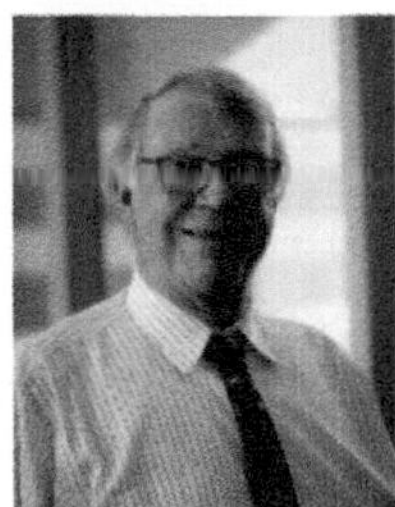

Robert J. Van Saun, DVM, MS, PhD
Editor

This issue of *Veterinary Clinics of North America: Food Animal Practice* continues the series of issues addressing metabolic diseases of ruminant animals. Previous issues were published in 1989, 2000, and 2013, all edited by Dr Thomas Herdt. I am honored to have been asked to be the guest editor for this issue given Dr Herdt was an important mentor during my graduate education in ruminant nutrition and metabolism. I owe much to him relative to my professional development.

Metabolic diseases continue to plague our domestic ruminants, leading to significant economic losses to farm enterprises as well as compromising animal health and welfare. Dr Jack Payne, who developed the Compton Metabolic Profile in the 1970s as a mechanism to evaluate metabolic health, characterized metabolic diseases as consequences of our own making in selecting animals to perform at current levels of productive efficiency. The lactating ruminant is to be greatly appreciated for what she can metabolically accomplish; however, success or failure here is critically dependent upon her ability to nutritionally support gestation and navigate metabolic adaptations around parturition in establishing and supporting her lactation. Unfortunately, our understanding and application of nutrition did not keep up with the advances of genetic selection that has led to these metabolic disease issues. This issue provides the most recent efforts of scientists in solving these metabolic issues and in providing practical preventive and therapeutic interventions.

I am again indebted to my colleagues in the American Association of Bovine Practitioners (AABP) and the American Association of Small Ruminant Practitioners (AASRP) for their suggestions for topical material to be included in developing this issue. Not only did these suggestions help define the scope of the issue but also individuals were willing to be contributors, making my work with this issue that much easier.

The issue leads off with my article reviewing current understanding of contributors to metabolic disease as related to disturbance of homeorhetic regulation in the transition

Vet Clin Food Anim 39 (2023) xi–xii
https://doi.org/10.1016/j.cvfa.2023.04.001
0749-0720/23/© 2023 Published by Elsevier Inc.

from pregnancy to lactation. This article is dedicated to two other mentors, Professors Dale Bauman and Alan Bell, who, during my Cornell graduate education, expanded my understanding of metabolism, nutrient partitioning, and implications to metabolic disease. It was Dale Bauman's seminal article in *Journal of Dairy Science* (1980) describing homeorhetic adaptation that set the stage for our greater appreciation of metabolic challenges during the transition from pregnancy to lactation. Metabolic disease research continues at Cornell and Michigan State and contributes significantly to this issue. Sabine Mann, Angel Abuelo, and Andreas Contreras collaborate to address new insights on the role of inflammation, immunity, and antioxidant status on transition metabolism as an underpinning of metabolic disease. Traditional metabolic disease concerns related to glucose, calcium, and magnesium homeostasis are addressed in articles authored by Jessica McArt, Sabine Mann, and Garrett Oetzel. Our ongoing challenges with calcium homeostasis are explored with new research on phosphorus metabolism as addressed in the article authored by Walter Grünberg. Josef Gross connects altered liver metabolism and fatty infiltration as a primary facilitator of metabolic disease, immunologic failure, and impaired reproductive performance in the transition ruminant. With the staging of metabolic disease addressed, the article by Matteo Mezzetti and Erminio Trevesi provides mechanisms for monitoring the success or failure of transition metabolic adaptation. John Roche's article addresses a challenge in managing the transition metabolism in a grazing environment, which would be inclusive of other ruminant species.

As this issue addresses metabolic disease of all ruminants, articles by Andrea Mongini and Jenna Bayne detail new perspectives on pregnancy toxemia management and therapeutic interventions in small ruminants. A range of metabolic diseases of beef cattle is described by Megan Hindman. Although not commonly considered a metabolic disease, Meredyth Jones makes the argument that urinary calculi of small ruminants is a metabolic disease. Collectively, these articles provide the practitioner with the most current research on underpinning mechanisms of metabolic disease as well as practical regimens for managing and preventing these diseases in ruminant animals.

This issue would not be the educational resource that it is without the dedicated efforts of all the authors. I am greatly indebted to the distinguished international scientists for their willingness and efforts to be contributors to this issue. I would also like to thank those individuals who accepted my invitation and served as independent reviewers of the articles. It is through the efforts of all these individuals that the information provided is of the highest quality.

Robert J. Van Saun, DVM, MS, PhD
Department of Veterinary and
Biomedical Sciences
College of Agricultural Sciences
Pennsylvania State University
108C Animal
Veterinary and Biomedical Sciences Building
University Park, PA 16802-3500, USA

E-mail address:
rjv10@psu.edu

Ruminant Metabolic Diseases: Perturbed Homeorhesis

Robert J. Van Saun, DVM, MS, PhD, DACT, DACVIM (Nutrition)

KEYWORDS

- Homeorhesis • Transition metabolism • Metabolic disease • Ruminant
- Inflammation

KEY POINTS

- Dysregulation of homeorhetic adaptations to nutrient partitioning results in risk for common metabolic diseases of ruminants.
- A simplistic perspective of disturbed homeostatic regulation of glucose, calcium, magnesium, or other essential nutrient does not completely explain metabolic disease pathogenesis and potential for preventive practices.
- Activated inflammation from physiologic stressors, pathogen exposure, adipose lipolysis, or other pro-inflammatory mediators are responsible for homeorhetic dysregulation.
- Transition management to minimize postpartum disease should be multipronged in addressing cow body condition, dry matter intake, sufficient nutrient intake, and reduction of inflammation initiators.

BACKGROUND

The modern dairy cow is often described as a high-performance metabolic machine given her ability to transform consumed feed into copious amounts of highly nutritious milk in support of the human population. Genetic selection used to achieve current levels of performance has challenged the cow's metabolic capabilities with nutritional strategies somewhat lagging. The mammary gland role in metabolic disease susceptibility is evidenced by studies comparing cows transitioning from pregnancy to calving with or without ensuing lactation. Canfield and Butler showed eliminating negative energy balance (NEB) associated with lactation by not milking cows following calving resulted in earlier return to reproductive cyclicity.[1] Mastectomized cows demonstrated lesser declines in serum vitamins A and E and phosphorus concentrations, more positive energy balance as indicated by lower nonesterified fatty acid (NEFA) concentration and no hypocalcemia compared with intact cows initiating a lactation.[2] Mastectomized cows did not experience reduction in peripheral blood

Department of Veterinary and Biomedical Sciences, College of Agricultural Sciences, Pennsylvania State University, 108 C Animal, Veterinary and Biomedical Sciences Building, University Park, PA 16802-3500, USA
E-mail address: rjv10@psu.edu

Vet Clin Food Anim 39 (2023) 185–201
https://doi.org/10.1016/j.cvfa.2023.02.001

T-lymphocyte populations, which would be associated with immune suppression, compared with intact cows and this response was not a result of cortisol secretion initiating parturition.[3] Metabolic and physiologic changes occurring as the cow shifts nutritional priorities from supporting pregnancy to sustaining lactation are associated with a complement of health issues experienced in the immediate postpartum period.[4,5] A plethora of studies have targeted these metabolic issues to better understand metabolic transition and impact on cow health, productivity, and reproduction.[5–10] This review discusses and integrates the various scientific perspectives on the origin of metabolic diseases in ruminants with emphasis on the critical period where the dam transitions from a state of pregnancy into one of lactation.

DEFINING THE TRANSITION PERIOD

The period where the ruminant animal physiologically changes from a non-lactating pregnant state to a nonpregnant lactating state is commonly termed the "transition period." Drackley directed focus on this transition period as the critical entity in dairy cattle production and defined it as the 3 weeks before and following calving.[7] Endocrine changes initiating parturition, lactogenesis, and galactopoiesis associated with metabolic modifications, directing nutrient partitioning and utilization relative to nutrient intake ultimately stage the cow's success or failure during early lactation.[11] Most of these metabolic and physiologic changes occur within this 6-week window; however, other studies have suggested an expanded timeframe of influence on postpartum performance.[12] Different nutrient supply levels during the dry period had no impact on postpartum performance, but overfeeding energy in the early weeks of the dry period (ie, far-off dry) had greater negative impact on postpartum metabolic status and health.[13–16]

Others have suggested that the period of interest relative to postpartum disease susceptibility should extend into the late lactation period as the end of lactation greatly influences body condition score (BCS) for the dry period and into early lactation.[17–19] This is critically important in cow management in grazing herds (see John Roche's article, "Transition Management in Grazing Systems – Pragmatism Before Precision," in this issue). The negative impact of excess BCS was first described as "fat cow syndrome."[20] This disease propagated much research into liver function during transition and the role of hepatic lipidosis in postpartum disease.[21–24] Cows with excess BCS experienced greater body condition loss in transition that was associated with greater oxidative stress, which may predispose the cow to metabolic disease.[25] Lipid mobilization, though an essential response to initiating lactation, has been recognized as a source of inflammatory mediators that could derail the metabolic adaptation to lactation.[26,27]

In spite of the volumes of published studies addressing metabolic complications and associated nutritional concerns of the transition cow over the ensuing decades, dairy cattle health surveys have not shown a significant change in metabolic disease prevalence (**Table 1**), though the data must be interpreted with caution as these were producer identified disease conditions.[28–31] Part of the problem is the confusion over transition period definitions, practicality and time constraints of suggested management practices, and differing recommendations from advisors.[32–34] Epidemiologic studies would indicate that more than 50% of calving dairy cows will experience one or more health events in the early postpartum period that increase early lactation involuntary culling, reduce productive efficiency, and impair reproductive performance.[35–37] This outcome underscores the problem with defining metabolic disease in simple terms with blood analyte associations.

Table 1
Percent of cows that were producer identified to have postpartum health conditions as reported in the National Animal Health Monitoring System reports from 1996, 2002, 2008, and 2014

Health Condition	1996	2002	2008	2014
Milk fever	5.9 ± 0.1	5.2 ± 0.1	4.9 ± 0.1	2.8 ± 0.2
Retained fetal membranes	7.8 ± 0.2	7.8 ± 0.2	7.8 ± 0.2	4.5 ± 0.4
Clinical mastitis	13.1 ± 0.3	14.7 ± 0.3	16.5 ± 0.5	24.8 ± 2.4
Displaced abomasum	2.0 ± 0.2	3.5 ± 0.1	3.5 ± 0.1	2.2 ± 0.2
Reproductive infertility[a]	11.6 ± 0.3	11.9 ± 0.3	12.9 ± 0.3	8.2 ± 0.5
Reproductive disease[b]	NR[c]	3.7 ± 0.2	4.6 ± 0.3	
Dystocia	NR	NR	NR	4.7 ± 0.7
Metritis	NR	NR	NR	6.9 ± 0.8
Lameness	10.5 ± 0.3	11.6 ± 0.3	14.0 ± 0.4	16.8 ± 1.6
Other diseases	2.2 ± 0.2	0.8 ± 0.1	0.6 ± 0.1	0.6 ± 0.3
Ketosis	NR	NR	NR	4.2 ± 0.5

Data are based on all operation sizes.
[a] Cow defined as being not pregnant by 150 d in milk.
[b] Includes dystocia and metritis in these reports.
[c] Not reported in the published report.

PERSPECTIVES ON METABOLIC DISEASE

Hypocalcemia had been recognized before the twentieth century and postpartum disease concerns were gaining much interest in middle decades of the century. Jack Payne, developer of the Compton Metabolic Profile test, first defined metabolic disease as a man-made consequence of high-production strain on the cow coupled with intensive systems of nutrition and husbandry.[38] The definition of production diseases was expanded by Sommer (cited by Rowlands[38]) to include the infectious diseases of mastitis and metritis as they were believed to be related to production level.[38] In contrast to the metabolic disease perspective touted by Payne where metabolic disease was "induced" by high production, current thinking would suggest high milk production reflects a state of cow health and lack of stress. This is not to state that the highly productive cow is not on the "metabolic edge" of potential derailment of health.

Classically, metabolic diseases are defined as those diseases where controls to maintain specific nutrient homeostasis have been lost. Common ruminant examples relative to calcium (Ca), phosphorus, magnesium (Mg), and glucose are hypocalcemia (eg, milk fever), hypophosphatemia (eg, downer cow), hypomagnesemia (eg, grass tetany/lactation tetany), hypoglycemia (eg, ketosis or pregnancy toxemia), respectively. Other articles in this issue will address details of these diseases and highlight their complex etiopathogenesis. Unfortunately, this perspective is taking an Occam's razor approach to metabolic diseases in assuming the simplest explanation is the correct one.

Intensified interest in dairy cow metabolic diseases stemmed from 1980s Cornell research identifying hypocalcemia to be associated with eight other postparturient diseases.[39] Curtis and colleagues recognized various postpartum metabolic diseases were interconnected and related to dry cow nutrition,[40] which then spurred intensive research addressing what became known as the "transition cow," though the concept could be applied to small ruminants in addressing pregnancy toxemia (see Andrea

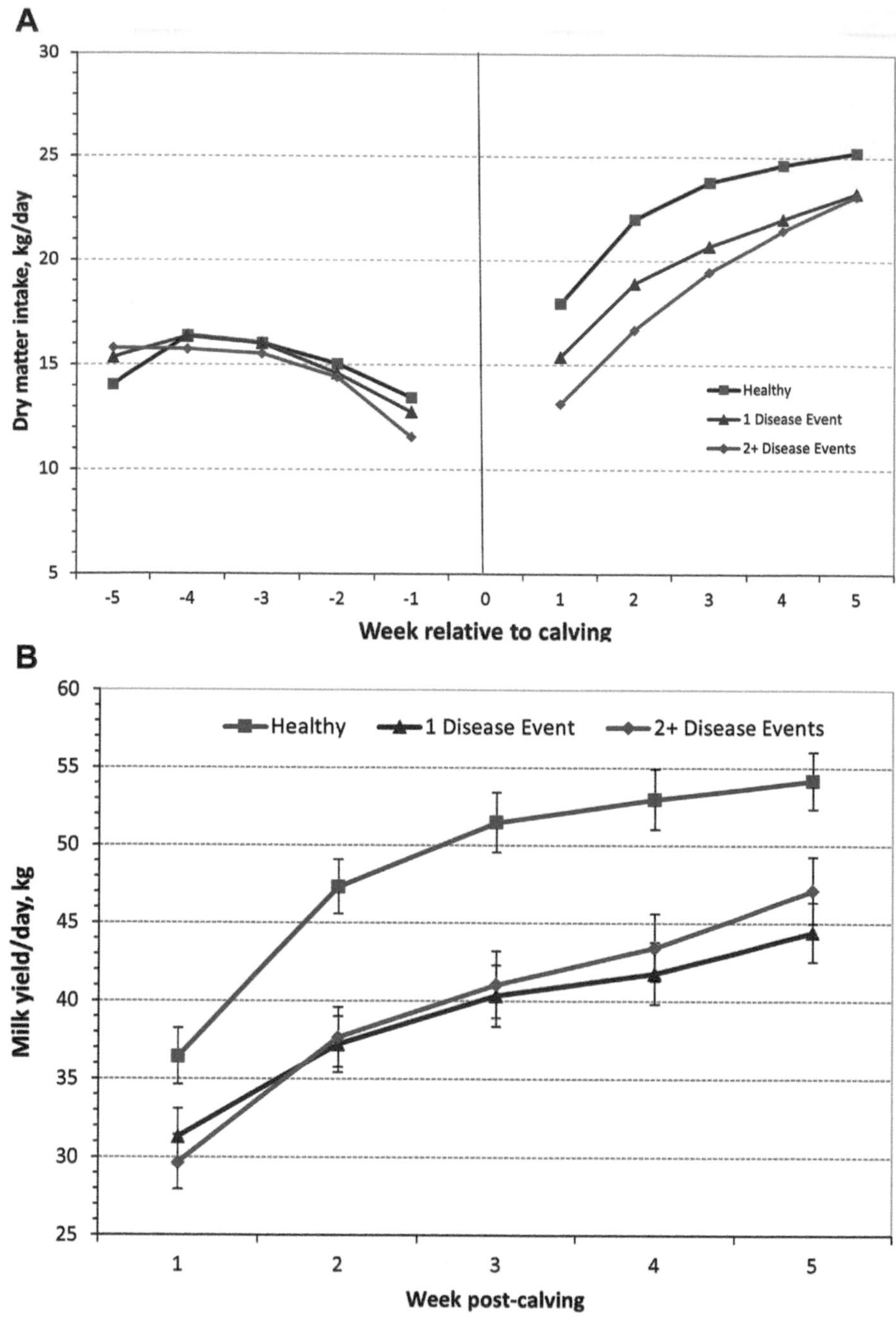

Fig. 1. Comparisons of prepartum and postpartum dry matter intake (*A*) and milk yield (*B*) for Holstein cows experiencing no disease events (*square*), 1 event (*triangle*), or 2 or more (*diamond*) events.

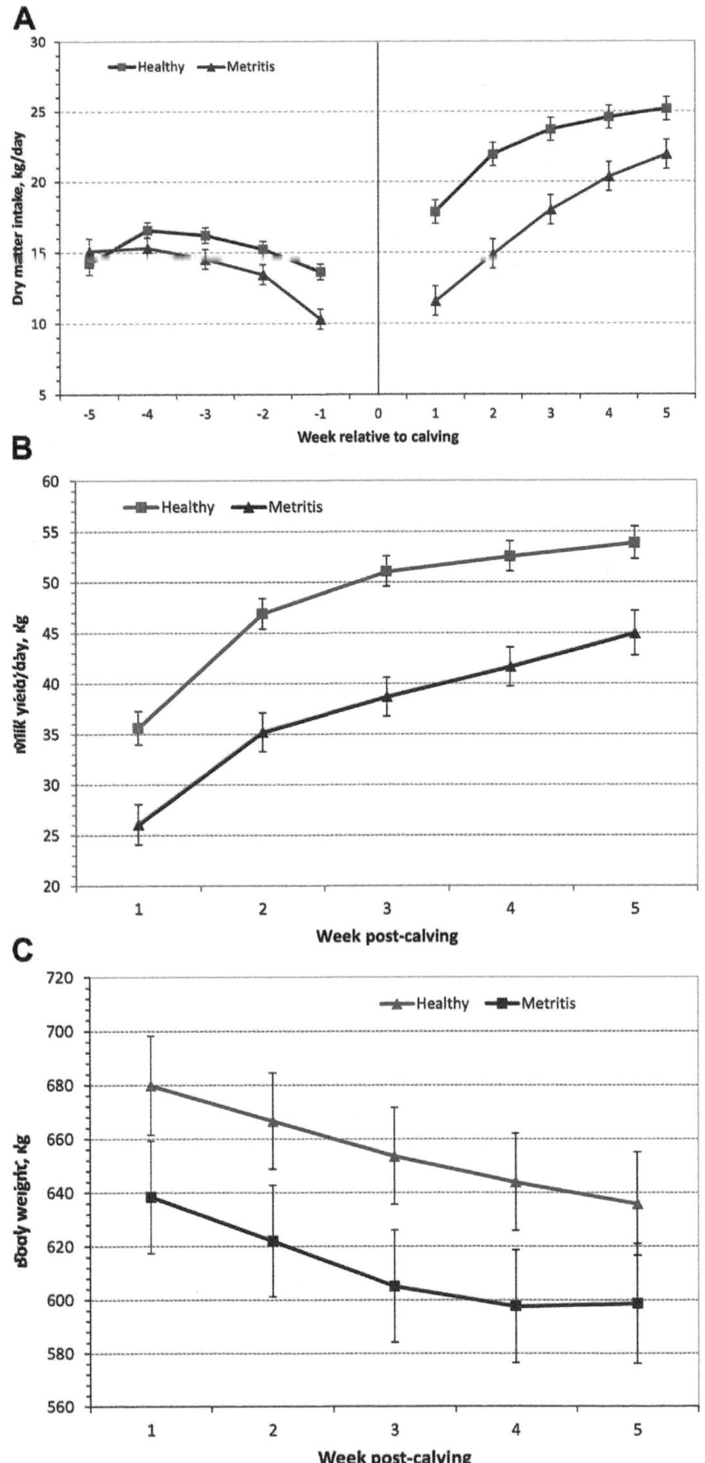

Fig. 2. Comparisons of prepartum and postpartum dry matter intake (*A*), milk yield (*B*), and postpartum body weight (*C*) for Holstein cows experiencing no disease events (*square*) with

Mongini and Robert J. Van Saun's article, "Pregnancy Toxemia in Sheep and Goats," in this issue) and similar postpartum disease conditions of ruminants.

At a transition cow symposium held at the 86th American Society of Animal Science annual meeting, Bell presented a paper that quantified the metabolic challenge of transition. Using data collected from Holstein cows, net uterine and mammary uptake of key metabolic fuels, glucose, amino acids, and fatty acids were calculated in support of pregnancy (last 2 weeks) and lactation (4 days in milk). These data showed a threefold, twofold, and nearly fourfold increase in glucose, amino acids, and fatty acids, respectively, uptake from late pregnancy to early lactation.[6] Critical to this perspective is acknowledging dry matter intake (DMI) is reduced by 25% to 30% during this period.[41] Homeorhetic control of these metabolic adaptations required in transitioning from a state of pregnancy to lactation seem to be the lynchpin to a ruminant's success or failure in this transition.[11,42,43] When homeorhetic controls are unable to maintain critical nutrient homeostasis in supporting productive functions, metabolic disease is a potential consequence.[5,43–45] These perspectives staged our initial understanding of transition cow diseases, and in the ensuing decades, underpinning metabolic and immunologic factors have been elucidated.

LYNCHPINS TO RUMINANT METABOLIC DISEASE

As metabolic diseases have been researched over the past 5 decades, one obvious conclusion has emerged: underlying cause(s) is/are complex with no simple solution to any disease process. Our understanding of metabolic disease is often reduced to focus on the key metabolite of interest leading to blood measurements of single analytes reflecting energy status (NEFA, β-hydroxybutyrate [BHB]), Ca, or Mg used in diagnostic or disease risk assessment. This "reductionist" perspective is limiting our understanding of underlying causes of metabolic disease, though a practical field approach. The use of metabolic profiling or multiple analyte indexes have been suggested to obtain a wider understanding of metabolic changes.[46,47] Newer diagnostic tools such as genomics, metabolomics, and proteomics are providing a much broader perspective on metabolic and immunologic modifications occurring during a disease process.[48] A "systems" approach to understanding metabolic disease is advocated.[49] This is more a research-based due to the sophisticated methodologies required and associated cost but may provide further insights as to underlying causes of metabolic disease and identify more robust biomarkers of disease or disease risks (see Matteo Mezzetti and Erminio Trevisi's article, "Methods of Evaluating the Potential Success or Failure of Transition Dairy Cows," in this issue).[46] The following are critical contributing factors leading to potential failure in the ruminant transition from pregnancy to lactation.

- *Hypocalcemia.* Hypocalcemia has been intensively researched as a metabolic disease entity itself as well as its association with other diseases, yet there is not a full understanding of mechanisms responsible for the pathogenesis.[50] Hypocalcemia impacts not only muscle function but also the immune response. Complexity here is demonstrated in animal performance responses identified relative to subclinical hypocalcemia.[51] Of interest is the observation that cows

cows diagnosed with metritis (*triangle*). Cows with metritis were not assessed relative to severity and may have had comorbidities. Prepartum intake was influenced by a disease by time interaction ($P = .02$), whereas postpartum intake was influenced by disease status ($P = .0002$) and its interaction with time ($P = .01$). Healthy cows had greater ($P = .0001$) milk yield. There was no disease effect or disease status by time effect on body weight.

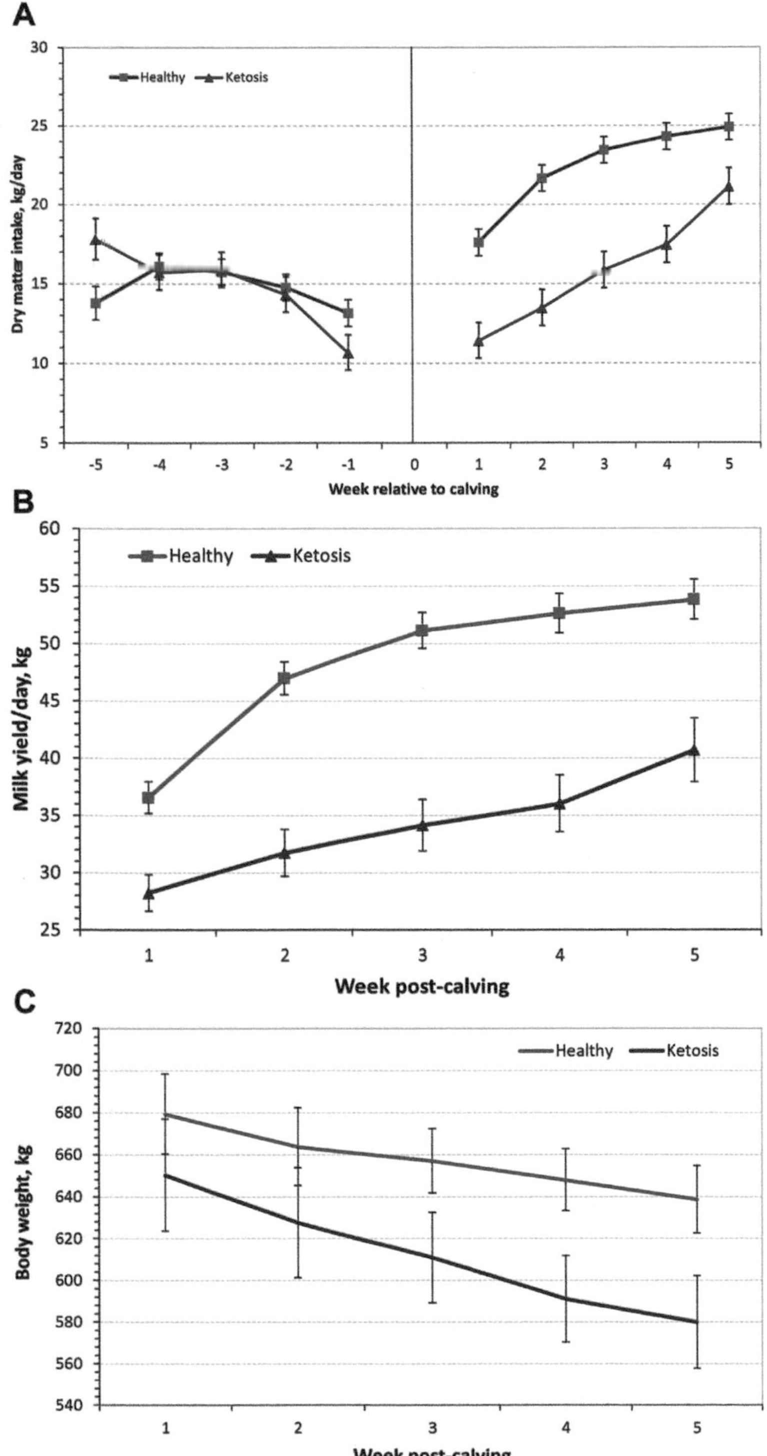

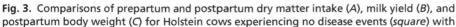

Fig. 3. Comparisons of prepartum and postpartum dry matter intake (*A*), milk yield (*B*), and postpartum body weight (*C*) for Holstein cows experiencing no disease events (*square*) with

experiencing transitory subclinical hypocalcemia had greater milk production compared with other subclinical hypocalcemia states. Does this suggest a transitory drop in blood calcium concentration is an important response to postpartum health and productivity? The Jessica A.A. McArt and Garrett R. Oetzel's article, "Considerations in the Diagnosis and Treatment of Early Lactation Calcium Disturbances," in this issue describe the states of eucalcemia and dyscalcemia relative to calcium homeorhesis.

- *Negative Energy Balance.* The initial metabolic disease focus was on energy metabolism addressing NEB and associated lipid mobilization.[17,21,24,44,52–54] Concerns of energy metabolism and NEB were related to the documented decline in DMI from late gestation through early lactation.[55] The severity of NEB as measured by NEFA concentration has been associated with greater postpartum disease risk[10]; however, evidence to suggest NEFA concentrations induce disease is limited. Similarly, infusing BHB does not induce disease conditions, though its elevated concentration is associated with disease risk.[56] Clearly, there is a more complex interaction of biomarkers leading to NEB-related disease such as ketosis (see Sabine Mann and Jessica A.A. McArt's article, "Hyperketonemia: a Marker of Disease, a Sign of a High-Producing Dairy Cow, or Both?" in this issue). Both NEFA and BHB do alter the cow's immune response.
- *Liver Metabolism.* The liver is the key metabolic organ of the body as it receives all absorbed nutrients from the alimentary tract. It is only second to the kidneys in terms of blood flow. In ruminants the liver is primarily responsible for maintaining blood glucose concentration through the process of gluconeogenesis primarily from propionate and amino acids. Much focus relative to metabolic disease has been on hepatic lipidosis and its impact on gluconeogenic capacity and its role in the inflammatory response. Liver function and disease are further discussed in the Josef J. Gross' article, "Hepatic Lipidosis in Ruminants," in this issue.
- *Dry Matter Intake.* An adequate consumption of feed that is nutritionally balanced is the foundation of good nutritional management practices. Bertics and colleagues suggested that maximizing DMI could mitigate perturbed metabolism and minimize hepatic fatty infiltration.[57] The role of DMI and its interaction with energy intake evolved into recommendations to minimize the late gestational DMI decline and controlling energy intake as the means to more successful postpartum metabolic status.[15,58]
- *Protein Status.* Dietary protein was also considered as a contributor given the potential of amino acids in supporting gluconeogenesis in early lactation.[59,60] Mobilization of labile protein occurs prepartum and can influence the cow's response to NEB.[61] Cows mobilizing less muscle had higher BHB concentrations potentially due to less glucose availability.[61] Amino acids also perform important metabolic roles in lipid transport, immune cell communication and function, export proteins, and inflammatory response. In spite of these multiple metabolic and physiologic roles, most transition cow studies showed no measurable cow production responses to dietary protein,[62,63] though a higher dietary protein

cows diagnosed with ketosis (*triangle*). Cows with ketosis may have had comorbidities. There was no disease effect or disease status by time effect on body weight. Prepartum intake was influenced by a disease by time interaction ($P = .0002$), whereas postpartum intake was influenced by disease status ($P < .0001$) and its interaction with time ($P < .0001$). Healthy cows had greater ($P = .0001$) milk yield. There was no disease effect or disease status by time effect on body weight.

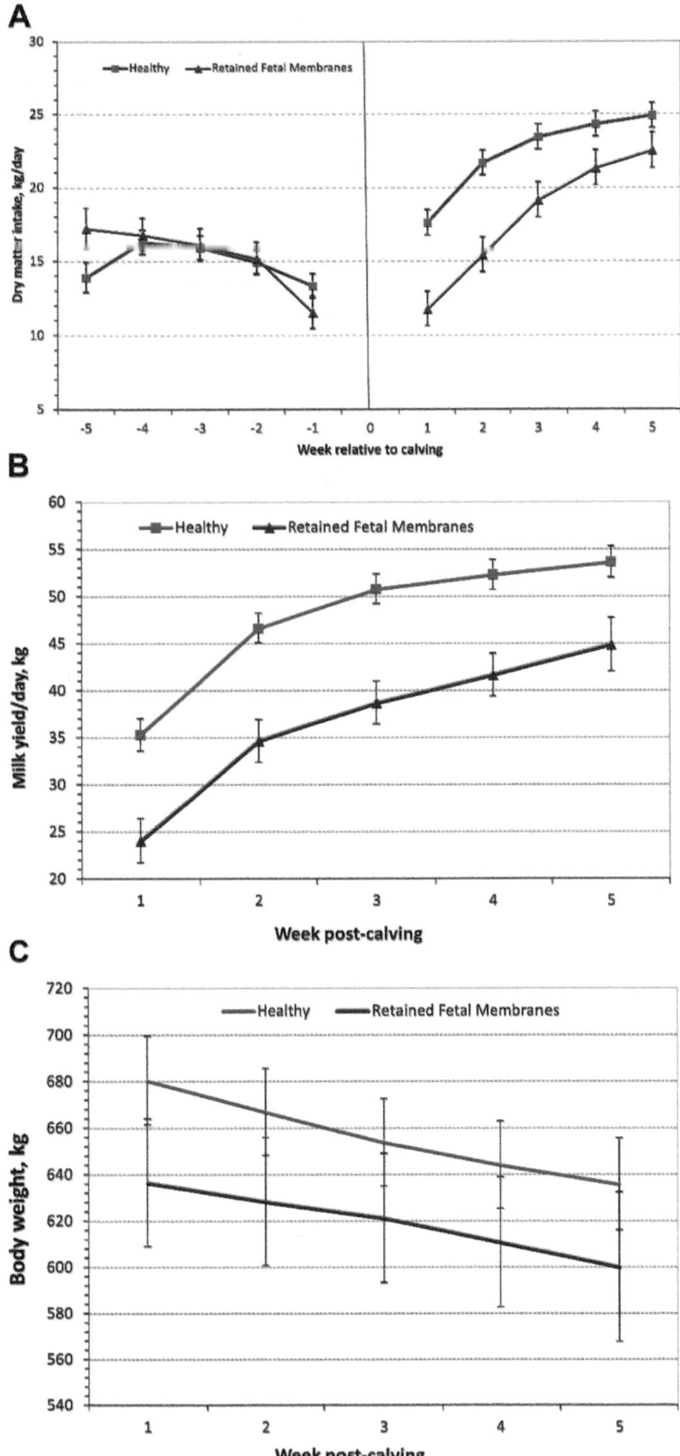

Fig. 4. Comparisons of prepartum and postpartum dry matter intake (*A*), milk yield (*B*), and postpartum body weight (*C*) for Holstein cows experiencing no disease events (*square*) with

content (14%) is recommended for springing heifers compared with mature cows.[64] The supplementation of rumen-protected methionine has shown promise in improving metabolic and immunologic health of the transition cow.[65,66]

- *Immune Response.* Beyond dysregulation of homeostasis as an underpinning issue with transition cow diseases, the recognition of altered immune response has been implicated in diseases of retained fetal membranes,[67] mastitis, and metritis.[68–71] Endocrine and glucocorticoid secretion around the time of calving are considered part of the underlying cause of immune suppression as well as the interaction of NEB with immune cell function.[68,71] Refer to the Angel Abuelo and colleagues' article, "Metabolic Factors at the Crossroads of Periparturient Immunity and Inflammation," in this issue for more detailed information on the role of immune activation and periparturient disease.
- *Other Mitigating Factors.* Cook and Nordlund have suggested most periparturient problems are linked not to nutritional mismanagement, but environmental stressors.[72] The number of pen moves disrupting group social hierarchy, comingling of primiparous and multiparous cows, overstocking, limited feed bunk space, water accessibility, and heat stress are just a few environmental issues that can further disturb metabolic adaptations during transition leading to greater disease risk.[72–74]

PERTURBED HOMEORHESIS: A NEW PERSPECTIVE

The concept of homeostasis defined as "maintaining a steady state" is one familiar to most as it is basic to teaching of biologic science. A seminal paper by Bauman and Currie brought attention to metabolic adaptations associated with physiologic states termed "homeorhesis." In contrast to homeostasis, homeorhesis is defined as the exquisite coordination of multiple tissues or organs in prioritizing essential nutrients in support of a given physiologic state. Homeorhetic initiation of lactation is controlled by growth hormone will induce a period of NEB accompanied by lipid mobilization.[43] The question here is whether or not excessive or prolonged NEB and lipolysis are the initiators of postpartum disease as suggested by current perspectives of NEFA and BHB concentrations and their association with periparturient diseases.

Much progress has been made in advancing our understanding of metabolic adaptations associated with metabolic diseases and transition cow management practices; however, we have not significantly impacted transition cow health events with the exception of hypocalcemia. In such a situation, it may be necessary to reassess our perspective. Activation of an inflammatory response has become a focal point of research in transition cow metabolism and dysregulation of homeorhesis.[27,75–79] Pro-inflammatory mediators have dramatic negative effects on intake[80–82] and prioritization of nutrients, especially glucose and amino acids, in support of the immune response.[83] Inflammatory response activation measured by increased pro-inflammatory mediators and hepatic release of acute phase proteins can result from lipomobilization (especially with excess BCS), tissue trauma, heat, and other stress responses, as well as endotoxins from inflammatory disease conditions (ie, rumen acidosis, lameness).[26,77,84–86]

cows diagnosed with retained fetal membrantes (*triangle*). Cows with retained fetal membranes may have had comorbidities. Prepartum intake was influenced by a disease by time interaction ($P = .008$), whereas postpartum intake was influenced by disease status ($P = .002$) and its interaction with time ($P = .01$). Healthy cows had greater ($P = .0001$) milk yield. There was no disease effect or disease status by time effect on body weight.

Liver function is adversely affected by an inflammatory state.[75,87] Overfeeding energy (150% of requirement) in the far-off prepartum diet was associated with inducing an inflammatory response and affecting liver function compared with cows fed 100% requirement independent of the close-up diet.[88] It would seem that activation of an inflammatory response and its impact on glucose utilization and diversion of amino acids to nonproductive purposes can provide a unifying model for dysregulation of metabolic adaptations during the transition period resulting in periparturient diseases.[79,89,90]

CLINICAL CASE OUTCOMES

Using cow performance data from two published feeding trials at Pennsylvania State University,[91,92] data on cow DMI, body weight change, milk production, and health events were obtained for 30 cows in each study (n = 60) over a 10-week period centered on calving. Twenty-three cows (38%) were identified as not having any adverse health event. Thirty-seven cows (62%) had one or more health events (mean: 1.8 events/cow; range: 1–5 events/cow). Health events were not gauged by severity but only if some treatment or diagnosis was recorded in herd health records. Health conditions of mastitis (n = 14), metritis (n = 12), ketosis (n = 11), retained fetal membranes (n = 10), and udder edema (n = 15) had sufficient numbers for comparisons.

Healthy cows had greater DMI in the 5-week postpartum compared with cows with 1 or 2+ disease events (**Fig. 1**A) and produced more milk (**Fig. 1**B). Although prepartum intake declined more for diseased cows compared with healthy, this was not significant nor was body weight different postpartum. In reviewing responses for specific diseases, these comparisons were more disparate. **Fig. 2** shows the cow responses between healthy cows and those having a diagnosis of metritis. The decline in prepartum intake (see **Fig. 2**A) is consistent with other reports.[93,94] Metritis-affected cows had significantly lower milk yield (see **Fig. 2**B) over the 5-week period, and the body weight (see **Fig. 2**C) was not statistically different. Healthy cows also showed a lesser decline in prepartum and markedly higher postpartum DMI compared with cows that would experience ketosis postpartum (**Fig. 3**A) consistent with other reports.[95,96] There was a significant difference in milk yield (**Fig. 3**B) and body weight at weeks 4 and 5 postpartum (**Fig. 3**C). Similar comparisons were made for cows with retained fetal membranes versus healthy cows (**Fig. 4**).Collectively, these cow responses demonstrate the loss of milk as the predominate effect of postpartum disease and not body weight. The calculated milk loss based on dietary energy intake differences underestimated observed milk production losses, not accounting for body condition losses providing some of the missing energy. These observations would be consistent with a lack of glucose to support milk yield most likely due to a pro-inflammatory process reducing intake and immune cell glucose consumption.

CLINICS CARE POINTS

- Ruminant animals undergo a highly coordinated metabolic adaptation to ensure there is sufficient glucose to support pregnancy and following parturition, lactation during a period of low dry matter intake supported by variable extent of lipolysis and labile protein mobilization
- Metabolic diseases are a consequence of dysregulation of these homeostatic mechanisms resulting in excessive lipid mobilization, hepatic fatty infiltration, and body protein depletion.

- Although specific blood analytes (ie, nonesterified fatty acid, β-hydroxybutyrate, calcium) are highly associated with postpartum disease risk, they may not directly induce disease.
- Underlying causes of ruminant metabolic diseases are not well characterized but are most likely related to an active pro-inflammatory response induced by many factors and contributing directly to reduced dry matter intake prepartum and postpartum.
- Management of the transition ruminant animal should focus on managing prepartum body condition score, intake stability, sufficient prepartum nutrient delivery, and minimizing potential inflammatory inducing conditions.

DISCLOSURES

Grant funding received from Pennsylvania Department of Agriculture, American Dairy Goat Association and, Zoetis.

REFERENCES

1. Canfield R, Butler W. Energy balance and pulsatile LH secretion in early postpartum dairy cattle. Domest Anim Endocrinol 1990;7:323–30.
2. Goff JP, Kimura K, Horst RL. Effect of mastectomy on milk fever, energy, and vitamins A, E, and β-carotene status at parturition. J Dairy Sci 2002;85:1427–36.
3. Kimura K, Goff JP, Kehrli ME Jr, et al. Effects of mastectomy on composition of peripheral blood mononuclear cell populations in periparturient dairy cows. J Dairy Sci 2002;85:1437–44.
4. Goff J, Horst R. Physiological changes at parturition and their relationship to metabolic disorders. J Dairy Sci 1997;80:1260–8.
5. Ingvartsen KL. Feeding- and management-related diseases in the transition cow: Physiological adaptation around calving and strategies to reduce feeding-related diseases. Anim Feed Sci Technol 2006;126:175–213.
6. Bell AW. Regulation of organic nutrient metabolism during transition from late pregnancy to early lactation. J Anim Sci 1995;73:2804–19.
7. Drackley JK. Biology of dairy cows during the transition period: The final frontier? J Dairy Sci 1999;82:2259–73.
8. Drackley JK, Dann HM, Douglas N, et al. Physiological and pathological adaptations in dairy cows that may increase susceptibility to periparturient diseases and disorders. Ital J Anim Sci 2005;4:323–44.
9. Grummer RR. Impact of changes in organic nutrient metabolism on feeding the transition dairy cow. J Anim Sci 1995;73:2820–33.
10. Wankhade PR, Manimaran A, Kumaresan A, et al. Metabolic and immunological changes in transition dairy cows: A review. Vet World 2017;10:1367–77.
11. Bauman DE, Currie WB. Partitioning of nutrients during pregnancy and lactation: a review of mechanisms involving homeostasis and homeorhesis. J Dairy Sci 1980;63:1514–29.
12. Daros RR, Weary DM, von Keyserlingk MAG. Invited review: Risk factors for transition period disease in intensive grazing and housed dairy cattle. J Dairy Sci 2022;105:4734–48.
13. Dann H, Litherland N, Underwood J, et al. Diets during far-off and close-up dry periods affect periparturient metabolism and lactation in multiparous cows. J Dairy Sci 2006;89:3563–77.

14. Douglas G, Overton T, Bateman H II, et al. Prepartal plane of nutrition, regardless of dietary energy source, affects periparturient metabolism and dry matter intake in Holstein cows. J Dairy Sci 2006;89:2141–57.
15. Janovick N, Boisclair Y, Drackley J. Prepartum dietary energy intake affects metabolism and health during the periparturient period in primiparous and multiparous Holstein cows. J Dairy Sci 2011;94:1385–400.
16. Dann H, Morin D, Bollero G, et al. Prepartum intake, postpartum induction of ketosis, and periparturient disorders affect the metabolic status of dairy cows. J Dairy Sci 2005;88:3249–61.
17. Barletta RV, Maturana Filho M, Carvalho PD, et al. Association of changes among body condition score during the transition period with NEFA and BHBA concentrations, milk production, fertility, and health of Holstein cows. Theriogenology 2017;104:30–6.
18. Roche JR, Kay JK, Friggens NC, et al. Assessing and managing body condition score for the prevention of metabolic disease in dairy cows. Vet Clin North Am Food Anim Pract 2013;29:323–36.
19. Roche JR, Macdonald KA, Schutz KE, et al. Calving body condition score affects indicators of health in grazing dairy cows. J Dairy Sci 2013;96:5811–25.
20. Morrow DA. Fat cow syndrome. J Dairy Sci 1976;59:1625–9.
21. Bobe G, Young J, Beitz D. Invited review: pathology, etiology, prevention, and treatment of fatty liver in dairy cows. J Dairy Sci 2004;87:3105–24.
22. Geelen MJ, Wensing T. Studies on hepatic lipidosis and coinciding health and fertility problems of high-producing dairy cows using the "Utrecht fatty liver model of dairy cows". A review. Vet Q 2006;28:90–104.
23. Hammon HM, Sturmer G, Schneider F, et al. Performance and metabolic and endocrine changes with emphasis on glucose metabolism in high-yielding dairy cows with high and low fat content in liver after calving. J Dairy Sci 2009;92:1554–66.
24. Grummer RR. Etiology of lipid-related metabolic disorders in periparturient dairy cows. J Dairy Sci 1993;76:3882–96.
25. Bernabucci U, Ronchi B, Lacetera N, et al. Influence of body condition score on relationships between metabolic status and oxidative stress in periparturient dairy cows. J Dairy Sci 2005;88:2017–26.
26. Alharthi A, Zhou Z, Lopreiato V, et al. Body condition score prior to parturition is associated with plasma and adipose tissue biomarkers of lipid metabolism and inflammation in Holstein cows. J Anim Sci Biotechnol 2018;9:12.
27. Sordillo LM, Raphael W. Significance of metabolic stress, lipid mobilization, and inflammation on transition cow disorders. Vet Clin North Am Food Anim Pract 2013;29:267–78.
28. USDA. In: Ft, editor. Part I: Reference of 1996 dairy management pracCNAHM. Collins, CO: USDA-APHIS-VS; 1996. p. 47.
29. USDA. In: Ft, editor. Part I: Reference of dairy health and management in the United StateVystem NAHM. Collins, CO: USDA:APHIS:VS,CEAH; 2002. p. 92.
30. USDA. Dairy 2007, Part I: reference of dairy cattle health and management practices in the United States. In: 2007 In: USDA-APHIS-VS C. Collins, CO: USDA-APHIS-VS, CEAH; 2007. p. 128.
31. USDA. Dairy 2014, Health and Management Practices on U.S. Dairy Operations. In: Ft, editor. 2014 In: USDA-APHIS-VS-CEAH-NAHMS. Collins, CO: USDA-APHIS-VS-CEAH-NAHMS; 2018. p. 216.
32. Mills KE, Weary DM, von Keyserlingk MAG. Identifying barriers to successful dairy cow transition management. J Dairy Sci 2020;103:1749–58.

33. Redfern EA, Sinclair LA, Robinson PA. Why isn't the transition period getting the attention it deserves? Farm advisors' opinions and experiences of managing dairy cow health in the transition period. Prev Vet Med 2021;194:105424. https://doi.org/10.1016/j.prevetmed.2021.105424.
34. Couto Serrenho R, Church C, McGee D, et al. Environment, nutrition, and management practices for far-off, close-up, and fresh cows on Canadian dairy farms-A retrospective descriptive study. J Dairy Sci 2022;105:1797–814.
35. Bigras-Poulin M, Meek A, Martin S, et al. Health problems in selected Ontario Holstein cows: frequency of occurrences, time to first diagnosis and associations. Prev Vet Med 1990;10:79–89.
36. LeBlanc S. Major advances in disease prevention in dairy cattle. J Dairy Sci 2006; 89:1267–79.
37. LeBlanc S. Monitoring metabolic health of dairy cattle in the transition period. J Reprod Dev 2010;56:S29–35.
38. Rowlands G. A review of variations in the concentrations of metabolites in the blood of beef and dairy cattle associated with physiology, nutrition and disease, with particular reference to the interpretation of metabolic profiles. World Rev Nutr Diet 1980;35:172–235.
39. Curtis C, Erb H, Sniffen C, et al. Association of parturient hypocalcemia with eight periparturient disorders in Holstein cows. Journal of the American Veterinary Association 1983;183:559–61.
40. Curtis C, Erb H, Sniffen C, et al. Epidemiology of parturient paresis: predisposing factors with emphasis on dry cow feeding and management. J Dairy Sci 1984;67: 817–25.
41. Hayirli A, Grummer R, Nordheim E, et al. Animal and dietary factors affecting feed intake during the prefresh transition period in Holsteins. J Dairy Sci 2002;85: 3430–43.
42. Baumgard LH, Collier RJ, Bauman DEA. 100-Year Review: Regulation of nutrient partitioning to support lactation. J Dairy Sci 2017;100:10353–66.
43. Roche JR, Bell AW, Overton TR, et al. Nutritional management of the transition cow in the 21st century – a paradigm shift in thinking. Anim Prod Sci 2013;53: 1000–23.
44. Herdt TH. Ruminant Adaptation to Negative Energy Balance. Vet Clin Food Anim Pract 2000;16:215–30.
45. Mulligan FJ, Doherty ML. Production diseases of the transition cow. Vet J 2008; 176:3–9.
46. Bertoni G, Trevisi E. Use of the liver activity index and other metabolic variables in the assessment of metabolic health in dairy herds. Vet Clin North Am Food Anim Pract 2013;29:413–31.
47. Van Saun R. Metabolic profiling in ruminant diagnostics. Vet Clin North Am Food Anim Pract 2023;39(1):49–71. In Press.
48. Ametaj BN, editor. Periparturient diseases of dairy cows: a systems biology approach. Cham, Switzerland: Springer International Publishing AG; 2017. p. 281.
49. Ametaj BN. Demystifying the Myths: Switching paradigms from reductionism to systems veterinary in approaching transition dairy cow diseases. In: Ametaj BN, editor. Periparturient diseases of dairy cows: a systems biology approach. Cham, Switzerland: Springer International Publishing AG; 2017. p. 9–30.
50. Dervishi E, Ametaj BN. Milk Fever: Reductionist versus Systems Veterinary Approach. In: Ametaj BN, editor. Periparturient diseases of dairy cows: a systems

biology approach. Cham, Switzerland: Springer International Publishing AG; 2017. p. 247–66.
51. McArt JAA, Neves RC. Association of transient, persistent, or delayed subclinical hypocalcemia with early lactation disease, removal, and milk yield in Holstein cows. J Dairy Sci 2020;103:690–701.
52. Arshad U, Santos JEP. Hepatic triacylglycerol associations with production and health in dairy cows. J Dairy Sci 2022;105:5393–409.
53. Nicola I, Chupin H, Roy JP, et al. Association between prepartum nonesterified fatty acid serum concentrations and postpartum diseases in dairy cows. J Dairy Sci 2022;105:9098–106.
54. van Knegsel AT, van den Brand H, Dijkstra J, et al. Effects of dietary energy source on energy balance, metabolites and reproduction variables in dairy cows in early lactation. Theriogenology 2007;68(Suppl 1):S274–80.
55. Grummer RR, Mashek DG, Hayirli A. Dry matter intake and energy balance in the transition period. Vet Clin North Am Food Anim Pract 2004;20:447–70.
56. Zarrin M, De Matteis L, Vernay M, et al. Long-term elevation of β-hydroxybutyrate in dairy cows through infusion: Effects on feed intake, milk production, and metabolism. J Dairy Sci 2013;96:2960–72.
57. Bertics SJ, Grummer RR, Cadorniga-Valino C, et al. Effect of prepartum dry matter intake on liver triglyceride concentration and early lactation. J Dairy Sci 1992; 75:1914–22.
58. Janovick N, Drackley J. Prepartum dietary management of energy intake affects postpartum intake and lactation performance by primiparous and multiparous Holstein cows. J Dairy Sci 2010;93:3086–102.
59. Overton T.R., Substrate utilization for hepatic gluconeogenesis in the transition dairy cow, 1998, Cornell Nutrition Conference for Feed Manufacturers, Proceedings of Cornell Nutrition Conference for Feed Manufacturers, Syracuse, NY, 237-246.
60. Bell AW, Burhans WS, Overton TR. Protein nutrition in late pregnancy, maternal protein reserves and lactation performance in dairy cows. Proc Nutr Soc 2000; 59:119–26.
61. van der Drift SGA, Houweling M, Schonewille JT, et al. Protein and fat mobilization and associations with serum beta-hydroxybutyrate concentrations in dairy cows. J Dairy Sci 2012;95:4911–20.
62. Robinson PH, Moorby JM, Arana M, et al. Influence of Close-up Dry Period Protein Supplementation on Productive and Reproductive Performance of Holstein Cows in Their Subsequent Lactation. J Dairy Sci 2001;84:2273–83.
63. Doepel L, Lapierre H, Kennelly JJ. Peripartum Performance and Metabolism of Dairy Cows in Response to Prepartum Energy and Protein Intake. J Dairy Sci 2002;85:2315–34.
64. Santos J, DePeters E, Jardon P, et al. Effect of prepartum dietary protein level on performance of primigravid and multiparous Holstein dairy cows. J Dairy Sci 2001;84:213–24.
65. Osorio JS, Ji P, Drackley JK, et al. Supplemental Smartamine M or MetaSmart during the transition period benefits postpartal cow performance and blood neutrophil function. J Dairy Sci 2013;96:6248–63.
66. Osorio JS, Trevisi E, Ji P, et al. Biomarkers of inflammation, metabolism, and oxidative stress in blood, liver, and milk reveal a better immunometabolic status in peripartal cows supplemented with Smartamine M or MetaSmart. J Dairy Sci 2014;97:7437–50.

67. Kimura K, Goff JP, Kerheli ME Jr, et al. Decreased Neutrophil Function as a Cause of Retained Placenta in Dairy Cattle. J Dairy Sci 2002;85:544–50.
68. Ingvartsen KL, Moyes K. Nutrition, immune function and health of dairy cattle. Animal 2013;7(Suppl 1):112–22.
69. LeBlanc SJ. Review: Relationships between metabolism and neutrophil function in dairy cows in the peripartum period. Animal 2020;14:s44–54.
70. Trevisi E, Minuti A. Assessment of the innate immune response in the periparturient cow. Res Vet Sci 2018;116:47–54.
71. Sordillo L.M., Immune dysfunction in periparturient dairy cows: evidence, causes and ramifications, Cornell Nutrition Conference for Feed Manufacturers, Proceedings paper from the conference, Syracuse, NY, 2014.
72. Cook NB, Nordlund KV. Behavioral needs of the transition cow and considerations for special needs facility design. Vet Clin North Am Food Anim Pract 2004;20:495–520.
73. McFarland DF, Tyson JT, Van Saun RJ. Nonnutritional factors influencing response to the nutritional program. Vet Clin North Am Food Anim Pract 2014; 30:745–64.
74. Proudfoot KL, Weary DM, LeBlanc SJ, et al. Exposure to an unpredictable and competitive social environment affects behavior and health of transition dairy cows. J Dairy Sci 2018;101:9309–20.
75. Bertoni G, Trevisi E, Han X, et al. Effects of inflammatory conditions on liver activity in puerperium period and consequences for performance in dairy cows. J Dairy Sci 2008;91:3300–10.
76. Bradford BJ, Swartz TH. Review: Following the smoke signals: inflammatory signaling in metabolic homeostasis and homeorhesis in dairy cattle. Animal 2020;14:s144–54.
77. Bradford BJ, Yuan K, Farney JK, et al. Invited review: Inflammation during the transition to lactation: New adventures with an old flame. J Dairy Sci 2015;98: 6631–50.
78. Trevisi E, Bertoni G, Lombardelli R, et al. Relation of inflammation and liver function with the plasma cortisol response to adrenocorticotropin in early lactating dairy cows. J Dairy Sci 2013;96:5712–22.
79. Horst EA, Kvidera SK, Baumgard LH. Invited review: The influence of immune activation on transition cow health and performance-A critical evaluation of traditional dogmas. J Dairy Sci 2021;104:8380–410.
80. Brown WE, Bradford BJ. Invited review: Mechanisms of hypophagia during disease. J Dairy Sci 2021;104:9418–36.
81. Szyszka O, Kyriazakis I. What is the relationship between level of infection and 'sickness behaviour' in cattle? Appl Anim Behav Sci 2013;147:1–10.
82. Kuhla B. Review: Pro-inflammatory cytokines and hypothalamic inflammation: implications for insufficient feed intake of transition dairy cows. Animal 2020;14: s65–77.
83. Kvidera SK, Horst EA, Abuajamieh M, et al. Glucose requirements of an activated immune system in lactating Holstein cows. J Dairy Sci 2017;100:2360–74.
84. Contreras GA, De Koster J, de Souza J, et al. Lipolysis modulates the biosynthesis of inflammatory lipid mediators derived from linoleic acid in adipose tissue of periparturient dairy cows. J Dairy Sci 2020;103:1944–55.
85. Koch F, Lamp O, Eslamizad M, et al. Metabolic Response to Heat Stress in Late-Pregnant and Early Lactation Dairy Cows: Implications to Liver-Muscle Crosstalk. PLoS One 2016;11:e0160912.

86. Eckel EF, Ametaj BN. Invited review: Role of bacterial endotoxins in the etiopathogenesis of periparturient diseases of transition dairy cows. J Dairy Sci 2016;99: 5967–90.
87. Ametaj B, Bradford B, Bobe G, et al. Strong relationships between mediators of the acute phase response and fatty liver in dairy cows. Can J Anim Sci 2005;85: 165–75.
88. Janovick NA, Trevisi E, Bertoni G, et al. Prepartum plane of energy intake affects serum biomarkers for inflammation and liver function during the periparturient period. J Dairy Sci 2023;106:168–80.
89. Moyes K. Triennial lactation symposium: Nutrient partitioning during intramammary inflammation: A key to severity of mastitis and risk of subsequent diseases? J Anim Sci 2015;93:5586–93.
90. Eckel EF, Ametaj BN. An Omics Approach to Transition Cow Immunity. In: Ametaj BN, editor. Periparturient diseases of dairy cows: a systems biology approach. Cham, Switzerland: Springer International Publishing AG; 2017. p. 31–50.
91. Ordway R, Ishler V, Varga G. Effects of sucrose supplementation on dry matter intake, milk yield, and blood metabolites of periparturient Holstein dairy cows. J Dairy Sci 2002;85:879–88.
92. Vallimont J, Varga G, Arieli A, et al. Effects of prepartum somatotropin and monensin on metabolism and production of periparturient Holstein dairy cows. J Dairy Sci 2001;84:2607–21.
93. Huzzey JM, Veira DM, Weary DM, et al. Prepartum behavior and dry matter intake identify dairy cows at risk for metritis. J Dairy Sci 2007;90:3220–33.
94. Perez-Baez J, Risco CA, Chebel RC, et al. Association of dry matter intake and energy balance prepartum and postpartum with health disorders postpartum: Part I. Calving disorders and metritis. J Dairy Sci 2019;102:9138–50.
95. Goldhawk C, Chapinal N, Veira DM, et al. Prepartum feeding behavior is an early indicator of subclinical ketosis. J Dairy Sci 2009;92:4971–7.
96. Perez-Baez J, Risco CA, Chebel RC, et al. Association of dry matter intake and energy balance prepartum and postpartum with health disorders postpartum: Part II. Ketosis and clinical mastitis. J Dairy Sci 2019;102:9151–64.

Metabolic Factors at the Crossroads of Periparturient Immunity and Inflammation

Angel Abuelo, DVM, MRes, MS (Vet Educ), PhD, Dip. DABVP (Dairy Practice), Dip. ECBHM, MRCVS[a],
Sabine Mann, Dr. med. vet., PhD, Dip. ACVPM (Epidemiology), Dip. ECBHM[b,*],
Genaro Andres Contreras, DVM, MS, PhD[a]

KEYWORDS

- Periparturient period • Periparturient inflammation
- Postpartum inflammatory dysregulation • Bovine immunometabolism
- Postpartum nutrient deficit

KEY POINTS

- Parturition and the onset of lactation trigger physiological inflammatory responses that are required for the transition from gestation into lactation.
- Periparturient hormonal milieu and reduced dry matter intake lead to nutrient and energy deficits.
- Postpartum immune function is altered by physiological processes associated with parturition, colostrogenesis, and lactogenesis, making the animal more susceptible to dysregulation and impaired efficacy.
- Postpartum metabolic rate increases the production of oxidants and reactive molecules, straining antioxidant reserves and thus increasing the risk for oxidative stress.

INTRODUCTION

The periparturient period of dairy cows, usually defined as 3 weeks before through 3 weeks after calving, is the lactation stage with the highest risk for health events.[1] The biological processes associated with colostrogenesis, parturition, and lactogenesis occur in this short window of time and demand intense changes in cows' metabolic and immune function.[2,3] A successful transition to a productive lactation requires a continuous supply of nutrients and energy substrates to fulfill these biological

[a] Department of Large Animal Clinical Sciences, College of Veterinary Medicine, Michigan State University, 736 Wilson Road, East Lansing, MI 48824, USA; [b] Department of Population Medicine and Diagnostic Sciences, College of Veterinary Medicine, Cornell University, 240 Farrier Road, Box 47, Ithaca, NY 14853, USA
* Corresponding author.
E-mail address: sm682@cornell.edu

Vet Clin Food Anim 39 (2023) 203–218
https://doi.org/10.1016/j.cvfa.2023.02.012 vetfood.theclinics.com
0749-0720/23/

demands. The transition also requires a functioning immune system that responds rapidly and effectively to tissue remodeling needs (eg, placental expulsion) and the continuous pathogen challenges associated with calving and management stressors. This article gives an overview of changes in bovine periparturient immune functions and immunometabolism, including leukocyte populations and bioenergetic dynamics. The authors also describe physiological and dysregulated inflammatory processes that link metabolic function and immunity in dairy cows during the immediate postpartum period and early lactation.

PERIPARTURIENT INNATE AND ADAPTIVE IMMUNITY

The biology of parturition and the onset of lactation include changes in innate and adaptive immunity that can affect the susceptibility to diseases in the periparturient cow.[4] However, not all cows experience drastic changes in circulating immune cell effector functions and many have higher disease resilience, suggesting the possibility of reducing immune impairment by improving management and genetic selection.[5] Inadequate immune system function during the periparturient period not only results in cows being more likely to become infected when exposed to pathogenic organisms but disease severity upon infection is also escalated. In the time around calving, the populations and functionality of circulating leukocytes change. Generally, the collective immune function of dairy cows starts to decline 2 to 3 weeks before calving and is not restored until about 4 weeks postcalving.[6] A study using mastectomized periparturient cows demonstrated that reductions in relevant leukocyte functions (eg, lymphocyte proliferation and secretion of interferon-γ and immunoglobulin (Ig) M by mitogen-stimulated leukocytes) during this period are partly due to the nutritional and metabolic demands imposed by the onset of lactation.[7]

Innate Immunity

Neutrophils represent the first line of cellular defense against invading pathogens and possess several microbicidal functions (**Fig. 1**). During parturition, cows exhibit a short period of neutrophilia, likely in response to the physiological peak in blood corticosteroid concentration, followed by neutropenia that lasts several days after calving, with cell counts lower than before parturition. This decline in blood neutrophil counts is likely due to the massive trafficking of these cells into the uterus following calving.[8] Although this effective migration of neutrophils to the uterus is needed for an immune response to pathogens, tissue clearance, and involution,[9] the decline in circulating cell counts may put cows at greater risk for other infections (ie, mastitis). In addition to shifts in blood neutrophil counts, their function is also impaired during the periparturient period. Neutrophils exhibit lower migration and microbicidal capacities (**Fig. 2**) during the periparturient period,[10] and this decrease in neutrophil function has been associated with the development of several diseases during this time.[11–14] Underlying reasons for the decrease in functionality may at least partially be due to the proinflammatory state that surrounds parturition, as this releases immature band neutrophils into the bloodstream. These immature neutrophils have inferior functions than mature segmented neutrophils, and their greater proportion could influence the response capacity of the circulating pool of neutrophils.

Other innate immune cells also exhibit changes around parturition. Circulating eosinophils decline by more than 50% due in part to heavy migration to the cervix at parturition following the drastic reduction in progesterone concentration.[8] Eosinophils play a role in resolving inflammatory conditions[15]; therefore, this reduction in blood counts can contribute to the exacerbated or dysregulated inflammatory responses

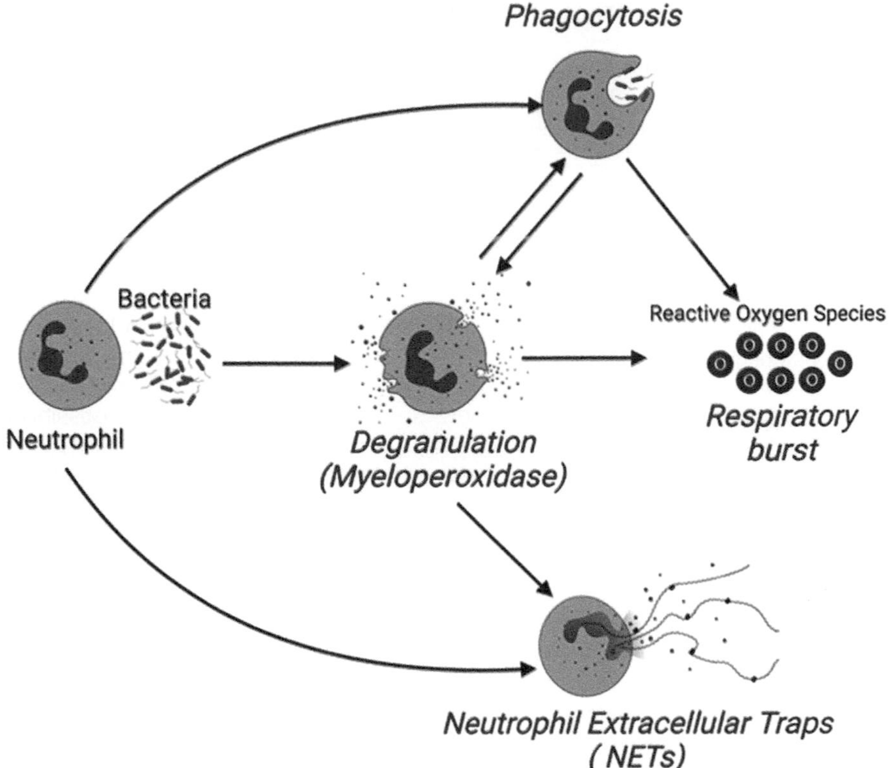

Fig. 1. *Neutrophils' bactericidal mechanisms.* Intracellular killing is the main bactericidal mechanism where the bacteria are engulfed and reactive oxygen species are produced through the oxidative burst to kill the bacteria. On activation, neutrophils can degranulate, releasing their granule content, which is rich in myeloperoxidase—an enzyme that catalyzes the formation of more reactive oxygen species. Neutrophils can also use extracellular bactericidal killing, where they release nuclear and granule contents, "trapping" and killing the microorganism through neutrophil extracellular traps (NETs). (Created with biorender.com.)

seen in periparturient cattle. Conversely, blood monocytes show a more proinflammatory response during the periparturient period, with increased production of inflammatory cytokines upon stimulation.[16,17]

Adaptive Immunity

The circulating populations of lymphocytes do not change markedly during the periparturient period, but lymphocyte functions decrease in a similar temporal fashion to neutrophil bactericidal capabilities.[6] Proliferation in response to stimuli is reduced from the 3 weeks prior up to 3 weeks after calving,[18] and this reduction is associated with a higher risk for clinical infections.[19] Similarly, there is a marked decline in circulating concentrations of IgG and IgM,[7] likely due to incorporating these Igs into colostrum rather than a decrease in B-cell function.

PERIPARTURIENT INFLAMMATION (FRIEND AND FOE)

Biological processes associated with calving and lactogenesis such as placental expulsion, uterine involution, and mobilization of energy stores require an

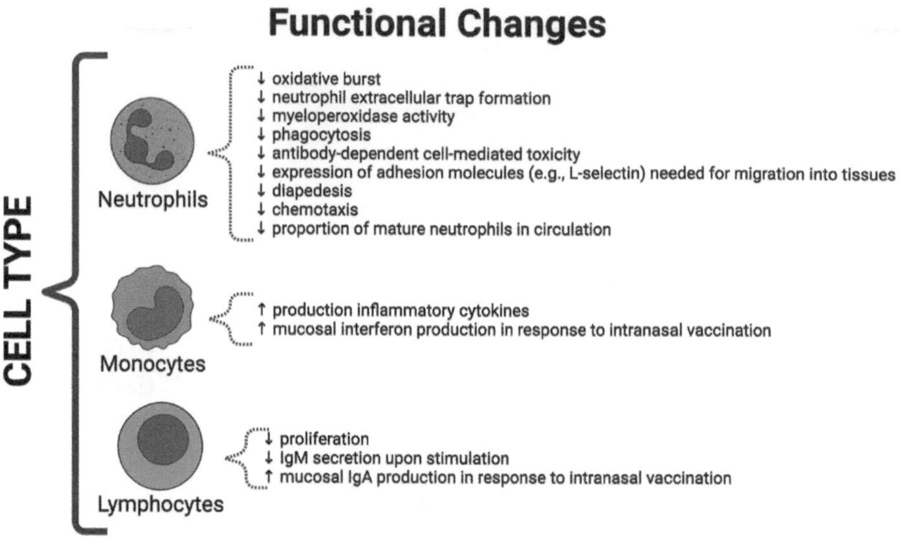

Functional Changes

CELL TYPE

Neutrophils
↓ oxidative burst
↓ neutrophil extracellular trap formation
↓ myeloperoxidase activity
↓ phagocytosis
↓ antibody-dependent cell-mediated toxicity
↓ expression of adhesion molecules (e.g., L-selectin) needed for migration into tissues
↓ diapedesis
↓ chemotaxis
↓ proportion of mature neutrophils in circulation

Monocytes
↑ production inflammatory cytokines
↑ mucosal interferon production in response to intranasal vaccination

Lymphocytes
↓ proliferation
↓ IgM secretion upon stimulation
↑ mucosal IgA production in response to intranasal vaccination

Fig. 2. Changes in blood immune cell functions during the transition period. Changes are described for 3 immune cell types: neutrophils,[11,12,18,102–105] monocytes,[17,106] and lymphocytes.[7,17,19,101] (Created with biorender.com.)

inflammatory process that executes the remodeling activity in organs such as the placenta, the postpartum uterus, and adipose tissues (ATs) required for uterine involution and fat mobilization.

Placental Expulsion

The detachment and expulsion of the placenta after delivery of the calf requires an inflammatory process that is driven by intense traffic of immune cells into the uterine caruncle.[20] The primary immune cells involved in placental expulsion include neutrophils, cytotoxic and helper T cells, and macrophages.[21,22] Neutrophils' phagocytic function is essential to remove apoptotic cells and trigger the inflammatory response to the caruncle area.[23] T cells are involved in recognizing the major histocompatibility complex I on the caruncle epithelium, a step necessary for identifying the placental cells as nonself.[24] Macrophages are continuously present in the uterine caruncle during gestation, exhibiting changes in their abundance and inflammatory phenotype as the pregnancy progresses and immediately after parturition.[25] Near calving, the number of macrophages in the caruncles increases initially with an antiinflammatory phenotype (ie, M2).[26] At the time of placental expulsion, the macrophage phenotype switches rapidly toward an inflammatory phenotype (ie, M1). Although the mechanism for this phenotype change is unclear, heavy neutrophil infiltration and activation in the uterine caruncle likely trigger macrophage proinflammatory polarization. M1 macrophages are effective in secreting enzymes that break down the extracellular matrix proteins that sustain the fetal-maternal epithelium linkage and facilitate the rapid expulsion of fetal membranes.[21] Cows that fail to release the fetal membranes exhibit a dysfunctional inflammatory response in the caruncles with reduced number of macrophages that present an M2 antiinflammatory phenotype.[27] Given the need for a rapid and effective inflammatory response in the uterine caruncle, the use of antiinflammatory drugs that target both cyclooxygenase (COX) 1 and COX2, such as flunixin meglumine, and corticoids is not recommended in dairy cows within 24 hours after calving, as these treatments increase the risk for stillbirths, retained placenta, and metritis.[28]

Uterine Involution and Bacterial Clearance

Following calf and placental expulsion, the cow's genital tract begins a rapid remodeling process that changes its size, a 10-fold reduction by 30 days after parturition, as well as anatomical and histological structures.[29] In healthy cows, uterine remodeling remnants are expelled as lochia during the first 2 weeks after calving, and by 30 days into lactation, the uterus and its endometrium are ready for a new pregnancy. The cycle of gestation and postpartum involution can be defined as a tissue damage and repair process.[30] Similar to what occurs in the caruncles, the muscular and mucosal layers of the uterus are gradually infiltrated with macrophages and neutrophils as parturition approaches, and their number further increases after delivery.[31] Chemoattractant cytokines (eg, monocyte chemoattractant protein-1) secreted by the myometrium drive macrophage infiltration into the uterus during and after the onset of term labor.[32] These mononuclear cells, in turn, recruit neutrophils to trigger the process of uterine involution that involves structural changes driven by extracellular matrix remodeling, the regeneration of the endometrium, and the replenishment of myometrial cells from uterine stem cells.[30] The involution process is only partially characterized in the bovine; however, a recent study demonstrates that dysregulation in immune cell trafficking and enhanced production of interleukin-1β (IL-1β) by epithelial cells in the endometrium may predispose to uterine disease.[33]

Increased immune cell trafficking into the uterus during the involution phase is also required for the clearance of bacterial contamination entering the uterine cavity during and after parturition, an event that occurs in more than 95% of cows.[34] Bacterial clearance is performed by phagocytic immune cells and the secretion of bactericidal and bacteriostatic peptides, including defensins and cathelicidins.[35,36]

Lipid Mobilization from Adipose Tissue

During the first 3 to 5 weeks post-partum, AT increases its rate of lipolysis and drastically reduces synthesis of new lipids (ie, lipogenesis) to offset the negative energy balance exhibited by nearly all fresh cows. Lipolysis is driven by low circulating insulin concentrations and increased growth hormone secretion post-partum.[37] After calving, cows' AT is also more responsive to catecholamines, the most important activators of lipolysis in adipocytes.[38] The primary outcome of enhanced lipolysis in AT is the release of nonesterified fatty acids (NEFA) and glycerol from adipocytes into circulation; however, AT lipolysis also involves a remodeling process characterized by an inflammatory response with immune cell infiltration.[39] Macrophages are the predominant immune cell type infiltrating the AT of postpartum cows, accounting for 5% to 7% of immune cell populations in fat.[40–43] When lipolysis is severe, such as when cows develop displaced abomasum and ketosis, macrophage infiltration is increased and can make up 20% of the cells in the stromal vascular fraction (ie, non-adipocytes) or 2% of the total number of cells in the AT.[40,43] Macrophage infiltration into the AT removes diglycerides, monoglycerides, and other lipolysis products that can cause lipotoxicity.[44,45] This assumed role likely explains the increased number of macrophages in the AT of cows undergoing rapid weight loss post-partum.[46,47] Although not shown in cows, macrophages recruit new fat cell progenitors.[45] Thus, a moderate infiltration of macrophages during postpartum lipolysis is beneficial for preventing lipotoxicity and promoting the replenishment of adipocyte populations following apoptosis or necrosis if lipolysis is elevated and protracted.[48]

PERIPARTURIENT DYSREGULATION OF IMMUNITY AND INFLAMMATION

General Principles of Immunometabolism

Immune cells require different nutrients when resting compared with their activated state. They undergo a so-called metabolic switch to fuel their respective functions, mainly through the use of glucose, with further contribution of lipids and amino acids. Nutrient requirements of the different immune cell types are best described in monogastrics.

Typically, immune cells increase their glucose requirements during activation; this is facilitated by an increase in the expression of a number of insulin-independent and insulin-dependent glucose transporters, as immune cells express the insulin receptor and respond to changes in insulin concentrations.[49] Energy is produced mainly by glycolysis and tricarboxylic acid cycle, and preference for this pathway depends on immune cell type.[50] Although the exact magnitude of glucose requirements is difficult to determine exactly in live animals, they are significant during acute immune activation. In a late-lactation cow model of acute immune activation using an intravenous lipopolysaccharide (LPS) challenge, additional glucose needs were estimated to exceed 1 kg over 12 hours.[51] It is well documented in monogastrics that immune cells need amino acids, specifically certain amino acids such as alanine, glutamine, serine, and threonine for cell activation and proliferation, as well as other amino acids for the production of antibodies (eg, branched chain amino acids), inflammatory mediators (eg, histamine from histidine), and cytotoxic substances (eg, nitric oxide from arginine).[52] In addition to glucose, immune cells use glutamine for their energetic and biosynthetic needs.[53]

Fatty acids are also an energy substrate for immune cells. Fatty acid β-oxidation is especially important in alternatively (ie, M2) activated macrophages. This mitochondrial process is more efficient energetically than glycolysis and supports the high energy requirements of macrophages during the remodeling and healing phases of inflammation.[54] In these macrophages, medium- and long-chain fatty acids are transported into the mitochondria for oxidation by carnitine palmitoyl transferase 1A; in contrast, short-chain fatty acids enter the organelle through passive diffusion.[55] Saturated fatty acids including palmitate and stearate are preferentially used for β-oxidation, although polyunsaturated fatty acids can be used as energy substrate.[55]

Calcium (Ca) is critical for immune cell functions, including chemotaxis, cytokine secretion, degranulation, and phagocytosis, due to its role as a second messenger.[56] The immune system also requires vitamins and trace minerals for adequate functioning. Key vitamins and minerals for optimal immune function include vitamins A, B complex (particularly B2, B6, B9, and B12), C, D, and E and copper, iron, magnesium, manganese, and selenium.[57] These substances can support immune cell function directly and through their role as cofactors in other proteins (eg, selenoproteins, superoxide dismutase, and so forth), either as part of the antioxidant defense system or via mechanisms distinct from antioxidant properties.[58]

Relevance of Innate Immune Activation and Inflammation on Postpartum Metabolic Status

The association between poor metabolic adaptation of the dairy cow during the transition period and inflammatory diseases has been well documented. As such, cows with early postpartum hyperketonemia (β-hydroxybutyrate [BHB] $\geq$ 1.2 mmol/L) had a 2- to 3-fold increased odds for metritis by 14 days in milk (DIM),[59–61] and cows diagnosed with endometritis at 28 DIM had approximately 2-fold greater BHB concentrations 2 weeks prior compared with controls.[13] Similarly, mastitis incidence in the first month post-partum, mainly due to gram-negative pathogens or showing no growth in milk bacteriological cultures, was greater in cows with BHB greater than 1.0 mmol/L in the first 3 DIM.[62] A meta-analysis showed clinical mastitis odds to be 1.6 times greater when cows were diagnosed with a BHB greater than or equal to 1.4 mmol/L post-partum.[61] Considering these associations, it is difficult to distinguish if metabolic diseases are at the root of greater disease risk in transition cows or if diseases cause a greater metabolic drain, as both directions are plausible explanations. When examining the effect that inflammation and activation of the innate immune system have on metabolism in controlled studies, an apparent effect can be seen. Yuan and colleagues[65] used subcutaneous infusion of recombinant tumor necrosis factor (TNF), a potent proinflammatory mediator, during the first 7 days post-partum and observed intake suppression and negative effects on water intake, milk yield, and components. Kushibiki and colleagues,[64] using a similar model but in midlactation cows, found intake and milk yield were depressed, and cows had higher NEFA concentrations, indicating an increase in lipolysis. Elsener and Bergeron[63] as well as Scott and colleagues[63] demonstrated that cows have a metabolic cost to immune activation by vaccination, with a drop in milk production often observed in dairy practice following herd vaccination. The direct metabolic cost of the activated immune system is exacerbated by the reduced nutrient intake stemming from intake suppression, as both go hand in hand.

In addition to indicators of energy metabolism, inflammation induces changes in amino acid and Ca concentrations. During the initial acute immune activation of post-partum cows challenged with intravenous LPS, circulating essential amino acid concentrations decrease further in concentration,[67] suggesting that amino acids are redirected to activated immune cells or hepatic metabolism to produce inflammatory mediators and acute phase proteins, respectively. Likewise, acute immune activation in fresh cows using LPS challenge models shows a transient decline in circulating Ca concentrations.[68] The mechanisms leading to the induction of hypocalcemia following immune activation are yet to be fully characterized but seem to be a protective evolutionarily conserved mechanism.[69]

Bovine Innate Immunity During the Peripartum Nutrient Deficit and Metabolic Status

Certain immune cell functions are impaired around the time of calving compared with control steers on the same diet.[6] All cows seem to experience some degree of transient immune dysfunction. With an increase in circulating estrogen, progesterone, and glucocorticoids, pregnancy itself dampens inflammatory response and certain immune cell functions before calving.[70] However, post-partum, a more severe nutrient deficit has been associated with higher disease risk and hyperinflammatory state in observational studies.[62,71] Observations by Huzzey and colleagues[66] and Hammon and colleagues[13] show that cows that go on to develop metritis postpartum are already showing depressed intake in the late prepartum period, suggesting a declining nutritional state during late gestation leads to a higher risk of disease. Negative nutrient balance is associated with a change in circulating metabolic indicators, as described earlier. Increased circulating ketone bodies, NEFA, and prooxidants and a decrease in circulating glucose, amino acids, and Ca concentrations are the hallmarks of this metabolic situation as detailed later.

Ketone bodies

To investigate the effect that ketone bodies have on the immune system, Zarrin and colleagues[75] infused late-lactation cows with BHB to reach a circulating concentration of 1.7 mmol/L. They then evaluated hyperketonemia effects on mammary gland immune response during an LPS challenge and showed that fewer immune cells were recruited to the mammary gland. Swartz and colleagues[65] used a *Streptococcus uberis* infection model and BHB intravenous infusions (BHB> 1.8 mmol/L) and found that hyperketonemic cows had higher bacterial numbers in infected quarters compared with cows not infused with BHB at the time of infection. Both studies suggest that innate defenses in the cow are altered by experimental elevation of BHB, which is supported by in vitro data of bovine immune cells.[72,73,74,77,78]

Nonesterified fatty acids

Elevated prepartum NEFA concentrations are associated with an increased risk of retained placenta, metritis, and mastitis.[76,79,80] This association may be related to NEFA's capacity to modulate immune cells' phenotype and inflammatory processes. For example, saturated fatty acids, such as palmitic acid, can activate the proinflammatory (M1) program in macrophages by binding to the toll-like receptor 4 and triggering the expression of nuclear factor κB (NF-κB).[81] The use of palmitic acid as energy substrate by mitochondria also generates reactive oxygen species (ROS) that in turn can polarize macrophages to M1.[82]

Glucose deficit

Although gluconeogenesis increases after calving, the enormous drain of glucose for mammary lactose synthesis explains why glucose concentrations are significantly lower post-partum.[83] In addition, intracellular glycogen storage of bovine immune cells, a readily available form of glucose, decreases in the immediate postpartum period.[84,85] This state of reduced glucose availability is accompanied by lower circulating concentrations of insulin and a markedly reduced metabolic response to acute inflammation in fresh cows,[67] suggesting the redirection of glucose toward an activated immune system is far reduced in magnitude during the time of energy deficit compared with late lactation and likely directly affects immune cell function.[49]

Protein deficit

Effects of protein malnutrition (ie, amino acid deficiencies) have been best described in human medicine, where an increased risk and severity of infections was demonstrated.[81] Glutamine plays a predominant role in immune cell metabolism. Circulating essential amino acid concentrations decline in the immediate postpartum period in dairy cattle.[86,87] Together with glutamate, phenylalanine, and methionine, glutamine is the amino acid with the most significant decline (approximately 25%) from late pregnancy to early lactation.[87] In vitro studies using bovine endometrial cultures supplemented with different amounts of glutamine demonstrate an immunomodulatory effect of this amino acid.[88] Cows supplemented in the peripartum period with rumen-protected methionine showed greater phagocytosis and oxidative burst capacity of neutrophils and greater phagocytosis of monocytes compared with unsupplemented cows.[89]

Calcium deficit and supplementation

As described earlier, Ca is an essential mineral for immune cell activation. A lack of available Ca due to postpartum hypocalcemia leads to impaired innate immune function, including a reduction in neutrophil phagocytosis and a blunted response to antigen activation of mononuclear cells.[56,90] Blanket Ca supplementation during inflammation-induced hypocalcemia is discouraged in other species due to a demonstrated increase in mortality.[91,92] Recent investigations on the effect of Ca supplementation in healthy cows[93] and a model of acute immune activation[68] in dairy cows have not conclusively shown a detrimental effect, but the effects of supplementation during naturally occurring diseases have not been described.

Prooxidants and oxidative stress and effect of antioxidants

Cows produce excessive amounts of ROS during the periparturient period due to increased metabolism, dysregulated inflammation and immune responses, and stress.[94] This increase in ROS production can lead to oxidative stress (ie, oxidative damage to macromolecules such as cell membrane lipids), which compromises the functional capacity of immune cell populations.[95] Under oxidative stress conditions, neutrophils have a reduced ability to phagocytose and kill bacteria. Also, oxidative stress activates the proinflammatory transcription factor NF-κB, releasing proinflammatory cytokines (ie, IL-6, IL-1β, TNF) and lipid mediators (prostaglandins, leukotrienes, and thromboxanes) that can cause aberrant inflammation. Moreover, immune cells respond to these inflammatory mediators by increasing ROS production that can escalate oxidative stress further. Thus, cows suffering from oxidative stress succumb to increased incidence and severity of metabolic and infectious diseases during early lactation.

Supplementation of periparturient cows with micronutrients that support antioxidant defenses, such as vitamins and trace minerals, can help reduce disease incidence and severity, as well as productivity.[96] Dietary requirements of these micronutrients for counteracting oxidative stress and improving immune function may be greater than the requirements to avoid deficiencies as judged by traditional methods.[97] Nevertheless, excessive antioxidant supplementation can also potentially have deleterious effects,[98,99,100] and establishing supplementation guidelines for optimal health is still an active area of research.

Postpartum Inflammation, Antiinflammatory Therapy, and Metabolic Effects

Inflammation's effects on metabolism and nutrient needs during times of nutrient scarcity explain the interest in metabolic and production effects of reducing or preventing inflammation in the postpartum period. Despite ongoing research efforts on the effect of different antiinflammatory compounds (recently reviewed by Bradford and Swartz),[106] there is no clear consensus on the metabolic effects of such treatments. This lack of response is likely due to the different steps in the inflammatory cascade affected by different compounds, use of different dosages and delivery forms, and a lack of understanding of the degree to which individual animals benefit from such interventions in studies applying blanket therapy. Currently, no antiinflammatory medication is licensed in the United States to alter metabolism or milk production in cattle.

SUMMARY

Despite significant advances in management, nutrition, and preventive medicine, the periparturient period continues to be the lactation stage with the highest risk for diseases in dairy cows. It is also a critical time point that influences lactation and reproductive efficiency. Our current understanding of the biology of the periparturient dairy cow highlights the need for nutritional and medical management that supports a balanced and effective immune response. Successful completion of physiological processes unique to the periparturient period, such as parturition, placental expulsion, and uterine involution, requires an inflammatory response with a strong initiation phase and a rapid resolution stage that minimizes tissue damage and systemic responses. Immune activation, including inflammation, is a process of intensive nutrient use during a time of already precarious supply, further challenging the balance of energy, protein, and microminerals. This article provides an overview of the underlying physiology linking metabolic function and immunity in periparturient dairy cows to disease risk.

CLINICS CARE POINTS

- The periparturient period includes physiological inflammatory processes such as placental expulsion, uterine involution, and AT remodeling that require a robust, effective, and fast-resolving inflammation.
- Despite the need for effective inflammatory responses for maintaining health, many periparturient cows experience exacerbated inflammation that hamper their immune responses and increase their disease risk.
- Immune activation requires nutrients that exacerbate the already precarious metabolic situation of the postpartum cow.
- There is a direct immunomodulatory effect of certain metabolites, nutrients, and minerals that is typically altered around the time of calving.

DISCLOSURE

The authors have nothing to disclose.

ACKNOWLEDGMENTS

The authors are supported by USDA-National Institute of Food and Agriculture (Washington, DC) competitive grants 2018-67015-28302 and 2022-67015-36350, the Michigan Alliance for Animal Agriculture (East Lansing, MI) awards AA19-002 and AA19-016 to A. Abuelo; USDA-National Institute of Food and Agriculture (Washington, DC) competitive grant 2019-67015-29834 to S. Mann; and USDA-National Institute of Food and Agriculture (Washington, DC) competitive grants 2019-67015-29443 and 2021-67015-34563 and the Michigan Alliance for Animal Agriculture (East Lansing MI) award AA21–154 to G.A. Contreras.

REFERENCES

1. Ingvartsen KL, Dewhurst RJ, Friggens NC. On the relationship between lactational performance and health: is it yield or metabolic imbalance that cause production diseases in dairy cattle? A position paper. Livest Prod Sci 2003;83(2–3):277–308.
2. Bell AW. Regulation of organic nutrient metabolism during transition from late pregnancy to early lactation. J Anim Sci 1995;73(9):2804–19.
3. Ingvartsen KL, Moyes KM. Factors contributing to immunosuppression in the dairy cow during the periparturient period. Jpn J Vet Res 2015;63(Suppl 1):S15–24.
4. Aitken SL, Corl CM, Sordillo LM. Immunopathology of mastitis: insights into disease recognition and resolution. J Mammary Gland Biol Neoplasia 2011;16(4):291–304.
5. Piccinini R, Binda E, Belotti M, et al. The evaluation of non-specific immune status of heifers in field conditions during the periparturient period. Vet Res 2004;35(5):539–50.
6. Goff JP, Horst RL. Physiological Changes at Parturition and Their Relationship to Metabolic Disorders. J Dairy Sci 1997;80(7):1260–8.

7. Nonnecke BJ, Kimura K, Goff JP, et al. Effects of the mammary gland on functional capacities of blood mononuclear leukocyte populations from periparturient cows. J Dairy Sci 2003;86(7):2359–68.
8. Van Engelen E, De Groot MW, Breeveld-Dwarkasing VNA, et al. Cervical ripening and parturition in cows are driven by a cascade of pro-inflammatory cytokines. Reprod Domest Anim 2009;44(5):834–41.
9. Pascottini OB, LeBlanc SJ. Modulation of immune function in the bovine uterus peripartum. Theriogenology 2020;150:193–200.
10. Sordillo LM, Afseth G, Davies G, et al. Effects of recombinant granulocyte-macrophage colony-stimulating factor on bovine peripheral blood and mammary gland neutrophil function in vitro. Can J Vet Res 1992;56(1):16–21.
11. Kehrli ME Jr, Nonnecke ME, Roth JA. Alterations of bovine neutrophil function during the periparturient period. Am J Vet Res 1989;50:207–14.
12. Cai TQ, Weston PG, Lund LA, et al. Association between neutrophil functions and periparturient disorders in cows. Am J Vet Res 1994;55(7):934–43.
13. Hammon DS, Evjen IM, Dhiman TR, et al. Neutrophil function and energy status in Holstein cows with uterine health disorders. Vet Immunol Immunopathol 2006; 113(1–2):21–9.
14. Bassel LL, Caswell JL. Bovine neutrophils in health and disease. Cell Tissue Res 2018;371(3):617–37.
15. Isobe Y, Kato T, Arita M. Emerging Roles of Eosinophils and Eosinophil-Derived Lipid Mediators in the Resolution of Inflammation. Review. Front Immunol 2012; 3. https://doi.org/10.3389/fimmu.2012.00270.
16. Sordillo LM, Pighetti GM, Davis MR. Enhanced production of bovine tumor necrosis factor-alpha during the periparturient period. Vet Immunol Immunopathol 1995;49(3):263–70.
17. Cortese VS, Woolums A, Hurley DJ, et al. Comparison of interferon and bovine herpesvirus-1-specific IgA levels in nasal secretions of dairy cattle administered an intranasal modified live viral vaccine prior to calving or on the day of calving. Vet Immunol Immunopathol 2017;187:35–41.
18. Saad AM, Concha C, Astrom G. Alterations in neutrophil phagocytosis and lymphocyte blastogenesis in dairy cows around parturition. Zentralblatt fur Veterinarmedizin Reihe B Journal of veterinary Medicine Series B 1989;36(5): 337–45.
19. Catalani E, Amadori M, Vitali A, et al. Short communication: Lymphoproliferative response to lipopolysaccharide and incidence of infections in periparturient dairy cows. J Dairy Sci 2013;96(11):7077–81.
20. Attupuram NM, Kumaresan A, Narayanan K, et al. Cellular and molecular mechanisms involved in placental separation in the bovine: A review. Mol Reprod Dev 2016;83(4):287–97.
21. Hansen PJ. Physiology and Endocrinology Symposium: maternal immunological adjustments to pregnancy and parturition in ruminants and possible implications for postpartum uterine health: is there a prepartum-postpartum nexus? J Anim Sci 2013;91(4):1639–49.
22. Nancy P, Erlebacher A. T cell behavior at the maternal-fetal interface. Int J Dev Biol 2014;58(2–4):189–98.
23. Kimura K, Goff JP, Kehrli ME Jr, et al. Decreased neutrophil function as a cause of retained placenta in dairy cattle. J Dairy Sci 2002;85(3):544–50.
24. Davies CJ, Hill JR, Edwards JL, et al. Major histocompatibility antigen expression on the bovine placenta: its relationship to abnormal pregnancies and retained placenta. Anim Reprod Sci 2004;82-83:267–80.

25. Miyoshi M, Sawamukai Y. Specific localization of macrophages in pregnant bovine caruncles. Reprod Domest Anim 2004;39(3):125–8.
26. Oliveira LJ, McClellan S, Hansen PJ. Differentiation of the endometrial macrophage during pregnancy in the cow. PLoS One 2010;5(10):e13213.
27. Nelli RK, De Koster J, Roberts JN, et al. Impact of uterine macrophage phenotype on placental retention in dairy cows. Theriogenology 2019;127:145–52.
28. Newby NC, Leslie KE, Dingwell HDP, et al. The effects of periparturient administration of flunixin meglumine on the health and production of dairy cattle. J Dairy Sci 2017;100(1):582–7.
29. Sheldon IM. The postpartum uterus. Vet Clin North Am Food Anim Pract 2004; 20(3):569–91.
30. Spooner MK, Lenis YY, Watson R, et al. The role of stem cells in uterine involution. Reproduction 2021;161(3):R61–77.
31. Shynlova O, Nedd-Roderique T, Li Y, et al. Myometrial immune cells contribute to term parturition, preterm labour and post-partum involution in mice. J Cell Mol Med 2013;17(1):90–102.
32. Shynlova O, Tsui P, Dorogin A, et al. Monocyte chemoattractant protein-1 (CCL-2) integrates mechanical and endocrine signals that mediate term and preterm labor. J Immunol 2008;181(2):1470–9.
33. Kelly P, Meade KG, O'Farrelly C. Non-canonical inflammasome-mediated IL-1β production by primary endometrial epithelial and stromal fibroblast cells is NLRP3 and caspase-4 dependent. Front Immunol 2019;10:102.
34. Sheldon IM, Dobson H. Postpartum uterine health in cattle. Anim Reprod Sci 2004;82-83:295–306.
35. Alan E, Liman N. Immunohistochemical localization of beta defensins in the endometrium of rat uterus during the postpartum involution period. Vet Res Commun 2012;36(3):173–85.
36. Merriman KE, Martinez N, Rodney Harris RM, et al. Neutrophil β-defensin gene expression of postpartum dairy cows is altered by prepartum dietary cation-anion difference. J Dairy Sci 2019;102(12):11636–51.
37. Bradford BJ, Yuan K, Farney JK, et al. Invited review: Inflammation during the transition to lactation: New adventures with an old flame. J Dairy Sci 2015; 98(10):6631–50.
38. Arner P, Langin D. Lipolysis in lipid turnover, cancer cachexia, and obesity-induced insulin resistance. Trends Endocrinol Metab 2014;25(5):255–62.
39. Contreras GA, Strieder-Barboza C, Raphael W. Adipose tissue lipolysis and remodeling during the transition period of dairy cows. J Anim Sci Biotechnol 2017; 8(1):41.
40. Haussler S, Germeroth D, Laubenthal L, et al. Short Communication: Immunohistochemical localization of the immune cell marker CD68 in bovine adipose tissue: impact of tissue alterations and excessive fat accumulation in dairy cows. Vet Immunol Immunopathol 2017. https://doi.org/10.1016/j.vetimm.2016.12.005.
41. Akter S, Haussler S, Germeroth D, et al. Immunohistochemical characterization of phagocytic immune cell infiltration into different adipose tissue depots of dairy cows during early lactation. J Dairy Sci 2012;95(6):3032–44.
42. Contreras GA, Thelen K, Schmidt S, et al. Adipose tissue remodeling in late-lactation dairy cows during feed restriction-induced negative energy balance. J Dairy Sci 2016;99. https://doi.org/10.3168/jds.2016-11552.
43. Contreras GA, Kabara E, Brester J, et al. Macrophage infiltration in the omental and subcutaneous adipose tissues of dairy cows with displaced abomasum. J Dairy Sci 2015;98(9):6176–87.

44. Aouadi M, Vangala P, Yawe JC, et al. Lipid storage by adipose tissue macrophages regulates systemic glucose tolerance. Am J Physiol Endocrinol Metab 2014;307(4):E374–83.
45. Lee YH, Petkova AP, Granneman JG. Identification of an adipogenic niche for adipose tissue remodeling and restoration. Cell Metabol 2013;18(3):355–67.
46. Newman AW, Miller A, Leal Yepes FA, et al. The effect of the transition period and postpartum body weight loss on macrophage infiltrates in bovine subcutaneous adipose tissue. J Dairy Sci 2019;102(2):1693–701.
47. De Koster J, Strieder-Barboza C, de Souza J, et al. Short communication: Effects of body fat mobilization on macrophage infiltration in adipose tissue of early lactation dairy cows. J Dairy Sci 2018;101(8):7608–13.
48. Sun K, Kusminski CM, Scherer PE. Adipose tissue remodeling and obesity. J Clin Invest 2011;121(6):2094–101.
49. Calder PC, Dimitriadis G, Newsholme P. Glucose metabolism in lymphoid and inflammatory cells and tissues. Curr Opin Clin Nutr Metab Care 2007;10(4): 531–40.
50. Pearce Erika L, Pearce Edward J. Metabolic Pathways in Immune Cell Activation and Quiescence. Immunity 2013;38(4):633–43.
51. Kvidera SK, Horst EA, Abuajamieh M, et al. Glucose requirements of an activated immune system in lactating Holstein cows. J Dairy Sci 2017. https://doi.org/10.3168/jds.2016-12001.
52. Li P, Yin Y-L, Li D, et al. Amino acids and immune function. Br J Nutr 2007;98(2): 237–52.
53. Song W, Li D, Tao L, et al. Solute carrier transporters: the metabolic gatekeepers of immune cells. Acta Pharm Sin B 2020;10(1):61–78.
54. Namgaladze D, Brune B. Macrophage fatty acid oxidation and its roles in macrophage polarization and fatty acid-induced inflammation. Biochim Biophys Acta 2016;1861(11):1796–807.
55. Mehta MM, Weinberg SE, Chandel NS. Mitochondrial control of immunity: beyond ATP. Nat Rev Immunol 2017;17(10):608–20.
56. Kimura K, Reinhardt TA, Goff JP. Parturition and hypocalcemia blunts calcium signals in immune cells of dairy cattle. J Dairy Sci 2006;89(7):2588–95.
57. Spears JW, Weiss WP. Role of antioxidants and trace elements in health and immunity of transition dairy cows. Vet J 2008;176(1):70–6.
58. Sordillo LM. Selenium-dependent regulation of oxidative stress and immunity in periparturient dairy cattle. Vet Med Int 2013;2013:154045.
59. Duffield TF, Lissemore KD, McBride BW, et al. Impact of hyperketonemia in early lactation dairy cows on health and production. J Dairy Sci 2009;92(2):571–80.
60. Suthar VS, Canelas-Raposo J, Deniz A, et al. Prevalence of subclinical ketosis and relationships with postpartum diseases in European dairy cows. J Dairy Sci 2013;96(5):2925–38.
61. Raboisson D, Mounie M, Maigne E. Diseases, reproductive performance, and changes in milk production associated with subclinical ketosis in dairy cows: a meta-analysis and review. J Dairy Sci 2014;97(12):7547–63.
62. Janosi S, Kulcsar M, Korodi P, et al. Energy imbalance related predisposition to mastitis in group-fed high-producing postpartum dairy cows. Acta Vet Hung 2003;51(3):409–24.
63. Yuan K., Farney J.K., Mamedova L.K., et al., TNFalpha altered inflammatory responses, impaired health and productivity, but did not affect glucose or lipid metabolism in early-lactation dairy cows, *PLoS One*, 8 (11), 2013, e80316, doi:10.1371/journal.pone.0080316.

64. Kushibiki S, Hodate K, Shingu H, et al. Metabolic and Lactational Responses during Recombinant Bovine Tumor Necrosis Factor-alpha; Treatment in Lactating Cows. J Dairy Sci 2003;86(3):819–27.
65. Bergeron R, Elsener J. Comparison of postvaccinal milk drop in dairy cattle vaccinated with one of two different commercial vaccines. Vet Ther 2008;9(2): 141–6.
66. Scott HM, Atkins G, Willows B, McGregor R. Effects of 2 commercially-available 9-way killed vaccines on milk production and rectal temperature in Holstein-Friesian dairy cows. Can Vet J 2001;42(10):793–8.
67. Chandler TL, Westhoff TA, Overton TR, et al. Lipopolysaccharide challenge following intravenous amino acid infusion in postpartum dairy cows: I. Production, metabolic, and hormonal responses. J Dairy Sci 2022. https://doi.org/10.3168/jds.2021-21226.
68. Chandler TL, Westhoff TA, Behling-Kelly E, et al. Eucalcemia during lipopolysaccharide challenge in postpartum dairy cows: I. Clinical, inflammatory, and metabolic response. J Dairy Sci 2023. https://doi.org/10.3168/jds.2022-22774.
69. Eckel EF, Ametaj BN. Invited review: Role of bacterial endotoxins in the etiopathogenesis of periparturient diseases of transition dairy cows. J Dairy Sci 2016; 99(8):5967–90.
70. Robinson DP, Klein SL. Pregnancy and pregnancy-associated hormones alter immune responses and disease pathogenesis. Horm Behav 2012;62(3):263–71.
71. Esposito G, Irons PC, Webb EC, et al. Interactions between negative energy balance, metabolic diseases, uterine health and immune response in transition dairy cows. Anim Reprod Sci 2014;144(3–4):60–71.
72. Huzzey JM, Veira DM, Weary DM, von Keyserlingk MA. Prepartum behavior and dry matter intake identify dairy cows at risk for metritis. J Dairy Sci 2007;90(7): 3220–33. https://doi.org/10.3168/jds.2006-807.
73. Hoeben D, Heyneman R, Burvenich C. Elevated levels of beta-hydroxybutyric acid in periparturient cows and in vitro effect on respiratory burst activity of bovine neutrophils. Vet Immunol Immunopathol 1997;58(2):165–70.
74. Swartz TH, Bradford BJ, Mamedova LK. Connecting Metabolism to Mastitis: Hyperketonemia Impaired Mammary Gland Defenses During a *Streptococcus uberis* Challenge in Dairy Cattle. Front Immunol 2021;12:700278. https://doi.org/10.3389/fimmu.2021.700278.
75. Zarrin M, Wellnitz O, van Dorland HA, et al. Induced hyperketonemia affects the mammary immune response during lipopolysaccharide challenge in dairy cows. J Dairy Sci 2014;97(1):330–9.
76. Dubuc J, Duffield TF, Leslie KE, et al. Risk factors for postpartum uterine diseases in dairy cows. J Dairy Sci 2010;93(12):5764–71.
77. Sato S, Suzuki T, Okada K. Suppression of mitogenic response of bovine peripheral blood lymphocytes by ketone bodies. J Vet Med Sci 1995;57(1):183–5.
78. Grinberg N, Elazar S, Rosenshine I, et al. Beta-hydroxybutyrate abrogates formation of bovine neutrophil extracellular traps and bactericidal activity against mammary pathogenic Escherichia coli. Infect Immun 2008;76(6):2802–7.
79. Ospina PA, Nydam DV, Stokol T, et al. Associations of elevated nonesterified fatty acids and beta-hydroxybutyrate concentrations with early lactation reproductive performance and milk production in transition dairy cattle in the northeastern United States. J Dairy Sci 2010;93(4):1596–603.
80. Chapinal N, Carson M, Duffield TF, et al. The association of serum metabolites with clinical disease during the transition period. J Dairy Sci 2011;94(10): 4897–903.

81. Korbecki J, Bajdak-Rusinek K. The effect of palmitic acid on inflammatory response in macrophages: an overview of molecular mechanisms. Inflamm Res 2019;68(11):915–32.
82. Abou-Rjeileh U, Contreras GA. Redox regulation of lipid mobilization in adipose tissues. Antioxidants 2021;10(7). https://doi.org/10.3390/antiox10071090.
83. Mann S, Yepes FA, Duplessis M, et al. Dry period plane of energy: effects on glucose tolerance in transition dairy cows. J Dairy Sci 2016;99(1):701–17.
84. Galvao KN, Flaminio MJ, Brittin SB, et al. Association between uterine disease and indicators of neutrophil and systemic energy status in lactating Holstein cows. J Dairy Sci 2010;93(7):2926–37.
85. Mann S, Sipka A, Leal Yepes FA, et al. Nutrient-sensing kinase signaling in bovine immune cells is altered during the postpartum nutrient deficit: a possible role in transition cow inflammatory response. J Dairy Sci 2018;101. https://doi.org/10.3168/jds.2018-14549.
86. Dalbach KF, Larsen M, Raun BM, et al. Effects of supplementation with 2-hydroxy-4-(methylthio)-butanoic acid isopropyl ester on splanchnic amino acid metabolism and essential amino acid mobilization in postpartum transition Holstein cows. J Dairy Sci 2011;94(8):3913–27.
87. Meijer GA, Van der Meulen J, Bakker JG, et al. Free amino acids in plasma and muscle of high yielding dairy cows in early lactation. J Dairy Sci 1995;78(5):1131–41.
88. Noleto PG, Saut JP, Sheldon IM. Short communication: glutamine modulates inflammatory responses to lipopolysaccharide in ex vivo bovine endometrium. J Dairy Sci 2017;100(3):2207–12.
89. Vailati-Riboni M, Zhou Z, Jacometo CB, et al. Supplementation with rumen-protected methionine or choline during the transition period influences whole-blood immune response in periparturient dairy cows. J Dairy Sci 2017;100(5):3958–68.
90. Martinez N, Risco CA, Lima FS, et al. Evaluation of peripartal calcium status, energetic profile, and neutrophil function in dairy cows at low or high risk of developing uterine disease. J Dairy Sci 2012;95(12):7158–72.
91. Malcolm DS, Zaloga GP, Holaday JW. Calcium administration increases the mortality of endotoxic shock in rats. Crit Care Med 1989;17(9):900–3.
92. Zaloga GP, Sager A, Black KW, et al. Low dose calcium administration increases mortality during septic peritonitis in rats. Circ Shock 1992;37(3):226–9.
93. Serrenho RC, Morrison E, Bruinje TC, et al. Assessment of systemic inflammation following oral cal cium supplementation in postpartum dairy cows—A randomized controlled trial. J Dairy Sci 2022;105(Supplement 1):84. Abstracts of the 2022 American Dairy Science Association Annual Meeting.
94. Abuelo A, Hernandez J, Benedito JL, et al. Redox Biology in Transition Periods of Dairy Cattle: Role in the Health of Periparturient and Neonatal Animals. Antioxidants 2019;8(1):20.
95. Cuervo W, Sordillo LM, Abuelo A. Oxidative stress compromises lymphocyte function in neonatal dairy calves. Antioxidants 2021;10(2):255.
96. Abuelo A, Hernandez J, Benedito JL, et al. The importance of the oxidative status of dairy cattle in the periparturient period: revisiting antioxidant supplementation. J Anim Physiol Anim Nutr 2015;99(6):1003–16.
97. Overton TR, Yasui T. Practical applications of trace minerals for dairy cattle. J Anim Sci 2014;92(2):416–26.
98. Bouwstra RJ, Nielen M, Stegeman JA, et al. Vitamin E supplementation during the dry period in dairy cattle. Part I: adverse effect on incidence of mastitis

postpartum in a double-blind randomized field trial. J Dairy Sci 2010;93(12):5684–95.
99. Bradford BJ, Swartz TH. Review: Following the smoke signals: inflammatory signaling in metabolic homeostasis and homeorhesis in dairy cattle. Animal 2020;14(S1):s144–54.
100. Bouwstra RJ, Nielen M, Newbold JR, et al. Vitamin E supplementation during the dry period in dairy cattle. Part II: oxidative stress following vitamin E supplementation may increase clinical mastitis incidence postpartum. J Dairy Sci 2010;93(12):5696–706.
101. Kehrli ME Jr, Nonnecke BJ, Roth JA. Alterations in bovine lymphocyte function during the periparturient period. Article. Am J Vet Res 1989;50(2):215–20.
102. Stevens MG, Peelman LJ, De Spiegeleer B, et al. Differential gene expression of the toll-like receptor-4 cascade and neutrophil function in early- and mid-lactating dairy cows. J Dairy Sci 2011;94(3):1277–88.
103. Xie L, Ma Y, Opsomer G, et al. Neutrophil extracellular traps in cattle health and disease. Res Vet Sci 2021;139:4–10.
104. Tan X, Li WW, Guo J, et al. Down-regulation of NOD1 in neutrophils of periparturient dairy cows. Vet Immunol Immunopathol 2012;150(1–2):133–9.
105. Guidry AJ, Paape MJ. Effect of bovine neutrophil maturity on phagocytosis. Am J Vet Res 1976;37(6):703–5.
106. Galvao KN, Felippe MJ, Brittin SB, et al. Evaluation of cytokine expression by blood monocytes of lactating Holstein cows with or without postpartum uterine disease. Theriogenology 2012;77(2):356–72.

Methods of Evaluating the Potential Success or Failure of Transition Dairy Cows

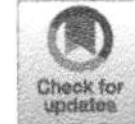

Matteo Mezzetti, PhD, Erminio Trevisi, PhD*

KEYWORDS

- Metabolic profile • Peripartum • Subclinical disorders • Immune functions
- Oxidative stress

KEY POINTS

- Failure of metabolic adaptation to the transition period increases the susceptibility of dairy cows to diseases and impairs performances during the following lactation.
- Plasma analyte trends during dry period (or even late lactation phase) serve as predictive markers for a bad transition.
- Plasma analyte trends during postpartum and early lactation phases, allows for monitoring of successful homeostasis recovery after calving.
- Improving current methods for applying metabolic profiling to transition dairy cows could increase the robustness of metabolic markers based on plasma analytes aimed at preventing disease onset.

INTRODUCTION TO METABOLIC PROFILING IN TRANSITION DAIRY COWS

Transition to calving has been widely documented as the most challenging physiologic phase for dairy cows. Sudden metabolic shifts accompanying parturition often exceed body homeorhetic capacity, resulting in a physiologic imbalance (PI) condition that is closely related to the risk of developing several metabolic and infectious disorders.[1] Early monitoring of the failure of metabolic adaptation to calving represents the most effective measure for allowing a prompt intervention on transition dairy cows, preventing deleterious effects on performances, such as reduced milk yield and fertility, as well as animal health and welfare issues driven by multiple disorders during the following lactation.

In living animals, alteration in the endocrine, immune, and metabolic assets are finely reflected by trends in blood analyte concentrations. Detecting any shift from "normal" trends in the blood analytes potentially reveals an abnormal condition. Blood

Department of Animal Sciences, Food and Nutrition (DIANA), Facoltà di Scienze Agrarie, Alimentari e Ambientali, Università Cattolica del Sacro Cuore, Piacenza 29122, Italy
* Corresponding author.
E-mail address: erminio.trevisi@unicatt.it

Vet Clin Food Anim 39 (2023) 219–239
https://doi.org/10.1016/j.cvfa.2023.02.008 vetfood.theclinics.com

could be divided into several analytical fractions but serum and plasma have the greatest relevance for clinical biochemistry. Plasma prevails in most analytical laboratories due to easier handling of samples (no clotting time required) and wider range of analytes assessable (ie, albumin, albumin-globulin ratio and potassium).[2–4] Thus, clinical biochemistry defines several pathologic thresholds for specific plasma analytes (named biomarkers) to reveal the progression of "subclinical" diseases (SCD).[1] These are often not reflected by any specific clinical signs but impart detrimental effects on performance and health status of the sick animal. This approach finds its widest application in dairy cows at their transition to calving, when the incidence of SCD is known to be highest across the whole lactation cycle.[5]

The wider application of metabolic profiling (MP), or the assessment of multiple plasma analytes as a benchmark for metabolic pathways, is currently less clear and accepted in farm animals. Because all the farm animals within a herd face the same feed, management, and environmental changes, assessing multiple plasma analytes on a group of cows undergoing the same phase of the lactation cycle has the potential to reflect their nutritional status, stress, and welfare condition.[6] Applying an expanded MP (ie, including inflammation and redox balance biomarkers) to the transition cows could (1) provide a deeper view on the cause of any pathologic condition affecting them, aimed at increasing the effectiveness and timely application of any treatment[7] and (2) provide a detailed feedback on the management practices adopted in a farm during this challenging phase based on animal responses.[6,8,9]

Despite this great potential, applying MP to transition cows is still hindered by several limitations. In fact, results obtained through MP are highly dependent on the protocol adopted by individual analytical laboratories, due to the lack of an accepted standard procedure for its application. This review is aimed at exploring the diagnostic power of MP in assessing the failure or success of dairy cows' adaptation to the peri-parturient phase, focusing on the state of the art of this technique, the definition of standard procedures for sample collection and handling, data analysis, and interpretation of analyte trends during the transition phase.

BLOOD SAMPLING TIMING STRATEGIES

In dairy cows, a "classical" transition period is defined as being between 21 days before and 21 days after parturition because most of the physiologic changes affecting hormonal patterns and nutrient redistribution take place within this time frame.[1] In practical situations, plasma samples reflecting dairy cows' adaptation to this phase could be obtained through collecting blood samples between 3 and 7 days postpartum.[10–12]

A more comprehensive approach for collecting blood samples aimed at monitoring dairy cows' adaptation to the new lactation would be extended to sampling during the dry period (from 60 to 10 days before expected calving date), early lactation (from 10 to 100 days in milk [DIM]), and midlate lactation phase (from 90 to 215 DIM). Besides providing an overview on management practices adopted in a commercial dairy farm during the whole lactation cycle, expanding the time frame for blood sample collection beyond the "classical" transition period improves the detection of analyte trends:

- Predicting an impaired adaptation to transition period challenges (for samples collected during the dry or even late lactation phases) or
- Reflecting a delayed recovery of homeostatic conditions after calving (for samples collected during the early lactation phase).

Trends related to altered immune system functions impart the greatest importance in this respect. On one hand, altered immune function before calving boosts severity of metabolic changes faced by dairy cows during the transition period,[13] detrimentally affecting adaptation to the new lactation through predisposing them at developing PI conditions.[1] On the other hand, delayed recovery of homeostatic condition for acute phase proteins (APP, both positive and negative) after calving have been related to long-term side-effects on lactation performance.[14]

REFERENCE INTERVAL CALCULATION FOR PLASMA ANALYTES IN TRANSITION COWS: AN OPEN ISSUE

Whatever the objective for performing an MP on a commercial farm, interpretation of measured analytes requires suitable reference intervals (RIs) reflecting optimal metabolic conditions for dairy cows within defined lactation cycle phase. At present, extrapolating the approach adopted in human clinical biochemistry for the definition of RI for plasma analytes to dairy cows is hindered by some limitations.[12]

The criteria used for reference individuals' recruitment potentially affect the resulting RI. For transition cows, including an SCD screening based on pathologic thresholds for plasma biomarkers (ie, β-hydroxybutyrate [BHB], Ca, and haptoglobin) before the reference individual's selection is of great importance in defining the RI. Limiting the selection to "healthy individuals" defined as animals showing no clinical diseases could result in inaccurate prediction of physiologic conditions for the population.[12] Furthermore, prevailing conditions characterizing the sampling area (ie, cow genetic merit, farm management and veterinary practices, diet composition, environmental conditions, and so forth) potentially affect plasma analyte trends (and the resulting RI) through altered welfare condition of reference individuals. Thus, despite several sets of RI having been suggested for the dry period,[10,12,15,16] postpartum phase,[10–12] early lactation,[9,11,12,15,17] and midlate lactation period,[12,17] utilizing these RI sets in farms having different operative conditions potentially leads to inaccurate interpretation of results.

Performing a preliminary welfare assessment considering multiple operative aspects at the farm level (as those proposed by Premi and colleagues[12]) has the potential to classify farms into different "welfare classes." Plasma analyte trends detected within each class could be used for calculating specific RI sets, and the most suitable one could be chosen for interpreting results obtained under similar operative conditions. Ideally, RI obtained in the highest welfare classes should be considered as the "gold standard" for plasma analytes of dairy cows raised under a certain breeding system.

BLOOD SAMPLING PROCEDURES

Defining Sample Size

Lowering the number of samples is a fundamental point for reducing costs related to MP. The first step for quantifying the minimum sample size is defining the investigation aim we want to perform. When MP is aimed at assessing the cause behind a pathologic condition, then a small sample of sick animals should be selected for the blood analysis. When the aim is assessing proper dairy cow adaptation to specific lactation cycle phases, then MP evaluation should be referred to the herd level. Despite no recognized standards exist on the minimum number of animals to be sampled for this purpose, guidelines provided by Herdt for evaluating nutritional status of dairy cows through plasma analytes[8] could be adopted. Thus, representative samples should consider 10% of the animals included in each group (at least 7 animals/group) bleed at a single time. Despite that, transition period management practiced on modern dairy farms consists of animals flowing successively into different groups, where consistency varies markedly based on the average calving rate. Thus, strictly applying the general standard to transition groups potentially results in an insufficient sample size. Kerwin and colleagues[18] proposed a sample of 12 to 24 cows/farm to be considered as an appropriate sample size for applying MP screening to transition cows. Sample should include one-third primiparous and two-thirds multiparous cows, to be bleed successively in the far off, close-up, fresh, and early lactation groups.

Bleeding Procedures, Samples Handling and Analysis

The gold standard for bleeding a cow to obtain plasma is by jugular venipuncture because collecting samples from the coccygeal vein increases the risk of obtaining hemolyzed samples and several analytes (ie, glucose, Ca, P, and K) could be affected by the mammary metabolism. Despite that, adopting other sampling sites (ie, coccygeal, or mammary veins) could be acceptable when suitable RIs are defined for analytes determined under the same condition. Heparinized vacuum tubes should be used for bleeding because other anticoagulants affect analytical results for several plasma analytes.[19] Performing bleedings before rumen fermentations reached their daily peak (ie, immediately before or at the time of first feeding) and minimizing acute stress conditions related to restraining animals, are pivotal for avoiding alteration of plasma analytes trends.[20] In modern dairy farms adopting a total mixed ration (TMR) system associated with headlocks along the feeding line, both requirements could be met by locking the animals and performing bleedings during the daily TMR distribution. Standard methods for handling samples between collection and analysis (including storage time and temperature) have been described by Calamari and colleagues[6]

Available methods for plasma tests desired in the MP are based on automated or semiautomated analyzers, which come at high cost. Alternative analytical methods based on dry chemistry or infrared spectroscopy have been validated in humans to cope with costs and delays between sampling and result reporting.[21–24] Despite several efforts having been made for extending these methods to dairy cows,[6] accuracy and repeatability of results limit their use to a subset of plasma analytes routinely included in an MP. In the last decades, a wide literature documented plasma analytes reflecting inflammatory condition and redox balance of dairy cows as promising biomarkers for assessing metabolic adaptation of the animal to the new lactation.[9,13,25] Reference analytical methods for assessing these analytes remain those performed with a clinical autoanalyzer. **Table 1** provides some examples of analytical methods for performing an expanded MP (ie, including inflammation and redox balance biomarkers) in dairy cows.

ASSESSING TRANSITION COWS' METABOLIC STATUS THROUGH PLASMA ANALYTE TRENDS

Punctual evaluation of dairy cows' adaptation to the transition period challenges within a herd rely on bleeding a representative sample of animals during the late lactation, the dry, the postpartum, the early and the midlate lactation phases. Blood samples should be analyzed individually for the packed cell volume and for the trends of plasma analytes reflecting the energy, protein and mineral metabolism, the kidney and liver function, the inflammatory status, and the redox balance. Within each phase of the lactation cycle, metabolic condition of each animal sampled should be evaluated through comparing analytes concentration with suitable RIs (ie, defined under operative conditions similar to those observed in the herd) and suspecting abnormal metabolic condition for analytes laying outside RI limits. Besides serving as a

Table 1
Intra-assay and interassay coefficient of variations, limit of quantification, analytical method, codes of commercial kits used, references for their validation in the bovine plasma, calibrators, and quality controls used for main plasma analytes determinable through a chemical auto analyzer

Parameter, UM	Method	Intra	Inter	LOQ	Kit	Reference	Calibrator	Quality control
Glucose, mmol/L	Trinder end point (glucose oxidase/ peroxidase)	1.33	0.75	0.1	182508401	-	Homemade bovine standard	Homemade bovine standard; SeraChem Control Level 1, 00181624121; Bov Asy Control 2, AN10263
Fructosamine, mmol/L	Colorimetric end kinetic metod	0.9	5.33	15	7080	-	Diagnostic Far Calibrator 7080s	Diagnostic Far Control N+P, 7510
NEFA, mmol/L	Enzymatic colorimetric method assay	2.27	5.00	0.01	NEFA-HR(2) R1 Set, 434-917952	-	NEFA standard, 270-77000[b]	Homemade bovine standard; SeraChem Control Level 1, 00181624121; Bov Asy Control 2, AN10263
BHB, mmol/L	Kinetic UV method	0.82	3.42	0.1	RB10073	-	BHB standard included in the kit	
Triglycerides, mmol/L	Enzymatic method (GPO-Trinder)	0.84	3.44	0.02	18255640	-	Homemade bovine standard	Homemade bovine standard; SeraChem Control Level 1, 00181624121; Bov Asy Control 2, AN10263
Urea, mmol/L	End point method (GLDH enzyme system)	1.14	1.23	0.01	182554401	-	Homemade bovine standard	
Creatinine, μmol/L	Colorimetric end point method	1.09	3.09	18	182555401	-	Homemade bovine standard	
Ca, mmol/L	Colorimetric end point method	0.93	1.86	0.2	182503401	-	Homemade bovine standard	
P, mmol/L	End point UV method	1.64	0.73	0.01	182512401	-	Homemade bovine standard	
Mg, mmol/L	Rate analysis, enzymatic methodology	1.00	1.65	0.02	182592401	-	Homemade bovine standard	
Na, mmol/L	Potentiometer method (Ion Selective Electrodes)	0.62	1.53	50	ISE Diluent, 00182534001;	-	ISE low calibrator, 00184692001; ISE high calibrator, 00184693001	
K, mmol/L		0.63	1.11	1.46	ISE Reference, 00182535001	-		
Cl, mmol/L		0.34	0.77	70	-	-		
Zn, mmol/L	Colorimetric method	1.76	3.83	0.5	439-149062	-	Bov Asy Control 2[c,d]	

(continued on next page)

Table 1 (*continued*)

Parameter, UM	Method	Intra	Inter	LOQ	Kit	Reference	Calibrator	Quality control
Total bilirubin, μmol/L	End point analysis	3.11	2.46	2	182546401	Shaw et al,[21] 1988	Bov Asy Control 2[d]	
AST, U/L	Kinetic analysis	1.78	3.55	1	182575401	-	No calibration is required	
GGT, U/L		2.27	4.42	2	182576401	-	No calibration is required	
ALP, U/L		0.77	3.52	2	182596401	-	ReferrIL E, 0018256300[a]	
Myeloperoxidase, U/L	Colorimetric method	1.83	8.60	10	-	SR et al,[22] 2000	No calibration is required	Homemade bovine standard; SeraChem Control Level 1, 00181624121
Total protein, g/L	Modified biuret methodology	1.07	2.87	10	182514401	-	Homemade bovine standard	Homemade bovine standard; SeraChem Control Level 1, 00181624121; Bov Asy Control 2, AN10263
Haptoglobin, g/L	Rate of oxidation of guaiacol from MetHB-Hp complex in presence of H_2O_2	3.64	3.50	0.01	-	Hahn et al,[23] 2010	No calibration is required	
Ceruloplasmin, μmol/L	P-phenylenediamine dihydrochloride oxidation	1.39	3.57	0.1	-	Lahmann et al,[24] 2013	Human plasma ceruloplasmin, A50143H[e,f]	
Albumin, g/L	Colorimetric end point method	1.20	3.41	16	182500401	-	Homemade bovine standard	
Cholesterol, mmol/L	Trinder end point (cholesterol oxidase/ peroxidase)	1.56	1.38	0.1	182505401	-	Homemade bovine standard	
Retinol, μmol/L		2.72	2.70	-	-		R7632	Homemade bovine standard;
Paraoxonase, U/mL	Kinetic photometric method	1.38	4.60	1.2	-	Mezzetti et al,[25] 2019	No calibration is required	Homemade bovine standard; SeraChem Control Level 1, 00181624121; Bov Asy Control 2, AN10263
Tocopherol, μmol/L		3.38	3.52	-	-		T3251	Homemade bovine standard;
β-Carotene, μmol/L		5.55	6.32	-	-		C4582	

FRAP, mmol/L	Colorimetric method	3.13	3.15	30	-	Manston et al,[26] 1975	TROLOX, 238813-1G[g]	Homemade bovine standard; SeraChem Control Level 1, 00181624121; Bov Asy Control 2, AN10263; TROLOX, 238813-1G8
Thiol groups, mmol/L	Colorimetric method	1.00	5.90	3.5	MC433	-	Calibrator SHp, MC.0309	Homemade bovine standard; SeraChem Control Level 1, 00181624121; Bov Asy Control 2, AN10263 Calibrator SHp, MC.0309
ROMt, mg H_2O_2/dL	Colorimetric method	1.40	2.93	3.2	MC0034	-	Calibrator d-ROMs, MC.030[h]	Homemade bovine standard SeraChem Control Level 1, 00181624121; Control Serum, MC0314; Calibrator d-ROMs, MC0304
AOPP, mmol/L		0.42	10.93	10	-	Wohlt et al,[27] 1984	Chloramine T trihydrate, 31224-250G10	Homemade bovine standard; SeraChem Control Level 1, 00181624121; Bov Asy Control 2, AN10263

Abbreviations: ALP, alkaline phosphatase; AOPP, advanced oxidation product of protein; AST, aspartate aminotransferase; BHB, β-Hydroxybutyrate; FRAP, ferric reducing antioxidant power; GGT, γ-glutamyl transferase; LOQ, limit of quantification; NEFA, nonesterified fatty acids; ROMt, total reactive oxygen metabolites.

[a] Instrumentation Laboratory Werfen, Milano, Italy.
[b] Wako Chemicals GmbH, neuss, Germany.
[c] Diacron International S.r.l., Grosseto, Italy.
[d] Megazyme, Wicklow, Ireland.
[e] Meridian Life Science, Memphis, USA.
[f] Thermo Scientific, Frederick, MD 2174, USA.
[g] Sigma-Aldrich Chemie GmbH, Steinheim, Germany.
[h] Carlo Erba, Rodano, Milano, Italy.

diagnostic tool for detecting the abnormal condition of an animal, this approach could be aimed at detecting the "smoke signals" highlighting managerial issues in specific phases of the lactation cycle. Thus, evaluation could be extended to the herd level through calculating the average herd value (AHV) for the concentration of each analyte and comparing AHVs to the RIs. Herd evaluation always requires care in the final interpretation of results, as the AHV is deeply affected by the individual contribution of each animal recruited in the initial sample. Thus, proportion of animals having abnormal values for a plasma analyte should be considered when AHV lays outside the RIs limits (ie, extending the evaluation to the herd level when abnormal values are detected at least on 50% of samples animals).

Individual Interpretation for Plasma Analytes

Packed cell volume (PCV) represents the percent of blood volume filled by erythrocytes and provides a measure of oxygen carrying capacity. Its trend, paired with those of albumin and hemoglobin have also been proposed as a long-term protein status biomarker in dairy cows.[26] Normal PCV trend across the lactation cycle is negatively related to milk yield (ie, higher in the dry and early postpartum than in the late lactation phase, and higher in the late lactation than in the early lactation phase) suggesting a modification of plasma volume driven by milk production, combined with differences in the erythopoiesis rate and erythrocyte halflife.[27,28]

Energy Metabolism Biomarkers

Glucose and Fructosamine. Glucose is the primary energy source for metabolic processes, whereas fructosamine is a stable ketoamine resulting from glucose glycation to protein molecules, finely reflecting fasting plasma glucose concentration within 1 to 3 weeks.[29,30] Trends of both analytes undergo a physiologic drop in the postpartum period, driven by the onset of galactopoietic processes and the activation of leukocytes to cope with calving-related insults.[12] As approaching the early and midlate lactation phases, both analytes gradually increase their plasma concentration. Compared with the midlate lactation, lower concentration of glucose could be found during the dry phase due to increased energy requirements driven by the gravid uterus combined to the lowered energy content of the dry ration.[31,32]

Nonesterified fatty acids, triglycerides, and β-hydroxybutyrate. Plasma nonesterified fatty acid (NEFA) concentration is proportional to the severity of body fat mobilization; triglycerides (TAG) reflect the ability of the liver in reesterifying NEFAs and exporting them through very low-density lipoproteins (VLDL), whereas BHB is released in the bloodstream when a NEFA overload impairs the β-oxidation process at the liver level.[33,34] Although, plasma BHB greater than 1.2 and 3.0 mmol/L are widely adopted as subclinical ketosis (SCK) and clinical ketosis thresholds, respectively,[35,36] plasma NEFA concentration could serve as diagnostic and prognostic biomarkers for a failure in homeorhetic adaptation to NEB, although proposed thresholds are still debated. Most of the thresholds have been defined on the risk of developing a specific disease condition and do not hold for all the aspects of cow biologic performances (ie, trends of other plasma analytes, feed intake, milk yield, and fertility), which are not discrete relative to thresholds but a continuum.

Both NEFA and BHB concentrations peak in the postpartum due to the NEB condition affecting dairy cows in this phase.[1,33] In this phase, the occurrence of SCK has been associated to increased disease incidence and impaired fertility, despite detecting plasma BHB greater than 0.9 mmol/L in postpartum having been associated to increase 305-mature equivalent milk yield.[18] Postpartum NEFA greater than 0.7 mmol/L have been proposed as a risk factor for developing ketosis and displaced abomasum in early lactation.[37–39] Recently, safety threshold for disease prevention has been lowered to 0.59 mmol/L, although decreased 305-mature equivalent milk yield were already documented when postpartum NEFA exceed 0.48 mmol/L.[18]

In early lactation, BHB level decreases and reflects ruminal production of butyric acid,[40] whereas NEFA progressively decreases as animals progress to the midlate lactation phase. Compared with late lactation, higher NEFA concentration could be found during the dry period, due to lower energy intake from the dry ration. Dry period NEFA concentration is commonly paired with the greatest TAG concentration, probably reflecting greater VLDL export and greater hepatic capability to reesterify circulating NEFA before calving compared with the postpartum phase.[41,42] Plasma NEFA greater than 0.3 mmol/L in the far off and greater than 0.5 mmol/L in the last week of gestation has been proposed as a risk factor for developing retained placenta, ketosis, displacement of abomasum, and metritis in early lactation.[37,39] Recently, a 0.17 mmol/L threshold has been proposed for prepartum NEFA concentration, where multiparous cows above this prepartum threshold had subsequent decreased 21-day pregnancy rate and increased risk of disorders.[18]

Protein Metabolism and Kidney Function Biomarkers

Urea and creatinine. Assessment of specific plasma analytes (ie, 3-methylhistidine) is required to effectively reflect protein turnover.[43] Despite that, quantifying plasma concentration in dairy cows is still expensive and time-consuming. Thus, valuable information on protein metabolism could be realized from urea and creatinine trends. Urea is synthesized in the liver from 2 sources: nitrogen deamination from amino acids and ammonia absorbed by the rumen.[44] Trends of plasma urea normally decline in the dry and postpartum phases, driven both by lower protein content of dry rations and low feed intake of postpartum cows compared with those in mid and late lactation.[45,46] Increased plasma urea during postpartum phase could be also observed under a severe NEB condition, due to the massive mobilization of muscle protein to face the energy deficit. Creatinine is related to phosphocreatine generated during normal muscular activity but interpretation of this plasma analyte is challenging. On one hand, plasma creatinine has been reported to reflect the amount of muscle mass in the body.[47] On the other hand, blood creatinine concentration reflects the kidneys' ability to remove it, and its elevation reflects an impaired glomerular filtration rate driven by stress events (ie, inflammation).[48,49] Both these interpretations are consistent with the trend of plasma creatinine across the lactation cycle. Highest concentration was reported in the dry phase, possibly reflecting a greater amount of muscle tissue in dry compared with lactating cows, or a transient impairment of kidney glomerular filtration rate driven by body fat mobilization and altered blood pressure during the late gestation phase.[50] Decrease of creatinine after parturition,[51] suggests both a reduced amount of muscle tissue (the mobilization of 13%–25% of body proteins occurs around calving[47]) and an improved glomerular filtration rate compared with the dry phase. Physiologic trends of PCV, glucose, fructosamine, NEFA, BHB, TAG, urea, and creatinine across the lactation cycle are shown in **Fig. 1**.

Mineral Metabolism Biomarkers

Calcium, phosphorus, and magnesium. Homeostatic regulation for these minerals is closely related to parathormone functioning.[1] In the postpartum phase, sequestration by the mammary gland exceeds reabsorption processes for Ca and P, leading to a physiologic reduction in their circulating pools, whereas Mg concentration is the lowest across the lactation cycle due to a lower absorption driven by altered rumen functions (ie, lowered feed intake and rumen motility postpartum).[52] In early lactation,

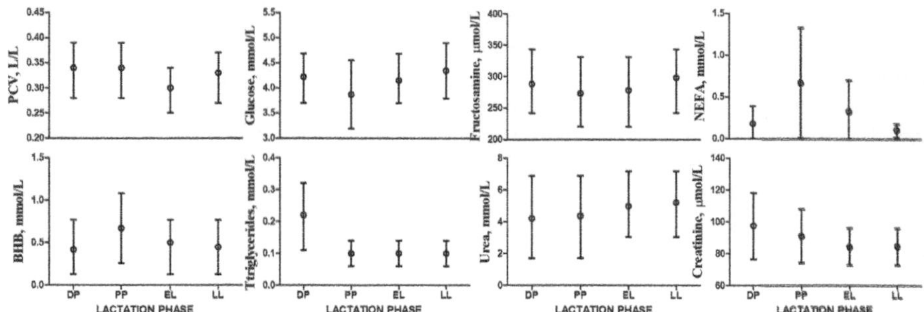

Fig. 1. Physiological trends of packed cell volume (PCV), glucose, fructosamine, NEFA, BHB, triglycerides, urea, and creatinine across the dry (DP; −30/−10 days from calving), postpartum (PP; 3/7 days from calving), early lactation (EL; 28/45 days from calving), and late lactation phases (LL; 160/305 days from calving) in Holstein dairy cows. Trend for each blood analyte within physiological phases have been defined through applying a bootstrap approach and a 95% confidence interval to a dataset including 361 healthy cows raised within 11 high welfare farms. (*Adapted from* Ref.[9])

plasma Ca concentration increases and remains stable thereafter, whereas P and Mg gradually increase throughout the lactation cycle phases.

Altered homeostatic conditions for plasma concentrations of these minerals could impair the ability of the animal to rise to its feet (as explained in more detail in another article in this issue). Postpartum, this pathologic condition is named "milk fever" and consists in a primary hypocalcemia (<1.92, <1.62, and < 0.87 mmol/L for stage I, II, and III, respectively) paired with a hypophosphatemic state (<1.2 and < 0.6 mmol/L, for stage I and II, respectively).[53,54] This condition could be driven by excessive dietary cation-anion difference (DCAD) load in the dry rations and inflammatory conditions,[55] and elevated parity order has been listed as a predisposing factor.

Lately in lactation (even in midlate lactation) secondary hypocalcemia could occur when excessive dietary cations and nonprotein nitrogen loads depress rumen Mg absorption postpartum. Then, hypomagnesemia state (<0.78 and < 0.66 mmol/L within 12 hours after calving for stage I and II, respectively)[54] depresses parathormone functioning.

Both primary and secondary hypocalcemia induce compensatory mechanism to preserve systemic anion–cation balance. In primary hypocalcemia, this consists in a secondary hypermagnesemia state (>1.23 and > 2.05 mmol/L for stage I and II, respectively) while secondary hypocalcemia commonly precedes a hyperphosphatemic state.[53]

Sodium, potassium, and chloride. Plasma electrolyte concentrations are quite stable across the lactation cycle phases because these minerals are involved in maintaining homeostasis in plasma membranes. Increased plasma concentration (hypernatremia) was only reported for Na and Cl before calving and in the postpartum phase due to impaired glomerular filtration rate and inflammatory conditions occurring around calving.[12] Pathologic conditions involving electrolytes equilibrium includes hypokalemia-driven flaccid paralysis (plasma K < 2.5 mmol/L),[54] occurring when the intracellular or extracellular K concentration decreases substantially, disrupting normal cell membrane potential and impairing several metabolic functions. Factors depleting intracellular K includes exaggerated renal excretion, prolonged fasting conditions (ie, those following a clinical ketosis status lasting longer than 5 days), and severe stressful conditions.[1]

Zinc and iron. Both Zn and Fe serve as substrates or cofactors in the activation of antioxidant enzymes (ie, superoxide dismutase, catalase), serving as secondary antioxidant systems.[56] In Holstein cows fed TMR diets lowest Zn concentration has been reported during lactation phase. Despite that, plasma concentration of Fe and Zn is significantly influenced by dietary supplementation and breeding system, and decreases under the acute phase response (APR) due to their sequestration in the liver aimed at preventing bacterial growth and the role exerted by transferrin (ie, Fe transport protein) as a negative acute phase protein.[9]

Physiologic trends of calcium, phosphorus, magnesium, sodium, potassium, chlorine, and zinc across the lactation cycle are shown in **Fig. 2**.

Liver Functions and Inflammation Biomarkers

Bilirubin results from the degradation of red blood cells. Its plasma concentration could be assumed as a cholestasis and liver function index because it reflects the efficiency of liver enzymes in removing it.[57] It peaks in postpartum, reflecting a transient impairment of liver function driven by the massive liver activities and the huge amounts of mobilized NEFA in this phase. Then, plasma bilirubin decreases from the early lactation until the dry phase, suggesting a gradual recovery of liver function.[12]

Hepatic enzymes. Both glutamate-oxalacetate transaminase (AST-GOT) and γ-glutamyl transferase (GGT) are involved in amino acid metabolism, whereas alkaline phosphatase (ALP) exerts a role in dephosphorylating compounds. Classically, increased plasma concentration of these enzymes serves as a cytolysis and liver damage biomarker,[57] whereas decreased ALP activity has been related to altered gut permeability.[58] Despite that, the AST-GOT phase trend is the only one overlapping

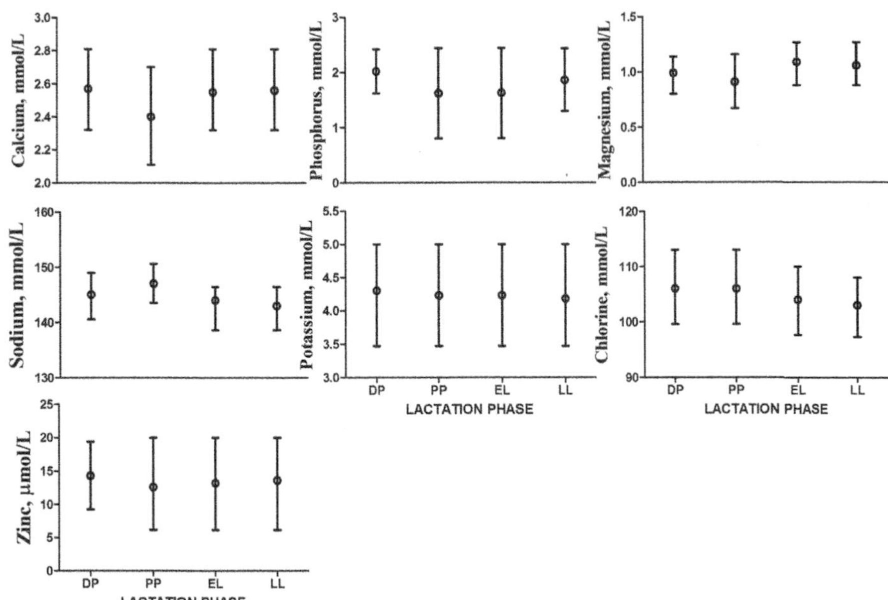

Fig. 2. Physiological trends of calcium, phosphorus, magnesium, sodium, potassium, chlorine, and zinc across the dry (DP; −30/−10 days from calving), postpartum (PP; 3/7 days from calving), early lactation (EL; 28/45 days from calving), and late lactation phases (LL; 160/305 days from calving) in Holstein dairy cows. Trend for each blood analyte within physiological phases have been defined through applying a bootstrap approach and a 95% confidence interval to a dataset including 361 healthy cows raised within 11 high welfare farms. (*Adapted from* Ref.[9])

that of bilirubin across the lactation cycle, as expected from a liver damage indicator. Conversely, ALP remains constant across the lactation cycle, whereas GGT has the highest plasma concentration at the end of lactation and during the dry phase, suggesting a longer half-life in the plasma fraction of this enzyme in respect of the AST-GOT.[12] AST-GOT has also been suggested as a muscle damage indicator and concentration higher than 100 U/L in the second week of lactation has been reported as a risk factor for displacement of the abomasum.[38]

Myeloperoxidase, total protein, and globulin. Myeloperoxidase (MPO) is involved in the generation of reactive oxygen species in activated neutrophils, thus serving as a reliable marker of inflammation.[59] It maintains stable concentration across the lactation cycle, peaking in the postpartum phase due to the activation of leukocytes occurring after calving.[12]

Total protein (albumin + globulin) and globulin have their highest plasma concentration in the early and late lactation phases, decreasing through dry phase and reaching a nadir in the postpartum phase. Lowered plasma protein reflects liver disease or acute infection and may be rarely related to immunodeficiency. Inadequate protein intake could be also considered as a cause when plasma protein deficit is generalized to the herd level. Heightened protein is found in paraproteinemia, leukemia or any condition causing an increase in immunoglobulins.

Acute phase proteins. Under an APR, the liver shifts protean synthesis in favor of positive APP, as haptoglobin and ceruloplasmin. The resultant is a reduced plasma concentration of albumin, retinol, and cholesterol (reflecting retinol binding protein and lipoproteins synthesis) and paraoxonase (PON), so named negative APPs.[1] Strongest APR conditions are found in the postpartum phase. Here, detecting plasma haptoglobin greater than 0.45 g/L has been associated to an increased disease incidence.[18] Thereafter, haptoglobin reach lower and more stable concentrations since the early lactation, whereas ceruloplasmin decreases and negative APPs increase gradually throughout the lactation cycle, serving as a longer lasting plasma biomarker relative to APR onset than haptoglobin.[12]

Physiologic trends of bilirubin, AST-GOT, GGT, MPO, protein, globulin, haptoglobin, ceruloplasmin, albumin, cholesterol, retinol, and PON across the lactation cycle are shown in **Fig. 3**.

Redox Balance Biomarkers

Antioxidant status. Several plasma analytes contribute to determining the body antioxidant capacity. Among vitamins, tocopherol (vitamin E) acts as a secondary antioxidant by reducing the chain propagation and amplification of lipid peroxidation, whereas β-carotene (provitamin A) exerts an indirect antioxidant action by maintaining other antioxidant molecules in their reduced form.[60] Concentration of other antioxidants is indirectly assessed through measuring antioxidant status of plasma against a reference substance, thus including heterogenous mixtures of compounds. Thiol groups (SHp) reflect the ability of glutathione peroxidase-1 in reducing hydroperoxides at the expense of albumin, lipoic acid, cysteine, and glutathione.[61] Ferric ion reducing antioxidant power (FRAP) provides a measurement of antioxidant power provided by bilirubin, uric acid, proteins, and vitamins C and E.[62] Oxygen reactive antioxidant capacity (ORAC) measures the antioxidant power of hydrosoluble antioxidants (ie, albumin and uric-acid) against reactive oxygen species.[63]

Plasma vitamin concentrations reach a nadir in the postpartum phase due to reduced feed intake and the depletion of circulating antioxidant systems driven by increased oxidative metabolism,[64] gradually increasing their plasma concentrations as cows approach the early lactation phase. In the dry phase, plasma tocopherol

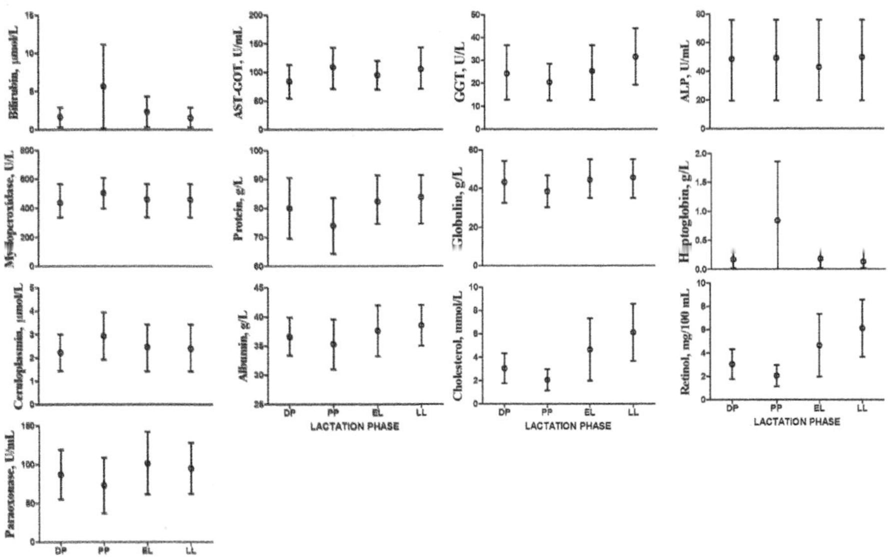

Fig. 3. Physiological trends of bilirubin, aspartate amino transferase (AST-GOT), gamma-glutamyl transferase (GGT), myeloperoxidase, protein, globulin, haptoglobin, ceruloplasmin, albumin, cholesterol, retinol, and paraoxonase across the dry (DP; −30/−10 days from calving), postpartum (PP; 3/7 days from calving), early lactation (EL; 28/45 days from calving), and late lactation phases (LL; 160/305 days from calving) in Holstein dairy cows. Trend for each blood analyte within physiological phases have been defined through applying a bootstrap approach and a 95% confidence interval to a dataset including 361 healthy cows raised within 11 high welfare farms. (*Adapted from* Ref.[9])

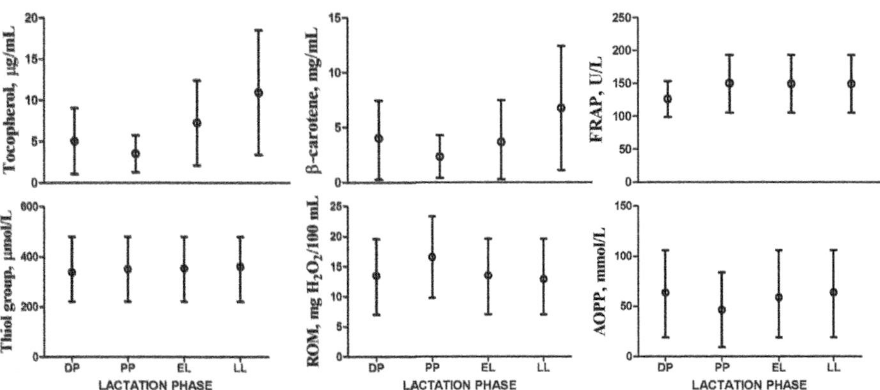

Fig. 4. Physiological trends of tocopherol, beta-carotene, FRAP, thiol group, ROMt and AOPP across the dry (DP; −30/−10 days from calving), postpartum (PP; 3/7 days from calving), early lactation (EL; 28/45 days from calving), and late lactation phases (LL; 160/305 days from calving) in Holstein dairy cows. Trend for each blood analyte within physiological phases have been defined through applying a bootstrap approach and a 95% confidence interval to a dataset including 361 healthy cows raised within 11 high welfare farms. (*Adapted from* Ref.[9])

Table 2
Ratios and indexes aimed at monitoring successful adaptation of dairy cows to the transition period challenges through aggregating plasma analyte trends

Item[1]	Biomarker	Interpretation	Reference
Ratios			
NEFA/albumin ratio (NAR)	Albumin fatty acids saturation	In humans, elevated NAR predisposes patients through developing diseases that include endothelial dysfunction in their pathology (ie, preeclampsia, coronary artery disease, type 2 diabetes), and impair antioxidant properties of albumin that includes Cu binding	[69,70]
Albumin/globulin ratio	Inflammation	Plasma albumin/globulin ratio of late lactating cows seems to predict the success of their adaptation to subsequent calving and lactation	Quiroz-Rocha et al,[10] 2009
Myeloperoxidase/paraoxonase ratio (MPR)	Mastitis	In humans, elevated MPR has been associated to dysfunctional high-density lipoprotein and risk stratification in coronary artery disease. In dairy cows, it has been associated to increased mastitis risk	[71,72]
ROMt/FRAP ROMt/ORAC	Integrated oxidant status	Provide a measurement of the redox balance of the body	[73]
Indexes			
{[(Albumin 5+Albumin 15+Albumin 30) + (Retinol 5+Retinol 15+Retinol 30) + (Cholesterol 5+Cholesterol 15+Cholesterol 30)]/9}[a]	Liver activity index (LAI)	Aimed at following up the successful adaptation of a dairy cow (within a sampled group) to the new lactation; aggregates the plasma albumin, cholesterol, and retinol concentrations measured 5, 15, and 30 d after calving. Optimal: >0.5 (higher is better)	Calamari et al,[6] 2016

[(Cholesterol RC + Albumin RC) – Bilirubin RC][b]	Liver functionality index (LFI)	Aimed at following up the successful adaptation of a dairy cow to the new lactation; aggregates the albumin, cholesterol, and bilirubin concentrations measured 3 and 28 d after calving. Optimal: >0 (higher is better)	68

[a] Analyte {*y*+*j*+*k*} = {[(Cow's analyte concentration at time y – Average analyte concentration in the sampled group)/Analyte standard deviation in the sampled group]+[(Cow's analyte concentration at time j – Average analyte concentration in the sampled group)/Analyte standard deviation in the sampled group]+[(Cow's analyte concentration at time *k* – Average analyte concentration in the sampled group)/Analyte standard deviation in the sampled group]}.

[b] Cholesterol RC = {[0.5*Cholesterol 3 DIM+0.5*(Cholesterol 28 DIM – Cholesterol 3 DIM)] –2.57}/0.43; Albumin RC = {[0.5*Albumin 3 DIM+0.5*(Albumin 28 DIM – Albumin 3 DIM)] –17.71}/1.08; Bilirubin RC = {[0.67*Bilirubin 3 DIM+0.33*(Bilirubin 28 DIM – Bilirubin 3 DIM)] –4.01}/1.21.

lower than 3 μmol/L has been related to a 9.4 times greater risk of having environmental mastitis within the first 7 DIM.[65] Concentration of SHp remains stable across the lactation cycle and FRAP maintains lower concentration in the dry than lactation phases, probably due to the upregulation of body antioxidant synthesis to cope with increased oxidative metabolisms during lactation.

Oxidant species and oxidative stress status biomarkers. Total reactive oxygen metabolites (ROMt), and reactive nitrogen species (RNS, ie, nitrite—NO_2, nitrate—NO_3, and nitric oxide—NOx) are the main oxidant species in dairy ruminants, originating from oxidative metabolisms occurring in the body (including immune cells functioning).[64] Plasma ROMt peak in the postpartum phase decreasing throughout the lactation cycle, whereas RNS trend is unknown.[66]

Advanced oxidation of protein products (AOPP) classically reflects protein oxidation driven by hypochlorous acid, thus representing a synthetic marker of oxidative stress caused by activated leukocytes through the respiratory burst.[66] Its plasma concentration drops in the postpartum phase, likely due to the primary contribution of albumin in facing oxidative damage in ruminants.[12] Thus, AOPP sensibility to serve as oxidative stress biomarker could be mitigated during APR conditions, as those physiologically affecting dairy cows during postpartum phase.

Physiologic trends of tocopherol, beta-carotene, FRAP, thiol group, ROM, and AOPP across the lactation cycle are shown in **Fig. 4**.

Ratios and Indexes

A strategy for evaluating specific metabolic functions could be combining plasma analyte trends in a calculation of indexes and ratios. Ratios (ie, NEFA/albumin ratio, albumin/globulin ratio) are widely used in human medicine, and potentially provide valuable information when extended to dairy cows,[13] whereas several indexes (mainly based on liver function and APR biomarkers) have been appositely developed for following up the successful adaptation of dairy cow to the new lactation.[9,67] State of the art on application of ratios and indexes to dairy cows, as well as the formulas used for their calculation and the interpretation of results are provided in **Table 2**.

SUMMARY

Assessing the proper adaptation of dairy cows to the transition period challenges though MP has enormous potential, as widely demonstrated by research in this field during the last decades. Despite this, high analytical costs, and the lack of any standardized procedure on its application in field conditions, limits its wide use. Developing standard methods for sample collection, handling and analysis, for results interpretation and for calculating suitable RIs for plasma analytes are key points for improving the accuracy and repeatability of results obtained through this technique. This (together with the reduction of costs and processing time that future development in analytical methods will hopefully provide us), could likely improve the robustness of currently available metabolic biomarkers in assessing the successful adaptation of dairy cows to the transition period challenges, making an extended MP as an essential tool to be implemented in any precision herd management context.

CLINICS CARE POINTS

To assess metabolic adaptation of dairy cows to the transition period challenge and to monitor the wellness state during the lactation through metabolic profiling:

- Select representative samples of animals undergoing the main phases of the lactation cycle: 10% of animals (at least 7) included in the dry (from 60 to 10 days before expected calving date), postpartum (from 3 to 7 days in milk [DIM]), early lactation (from 10 to 100 DIM), and midlate lactation groups (from 90 to 215 DIM)
- When transition cows flow successively in contiguous pen, then 12 to 24 cows/farm should be considered, including one-third primiparous and two-thirds multiparous cows, to be bleed successively in the far off, close-up, postpartum and early lactation groups
- Collect blood samples within 30 minutes from daily TMR distribution by jugular venipuncture through heparinized vacuum tubes
- Take care during handling of the samples to avoid any alteration of blood analytes, and use a clinical autoanalyzer calibrated for bovine plasma to perform analysis
- Metabolic condition of each animal sampled should be evaluated through comparing analytes concentration with suitable reference intervals (ie, defined under operative conditions similar to those observed in the herd) and suspecting abnormal metabolic condition for analytes laying outside reference interval limits
- Evaluation could be extended to the herd level through calculating the average herd value (AHV) for the concentration of each analyte and comparing AHVs to the reference intervals

DISCLOSURE

The authors have nothing to disclose.

ACKNOWLEDGMENTS

Research in the Department of Animal Sciences, Food and Nutrition is supported in part by CREI (Romeo and Enrica Invernizzi Research Center of the Università Cattolica del S. Cuore funded by the “Fondazione Romeo ed Enrica Invernizzi”, Milan, Italy) and in part by the Ministero Italiano delle Politiche Agricole, Alimentari ed Ambientali (MIPAAF). A heartfelt thanks to Elena Castellani, Giorgia Lovotti, and Michele Premi for the precious contribution offered in figures and tables preparation.

REFERENCES

1. Mezzetti M., Carpenter G.A., Bradford B.J., et al., Metabolism and Inflammation in Dairy Cows. In: Production diseases in farm animals. 2023.
2. Hrubec TC, Whichard JM, Larsen CT, et al. Plasma Versus Serum: Specific Differences in Biochemical Analyte Values. J Avian Med Surg 2002;16(2):101–5.
3. Ladenson JH, Tsai L-MB, Michael JM, et al. Serum versus Heparinized Plasma for Eighteen Common Chemistry Tests: Is Serum the Appropriate Specimen? Am J Clin Pathol 1974;62(4):545–52.
4. Plebani M, Banfi G, Bernardini S, et al. Serum or plasma? An old question looking for new answers. Clin Chem Lab Med 2020;58(2):178–87.
5. Ingvartsen KL, Moyes K, Ingvartsen KL, et al. Nutrition, immune function and health of dairy cattle. Page in Animal. Animal 2013;7(s1):112–22.
6. Calamari L, Ferrari A, Minuti A, et al. Assessment of the main plasma parameters included in a metabolic profile of dairy cow based on Fourier Transform mid-infrared spectroscopy: preliminary results. BMC Vet Res 2016;12(1):4.
7. Clarke CJ, Haselden JN. Metabolic Profiling as a Tool for Understanding Mechanisms of Toxicity. Toxicol Pathol 2008;36(1):140–7.

8. Herdt TH. Variability Characteristics And Test Selection In Herdlevel Nutritional And Metabolic Profile Testing. Vet Clin North Am Food Anim Pract 2000;16(2): 387–403.
9. Bertoni G, Trevisi E. Use of the Liver Activity Index and Other Metabolic Variables in the Assessment of Metabolic Health in Dairy Herds. Vet Clin North Am Food Anim Pract 2013;29(2):413–31.
10. Quiroz-Rocha GF, LeBlanc SJ, Duffield TF, et al. Reference limits for biochemical and hematological analytes of dairy cows one week before and one week after parturition. Can Vet J 2009;50(4):383–8. Available at: http://www.ncbi.nlm.nih.gov/pubmed/19436445.
11. Moretti P, Paltrinieri S, Trevisi E, et al. Reference intervals for hematological and biochemical parameters, acute phase proteins and markers of oxidation in Holstein dairy cows around 3 and 30 days after calving. Res Vet Sci 2017;114: 322–31.
12. Premi M, Mezzetti M, Ferronato G, et al. Changes of Plasma Analytes Reflecting Metabolic Adaptation to the Different Stages of the Lactation Cycle in Healthy Multiparous Holstein Dairy Cows Raised in High-Welfare Conditions. Animals 2021;11(6):1714.
13. Cattaneo L, Lopreiato V, Piccioli-Cappelli F, et al. Plasma albumin-to-globulin ratio before dry-off as a possible index of inflammatory status and performance in the subsequent lactation in dairy cows. J Dairy Sci 2021;104(7):8228–42.
14. Trevisi E, Amadori M, Archetti I, et al. Inflammatory response and acute phase proteins in the transition period of high-yielding dairy cows. In: Vea F, editor. Acute phase protein/book 2. Croatia: InTech Rijeka; 2011. p. 355–80.
15. Bertoni G. Welfare, health and management of dairy cows. In: Piva G, Bertoni G, Masoero F, et al, editors. Recent progress in animal production science. Milan, Italy: FrancoAngeli; 1999. p. 59–78.
16. Brscic M, Cozzi G, Lora I, et al. Short communication: Reference limits for blood analytes in Holstein late-pregnant heifers and dry cows: Effects of parity, days relative to calving, and season. J Dairy Sci 2015;98(11):7886–92.
17. Cozzi G, Ravarotto L, Gottardo F, et al. Short communication: Reference values for blood parameters in Holstein dairy cows: Effects of parity, stage of lactation, and season of production. J Dairy Sci 2011;94(8):3895–901.
18. Kerwin AL, Burhans WS, Mann S, et al. Transition cow nutrition and management strategies of dairy herds in the northeastern United States: Part II—Associations of metabolic- and inflammation-related analytes with health, milk yield, and reproduction. J Dairy Sci 2022;105(6):5349–69.
19. Smith JC, Lewis S, Holbrook J, et al. Effect of heparin and citrate on measured concentrations of various analytes in plasma. Clin Chem 1987;33(6):814–6.
20. Jørgenrud B, Jäntti S, Mattila I, et al. The influence of sample collection methodology and sample preprocessing on the blood metabolic profile. Bioanalysis 2015;7(8):991–1006.
21. Shaw RA, Kotowich S, Leroux M, et al. Multianalyte Serum Analysis Using Mid-Infrared Spectroscopy. Ann Clin Biochem Int J Lab Med 1998;35(5):624–32.
22. SR A, Mantsch HH. Infrared Spectroscopy in Clinical and Diagnostic Analysis. In: MR A, editor. Encyclopedia of analytical chemistry. Chichester: John Wiley & Sons Ltd; 2000. p. 83–102.
23. Hahn H, Pallua JD, Pezzei C, et al. Infrared-Spectroscopy: A Non-Invasive Tool for Medical Diagnostics and Drug Analysis. Curr Med Chem 2010;17(26): 2956–66.

24. Lehmann S, Delaby C, Vialaret J, et al. Current and future use of "dried blood spot" analyses in clinical chemistry. Clin Chem Lab Med 2013;51(10):1897–909.
25. Mezzetti M, Minuti A, Piccioli-Cappelli F, et al. The role of altered immune function during the dry period in promoting the development of subclinical ketosis in early lactation. J Dairy Sci 2019;102(10):9241–58.
26. Manston R, Russell A, Dew S, et al. The influence of dietary protein upon blood composition in dairy cows. Vet Rec 1975;96(23):497–502.
27. Wohlt JE, Evans JL, Trout JR. Blood Constituents in Lactating Holstein Cows Influenced by Hematocrit, Sampling Site, and Diet Protein and Calcium. J Dairy Sci 1984;67(10):2236–46.
28. Shalit U, Maltz E, Silanikove N, et al. Water, Sodium, Potassium, and Chlorine Metabolism of Dairy Cows at the Onset of Lactation in Hot Weather. J Dairy Sci 1991;74(6):1874–83.
29. Caré S, Trevisi E, Minuti A, et al. Plasma fructosamine during the transition period and its relationship with energy metabolism and inflammation biomarkers in dairy cows. Livest Sci 2018;216:138–47.
30. Baker JR, O'Connor JP, Metcalf PA, et al. Clinical usefulness of estimation of serum fructosamine concentration as a screening test for diabetes mellitus. BMJ 1983;287(6396):863–7.
31. Bell AW, Bauman DE. Adaptations of glucose metabolism during pregnancy and lactation. J Mammary Gland Biol Neoplasia 1997;2(3):265–78.
32. Janovick NA, Boisclair YR, Drackley JK. Prepartum dietary energy intake affects metabolism and health during the periparturient period in primiparous and multiparous Holstein cows. J Dairy Sci 2011;94:1385–400.
33. Herdt TH. Ruminant adaptation to negative energy balance. Influences on the etiology of ketosis and fatty liver. Vet Clin North Am Food Anim Pract 2000;16(2):215–30.
34. Vazquez-Añon M, Bertics S, Luck M, et al. Peripartum Liver Triglyceride and Plasma Metabolites In Dairy Cows. J Dairy Sci 1994. https://doi.org/10.3168/jds.S0022-0302(94)77092-2.
35. Herdt TH, Stevens JB, Olson WG, et al. Blood concentrations of beta hydroxybutyrate in clinically normal Holstein-Friesian herds and in those with a high prevalence of clinical ketosis. Am J Vet Res 1981;42(3):503–6. Available at: http://www.ncbi.nlm.nih.gov/pubmed/7271015.
36. Duffield TF. Subclinical ketosis in lactating dairy cattle. Vet Clin North Am Food Anim Pract 2000;16(2):231–53.
37. LeBlanc SJ, Leslie KE, Duffield TF. Metabolic Predictors of Displaced Abomasum in Dairy Cattle. J Dairy Sci 2005;88(1):159–70.
38. Geishauser T, Leslie K, Duffield T. Metabolic Aspects in the Etiology of Displaced Abomasum. Vet Clin North Am Food Anim Pract 2000;16(2):255–65.
39. Ospina PA, Nydam DV, Stokol T, et al. Associations of elevated nonesterified fatty acids and β-hydroxybutyrate concentrations with early lactation reproductive performance and milk production in transition dairy cattle in the northeastern United States. J Dairy Sci 2010;93(4):1596–603.
40. Church DC. Nutrition. In: Digestive physiology and nutrition of ruminants, vol. 2, 2nd edition. Corvallis (OR): O & B Books, Inc.; 1979. p. 618.
41. Bertics SJ, Grummer RR, Cadorniga-Valino C, et al. Effect of Prepartum Dry Matter Intake on Liver Triglyceride Concentration and Early Lactation. J Dairy Sci 1992;75(7):1914–22.

42. Skaar TC, Grummer RR, Dentine MR, et al. Seasonal Effects of Prepartum and Postpartum Fat and Niacin Feeding on Lactation Performance and Lipid Metabolism. J Dairy Sci 1989;72(8):2028–38.
43. Kochlik B, Gerbracht C, Grune T, et al. The Influence of Dietary Habits and Meat Consumption on Plasma 3-Methylhistidine-A Potential Marker for Muscle Protein Turnover. Mol Nutr Food Res 2018;62(9):1701062.
44. Herdt TH. Gastrointestinal physiology and metabolism. In: Saunders WB, editor. Textbook of veterinary physiology. Amsterdam, The Netherlands: Elsevier; 2002. p. 222–4.
45. Marini JC, Van Amburgh ME. Nitrogen metabolism and recycling in Holstein heifers. J Anim Sci 2003;81(2):545–52.
46. Odensten MO, Chilliard Y, Holtenius K. Effects of two different feeding strategies during dry-off on metabolism in high-yielding dairy cows. J Dairy Sci 2005;88(6): 2072–82.
47. McCabe CJ, Boerman JP. Invited Review: Quantifying protein mobilization in dairy cows during the transition period. Appl Anim Sci 2020;36(3):389–96.
48. Cruz LAB, Barral-Netto M, Andrade BB. Distinct inflammatory profile underlies pathological increases in creatinine levels associated with Plasmodium vivax malaria clinical severity. In: Escalante AA, editor. PLoS Neglected Trop Dis 2018; 12(3):e0006306.
49. Zoccali C, Maio R, Tripepi G, et al. Inflammation as a mediator of the link between mild to moderate renal insufficiency and endothelial dysfunction in essential hypertension. J Am Soc Nephrol 2006;4(2):S64–8.
50. Thompson M, Ray U, Yu R, et al. Kidney Function as a Determinant of HDL and Triglyceride Concentrations in the Australian Population. J Clin Med 2016;5(3):35.
51. Kokkonen T, Taponen J, Anttila T, et al. Effect of Body Fatness and Glucogenic Supplement on Lipid and Protein Mobilization and Plasma Leptin in Dairy Cows. J Dairy Sci 2005;88(3):1127–41.
52. Calamari L, Soriani N, Panella G, et al. Rumination time around calving: an early signal to detect cows at greater risk of disease. J Dairy Sci 2014;97(6):3635–47.
53. Oetzel GK. Parturient paresis and hypocalcemia in ruminant livestock. Vet Clin North Am Food Anim Pract 1988;4(2):351–64.
54. Goff JP. Mineral disorders of the transition period: origin and control. In: Proceedings of the world buiatrics congress. France: Nice; 2006.
55. Trevisi E, Minuti A. Assessment of the innate immune response in the periparturient cow. Res Vet Sci 2018;116:47–54.
56. Jihye K, Young Ju K, Rena L, et al. Serum levels of zinc, calcium, and iron are associated with the risk of preeclampsia in pregnant women. Nutr Res 2012; 32(10):764–9.
57. Rodriguez-Jimenez S, Haerr KJ, Trevisi E, et al. Prepartal standing behavior as a parameter for early detection of postpartal subclinical ketosis associated with inflammation and liver function biomarkers in peripartal dairy cows. J Dairy Sci 2018;101(9):8224–35.
58. Minuti A, Ahmed S, Trevisi E, et al. Experimental acute rumen acidosis in sheep: consequences on clinical, rumen, and gastrointestinal permeability conditions and blood chemistry. J Anim Sci 2014;92(9):3966–77.
59. Faith M, Sukumaran A, Pulimood AB, et al. How reliable an indicator of inflammation is myeloperoxidase activity? Clin Chim Acta 2008;396(1–2):23–5.
60. Ghiselli A, Serafini M, Maiani G, et al. A fluorescence-based method for measuring total plasma antioxidant capability. Free Radic Biol Med 1995;18(1): 29–36.

61. Sordillo LM, Aitken SL. Impact of oxidative stress on the health and immune function of dairy cattle. Vet Immunol Immunopathol 2009;128(1–3):104–9.
62. Benzie IF, Strain JJ. The ferric reducing ability of plasma (FRAP) as a measure of "antioxidant power": the FRAP assay. Anal Biochem 1996;239(1):70–6.
63. Cao G, Prior RL. Measurement of oxygen radical absorbance capacity in biological samples. Methods Enzymol 1998;299:50–62.
64. Celi P. Oxidative stress in ruminants. In: Mandelker L, Vajdovich P, editors. Studies on veterinary medicine. Oxidative stress in applied basic research and clinical practice. Totowa, NJ: Humana Press; 2011. p. 191–231.
65. Weiss WP, Hogan JS, Todhunter DA, et al. Effect of Vitamin E Supplementation in Diets with a Low Concentration of Selenium on Mammary Gland Health of Dairy Cows. J Dairy Sci 1997;80(8):1728–37.
66. Celi P, Gabai G. Oxidant/antioxidant balance in animal nutrition and health: the role of protein oxidation. Front Vet Sci 2015;2(48). https://doi.org/10.3389/fvets.2015.00048.
67. Trevisi E, Amadori M, Cogrossi S, et al. Metabolic stress and inflammatory response in high-yielding, periparturient dairy cows. Res Vet Sci 2012;93(2):695–704.

Considerations in the Diagnosis and Treatment of Early Lactation Calcium Disturbances

Jessica A.A. McArt, DVM, PhD, DABVP (Dairy Practice)[a,*],
Garrett R. Oetzel, DVM, MS[b]

KEYWORDS

• Hypocalcemia • Dyscalcemia • Transient • Calcium supplementation

KEY POINTS

- High-yielding multiparous cows will often have low blood calcium concentrations at 1 day in milk (DIM) but regain eucalcemia by 4 DIM.
- Focus routine hypocalcemia monitoring on multiparous dyscalcemic cows with blood calcium concentrations <2.2 mmol/L at 4 DIM.
- Collect a blood sample from all cows with suspected clinical hypocalcemia before treatment and place it in a refrigerator; if a positive response to treatment is not apparent, submit for total calcium analysis to confirm the diagnosis.
- Cows with clinical hypocalcemia often require oral calcium supplementation beyond the initial bottle of intravenous calcium.
- There is minimal evidence to support the routine use of subcutaneous calcium as a prevention strategy for subclinical hypocalcemia, whereas older cows with high milk-producing potential benefit from oral calcium supplementation.

BACKGROUND

Milk fever, one of the most historically relevant diseases of modern dairy cows, was first mentioned in German literature in 1793.[1] Close to 100 years ago, the treatment of milk fever with intravenous calcium was initiated,[2] and this remains the treatment of choice by bovine practitioners to this day. Improvements in nutrition and transition cow management over recent decades have drastically reduced the incidence of milk

[a] Department of Population Medicine and Diagnostic Sciences, College of Veterinary Medicine, Cornell University, Ithaca, NY 14853, USA; [b] Department of Medical Sciences, School of Veterinary Medicine, University of Wisconsin, Madison 53706, USA
* Corresponding author.
E-mail address: jmcart@cornell.edu
Twitter: jmcartdvm (J.A.A.M.)

Vet Clin Food Anim 39 (2023) 241–259
https://doi.org/10.1016/j.cvfa.2023.02.009
vetfood.theclinics.com

fever, which we will subsequently term "clinical hypocalcemia", from around 5.8% to 2.8%.[3] The etiology of hypocalcemia, the importance of calcium in bodily functions, and the role of magnesium and phosphorus in this disorder have been well described and will not be reviewed here.[4–8] In addition, numerous studies have evaluated the effects of prepartum nutritional management of hypocalcemia, the summary of which is beyond the scope of this article, and we encourage review of the primary literature on this topic.[9,10]

As the incidence of clinical hypocalcemia has reduced, the attention of bovine practitioners and researchers has increasingly turned to subclinical hypocalcemia, a term defining a state of low blood calcium concentration without clinical signs of disease. The incidence of subclinical hypocalcemia is not trivial and depends on the exact definition of the term, which will be discussed in detail below. Although definitions and days in milk at diagnosis vary, subclinical hypocalcemia likely affects 25% to 50% of early lactation, multiparous cows.[11–13]

We would like to highlight that clinical hypocalcemia is a disease of postparturient dairy cows with a well-known clinical presentation. Subclinical hypocalcemia is, by definition, void of clinical signs, and thus not, on its own, a disease or disorder.

CLINICAL RELEVANCE–HYPOCALCEMIA AND DYSCALCEMIA

Following, we present a discussion of the relevance of hypocalcemia, both clinical and subclinical, with particular focus on postpartum calcium dynamics and dyscalcemia. Clinical relevance deals not only with how to evaluate an individual cow for hypocalcemia but also pertains to conversations with herd management teams regarding herd-level investigations, troubleshooting, and management as well as long-term impacts on health, production, and reproduction.

Clinical hypocalcemia: Arguably, the most classic clinical diagnosis of dairy cows, clinical hypocalcemia manifests as a recumbent cow soon after calving, often with cold ears due to loss of thermoregulation and an auto-auscultatory body position (ie, the cow appears to be listening to her own heart) due to muscle weakness and inability to raise the head. Stage 1 clinical hypocalcemia includes early clinical signs of hypocalcemia but with less severity and without recumbency. Details of the stages of clinical hypocalcemia and associated physical examination findings have been well documented elsewhere and are not reviewed further here.[14,15]

Most clinical hypocalcemia cases occur within 48 hours postpartum due to the immense draw of calcium at the initiation of lactation. Fortunately, this presentation is so characteristic that most practitioners and producers can diagnose and treat these cases appropriately.

As practitioners, we are often called for "outbreaks" of clinical hypocalcemia when multiple postparturient cows are found down over the course of a few days. Commonly, by the time a workup is conducted (including physical examinations and pre-treatment blood work), the outbreak has passed. Although many bovine veterinarians have experienced these outbreak-type situations, they happen infrequently enough that causes have not been identified. In our experience, these outbreaks are often due to (1) improper feeding and/or intake of a prepartum diet aimed at preventing clinical hypocalcemia; (2) an undetected change in the mineral content of the prepartum diet due to an error in feed ingredient inclusion or in the preparation of a custom mix; or (3) a delay in feed delivery to the maternity or the postpartum fresh pen, causing the feed bunk to be empty for multiple hours.

It is useful to remember that cows can develop clinical hypocalcemia at any stage of lactation when calcium absorption from the diet does not meet the demands of milk production. These mid-lactation cases are often more difficult to diagnose as clinical hypocalcemia slips lower on the differential list as lactation progresses. In our experience, mid-lactation, high-producing cows present with signs of clinical hypocalcemia due to one of four reasons: (1) the calcium content of the diet is inadequate to support lactation, often occurring due to an abrupt ration or mixing error; (2) feed delivery is delayed, and cows have an empty feed bunk for multiple hours; (3) the very early stages of a severe disease condition (eg, coliform mastitis or hemorrhagic bowel syndrome) that will soon become apparent; or (4) cows with an intense expression of estrus resulting in increased activity and little to no feed intake.

Although a short-term illness, postparturient cows with clinical hypocalcemia experience reduced milk production for 4 to 6 weeks following diagnosis.[16] In addition, clinical hypocalcemia has been associated with several subsequent diseases, most notably prolapsed uteri and retained placentas,[17,18] which often lead to metritis. The association of milk fever with subsequent uterine disease results in an indirect association of milk fever with reduced reproductive performance.[18] Conversely, mid-lactation cases of clinical hypocalcemia are quickly fixed, and although there is no evidence-based research to support our clinical impressions, these cows rebound to normal without subsequent consequences once appropriate calcium intake has been restored.

Subclinical hypocalcemia: By definition, subclinical hypocalcemia is the occurrence of blood calcium concentrations below a certain threshold without presence of clinical signs. The issue with this definition is that it is unclear—what is the threshold at which subclinical hypocalcemia occurs and when is being below this threshold detrimental? Is being under this threshold always associated with unfavorable outcomes, or is it at times indicative of a high-producing cow? This definition is made even more difficult during the periparturient period as numerous metabolic homeorhetic and homeostatic changes are occurring.

The first studies aimed at identifying subclinical hypocalcemia did so through the categorization of blood calcium concentrations in early lactation.[19–21] Subsequent research in large field trials aimed at improving characterization through the association of blood calcium concentrations with epidemiologically important outcomes, notably milk production, disease events, and reproductive success.[12,22–25] Unfortunately, these studies did not provide a consensus on a blood calcium cut point for which to diagnose subclinical hypocalcemia, nor did they agree on an optimal test DIM. However, a more recent investigation of blood calcium concentrations in early lactation led to the idea of "calcium dynamics", a term describing the change in calcium concentrations over the first few days in milk, which when occurring in specific patterns, is associated with positive or negative events.[13,26–28] A recent excellent review on clinical and subclinical hypocalcemia provides in-depth insight into the progression of subclinical hypocalcemia's definition as well as a summary of health and performance effects based on these varying definitions.[29]

The large and constant calcium draw at the initiation of lactation might lead to a period of calcium homeorhesis rather than homeostasis. Multiple studies investigating the association of blood calcium concentration in early lactation have shown that cows with low blood calcium concentrations at 1 day in milk (DIM; using the convention that the day of calving is 0 DIM) make more milk over the first few months of lactation than their normocalcemic counterparts.[13,30,31] It is not until 2 DIM for primiparous cows and 4 DIM for multiparous cows that having low blood calcium concentrations are detrimental, which leads to reduced milk yield and an increased risk of subsequent disease events.[13] The majority of work in this area has been conducted on multiparous cows, and additional studies are needed in primiparous cows to better understand these dynamics. Based on these DIM time points, multiparous cows can be classified into one of four calcium dynamic groups depending on whether they are above or below identified thresholds at 1 and 4 DIM: normocalcemic, transiently hypocalcemic, persistently hypocalcemic, or delayed hypocalcemic (**Fig. 1**).

As most scientific literature notes blood calcium concentrations using units of mmol/L and many diagnostic labs report results in mg/dL, **Box 1** shows the method to easily convert between the two units. Current evidence suggests a 1 DIM threshold of total calcium around 1.8 to 2.0 mmol/L with reasonable variation between studies, whereas a 4 DIM threshold of 2.2 mmol/L seems a common target.[13,31]

The exact cut points are not imperative to recognize; rather, we encourage an understanding of the importance of the direction of change of blood calcium concentrations over time between calving and 4 DIM. In this sense, we can further categorize early lactation calcium homeorhesis into two main groups: (1) eucalcemia, and (2) dyscalcemia (**Fig. 2**). Eucalcemic cows are either normocalcemic or transiently hypocalcemic and have good dry matter intake, good to high milk yield in early lactation, reduced risk of early lactation disease, and good reproductive outcomes. Dyscalcemic cows are either persistently hypocalcemic or delayed hypocalcemic and have reduced dry matter intake, reduced milk yield in early lactation, increased risk of early lactation disease, and reduced reproductive success.[13,31,32]

The clinical relevance of early lactation calcium homeorhesis is important on both the individual cow and herd levels. Individually, eucalcemic homeorhesis is associated with high milk production and no impairment in dry matter intake. Herds in which the majority of cows are eucalcemic tend to be extremely high-producing herds with a low incidence of early lactation disease and good reproductive success. However, no trials have been conducted to support this conclusion.

Cows with dyscalcemic homeorhesis (ie, persistent or delayed hypocalcemia) need our attention. Currently, the exact causes of a persistent or delayed state of hypocalcemia are unknown. Possible causes include impaired dry matter intake, excessive inflammation and immune activation, dysregulation of calcium metabolism, or a combination of these factors.[31,33,34] Dyscalcemic cows are not performing up to their potential, and although some overcome the early lactation obstacles and go on to successful lactations, these cows are more likely to be low producers needing increased resources for disease therapy and reproductive success. Herds with a high incidence of dyscalcemic cows likely have multiple management challenges that reduce cow comfort and access to a well-formulated diet. Again, these management areas are associated with numerous postpartum diseases, and we eagerly await the identification of the causes of dyscalcemia.

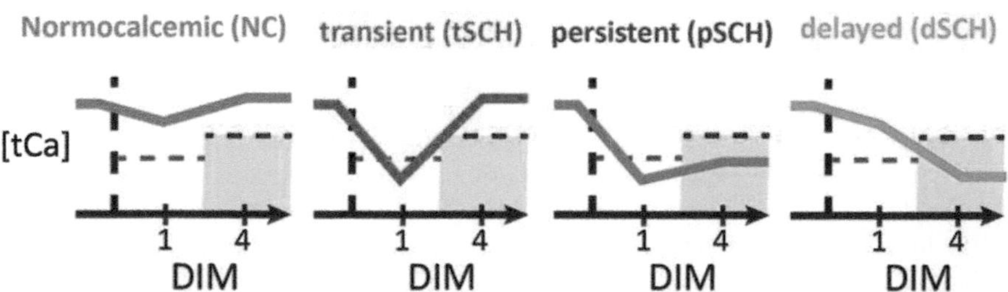

Fig. 1. Blood total calcium (tCa) concentrations of multiparous cows at 1 and 4 DIM displaying differences among calcium dynamic groups. This figure was created by J. A. Seminara with input from the authors.

Box 1
Conversion equation and quick estimation method for adjusting units of total calcium concentration from mg/dL to mmol/L

Conversion: 1 mg/dL calcium = 0.2495 mmol/L calcium
To quickly estimate calcium concentration in mmol/L: divide mg/dL by 4

Examples:	Calcium		
	mg/dL	mmol/L	Estimated mmol/L
	1.0	0.2495	0.25
	4.0	0.998	1.0
	6.0	1.497	1.5
	8.0	1.996	2.0
	10.0	2.495	2.5
	12.0	2.994	3.0
	14.0	3.493	3.5

Most diagnostic laboratories in the United States report total calcium concentration in mg/dL. However, standard international units of total calcium (mmol/L) are encouraged in published literature, and this can create confusion when reviewing primary literature sources for application to practice. Fortunately, the conversion of total calcium from mg/dL to mmol/L is quite simple, which is not the case for all analytes.

DIAGNOSIS–HOW AND WHEN TO TEST

Diagnosis of clinical and subclinical hypocalcemia, both on the individual cow and herd levels, can be completed using direct tests for blood calcium concentrations. Calcium is found in three major forms in the blood: bound to proteins such as albumin, free or ionized, and, to a much lesser extent, complexed to soluble anions such as citrate, phosphate, bicarbonate, and sulfate.[7] The total calcium concentration refers to the sum of all the above components, whereas ionized calcium refers to only the free or ionized portion. Ionized calcium makes up a little less than 50% of total calcium and can fluctuate slightly (~6%) during acidic conditions (increases slightly) versus alkaline conditions (decreases slightly).[7] Another commonly discussed variation in

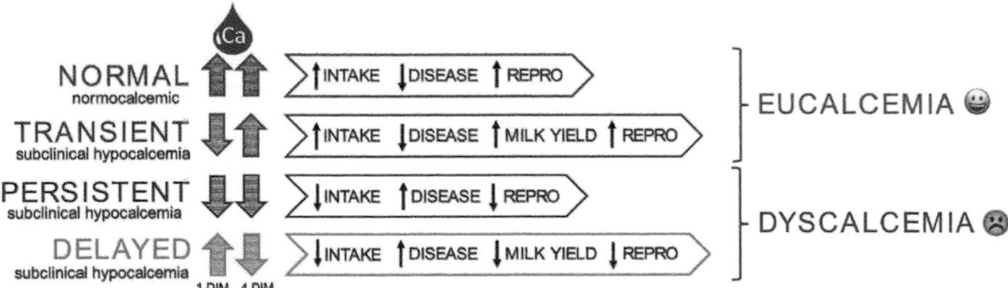

Fig. 2. Calcium dynamic groups based on blood total calcium concentrations of multiparous cows at 1 and 4 DIM and their association with dry matter intake, subsequent disease incidence, early lactation milk yield, and reproductive success. Taken together, normocalcemic and transiently hypocalcemic cows appear to adeptly regulate blood calcium concentrations in early lactation and are considered eucalcemic. On the other hand, cows with either persistent or delayed hypocalcemia are unable to increase or maintain their blood calcium concentrations, respectively, and are thus in a state of dyscalcemia. The factors leading to dyscalcemia are currently being investigated. This figure was created by C. R. Seely with input from the authors.

the ionized to total calcium ratio is the concentration of albumin. However, there is no evidence that hyper- or hypo-albuminemia should necessitate adjustment of calcium concentrations in cows, and recent evidence shows that albumin concentration in the immediate postpartum period does not vary between normocalcemic and subclinically hypocalcemic cows.[7,35]

Ionized calcium. Although ionized calcium is thought to have a greater biological relevance than total calcium, it requires special handling procedures to ensure there is no exposure to air and samples maintain electrolyte balance. Ion-selective electrode technologies (ie, blood gas analyzers) are largely employed for clinical use, which make testing for ionized calcium quite expensive, even for an individual cow, in addition to being logistically problematic. Cows must either be tested immediately after sample collection or have blood collected into heparin-balanced syringes, which are themselves not inexpensive. The improper collection leads to changes in sample pH, the most common of which is an increase in pH which falsely lowers ionized calcium concentrations.

Although there are several meters commercially available for on-farm ionized calcium measurement, only the i-STAT (Abbott, Abbott Park, IL) has been validated for use in cows.[36] The most commonly used cartridge for this point-of-care device on dairies is the CG8$^+$, which measures ionized calcium in addition to several other helpful (and some unhelpful) metabolites; however, at approximately $20 per cartridge (in addition to the purchase of a multi-thousand dollar machine) with a 1.5-minute analysis time, this devise is economically practical for only single cow analyses. In addition, these types of electronic point-of-care devices require constant recalibration and function within a narrow temperature range. It is important to note that while other commercial meters are advertised, none of these have undergone rigorous validation measures that prove utility for bovine practitioners or our patients. Some have been shown to be both inaccurate and/or imprecise in both published and unpublished testing.[36]

Given the economic and logistical difficulties when testing for ionized calcium, the only advantage to testing for this substance would occur if the information we gain is superior to that of total calcium analysis. Although the relationship between ionized and total calcium varies slightly in the few days following parturition, there is no evidence to support that knowledge of ionized calcium concentrations provides additional benefit over total calcium concentrations alone.

Total calcium. The benefit of total calcium is that it is easy to measure. Samples can be collected into non-anticoagulant (serum; red top) or lithium heparin (heparinized plasma; green top) tubes without consideration for special handling procedures. Practitioners should never utilize ethylenediaminetetraacetic acid (EDTA) (purple top) tubes for blood calcium analyses. EDTA chelates calcium and, if submitted for total calcium analysis, samples collected into EDTA tubes will produce a result that is incompatible with life. Fortunately, samples can remain for up to 6 hours at 22°C with minimal changes ($\leq$0.05 mmol/L) in the resulting total calcium concentration post-analysis.[37] In addition, and extremely practical for both practitioners and their clients, whole-blood samples can remain in non-anticoagulant or heparinized tubes for at least 14 days in a 4°C refrigerator without a change in total calcium concentration.[38] This has implications for testing individual cows as well as for herd-level monitoring, as discussed below.

Unfortunately, there are still no commercially available, accurate, logistically feasible, and economically viable on-farm testing methods for total calcium. Thus, practitioners are required to bring samples back to a central location for testing on benchtop analyzers or submission to diagnostic laboratories. Although less expensive than testing for ionized calcium, per sample costs range for total calcium analysis is from $5 to $15, plus the cost of the analyzer if needed. This lag time in resulting information is problematic for individual cow diagnosis and treatment decisions, but less so for herd-level monitoring. Although several groups have attempted to design and/or validate on-farm methods to test for total calcium, as of yet these methods are either inaccurate or not perfected to the point of utility.[39,40]

Clinical hypocalcemia. Most cases of clinical hypocalcemia are diagnosed via physical examination and confirmed by a positive and rapid response to treatment, as this is the primary differential for a recumbent multiparous cow with a history of parturition in the previous 48 hours. There are other notable differentials for cows with this history if the response to treatment is not adequate. For these reasons, direct testing of cows with clinical hypocalcemia is not often conducted.

Veterinarians should always collect a blood sample before treatment of cows with clinical hypocalcemia. They should also train farm employees to do the same. A pre-treatment blood sample is the only means of confirming the diagnosis of clinical hypocalcemia if the cow does not respond to treatment. As noted above, this sample can be placed in a 4°C refrigerator for up to 14 days. If the cow recovers after empirical treatment, throw the sample away; if she does not recover, submit it for macromineral analysis to rule in or out other differentials.

Cows with clinical hypocalcemia typically have blood total calcium concentrations <1.5 mmol/L, and, in our experience, most are <1.25 mmol/L. Interestingly, all cows with clinical hypocalcemia will have low blood calcium concentrations, but not all cows with low blood calcium concentrations will show signs of clinical hypocalcemia. After conducting numerous field trials in early lactation cows, we have noticed a small fraction of cows with blood calcium concentrations <1.5 mmol/L with a physically normal appearance. It is yet unknown why these cows do not suffer recumbency like their herd mates with clinical hypocalcemia.

Subclinical hypocalcemia. The issue with all subclinical ailments is that you do not know it exists until you test for them. Given the expense noted above for ionized calcium testing, and the fact that no epidemiologically based studies on subclinical hypocalcemia diagnosis have been conducted using this method, current diagnosis revolves around blood total calcium concentrations.

The first question a practitioner must answer when testing multiparous cows for subclinical hypocalcemia is "For what type of subclinical hypocalcemia am I testing?" If the goal is to detect the percentage of high-producing cows in the herd that is not limited by intake or management (ie, transient hypocalcemia), and compare this to the percentages of cows that are not adapting well to the initiation of lactation (ie, persistent or delayed hypocalcemia), then testing multiparous cows at 1 and 4 DIM is recommended. As mentioned earlier, the focus of this dual-day testing is to generally understand in which direction total calcium concentration is heading between 1 and 4 DIM, and ensuring total calcium is above a certain threshold by 4 DIM. However, this takes concerted effort as the same cows must be sampled at both 1 and 4 DIM, which makes testing individual cows as well as herd-level monitoring twice as laborious and expensive. Although academically it is interesting to understand the epidemiology of these different calcium dynamic groups and what causes them, from an on-farm application standpoint, the goal of testing is more likely to understand if a cow or cows are dyscalcemic. If this is the question a practitioner hopes to answer, total calcium concentrations should be measured at 4 DIM with a current threshold recommendation of 2.2 mmol/L.[13,31]

To date, only one study has assessed calcium dynamic groups in primiparous cows, and as noted above, dyscalcemia for these younger animals is thought to occur earlier in lactation, that is, at approximately 2 DIM.[13] Some second parity cows might also fit this pattern. More research is required to better describe calcium dynamics in younger cows.

Herd-level monitoring. Limited studies have assessed the herd-level incidence of eucalcemia or dyscalcemia; more field studies in this area will help us understand how our feeding and management practices can affect dyscalcemia and subsequently herd health, milk production, and reproduction. Investigation on herds enrolled in field trials shows an approximate range in the incidence of transient hypocalcemia of 20% to 40%, persistent hypocalcemia of 5% to 25%, and delayed hypocalcemia of 10% to 30%; dyscalcemia incidence was 20% to 60% in these studies.[13,31,41,42]

As for herd-level hyperketonemia monitoring, we recommend herd-level testing of multiparous cows on a routine basis (eg, once per month) to monitor dyscalcemia prevalence at 4 DIM and adjust management accordingly. The number of cows required for testing will vary based on the desired confidence around the resulting estimate, with sampling more cows allowing more certainty with the resulting outcome. Often, when weighing the expense of testing with the required confidence, sampling n = 12 cows is a reasonable start. The concept of precision and confidence around the testing prevalence estimate has been well described, and readers are encouraged to go to the primary literature for further explanation.[43–45]

One issue commonly encountered by practitioners is that there are not enough cows at 4 DIM on a given farm to provide a reasonable estimate. This can be overcome by repeated sampling on a regular basis (eg, every herd check) or training farm employees to sample cows at 4 DIM and place tubes in an appropriately working refrigerator. These samples can then be collected at the next herd check or brought to a clinic when the target number of samples has been collected. This provides a rolling prevalence, with a small lag in results, but is an excellent approach to identifying areas for opportunity on smaller herds.

THERAPEUTIC OPTIONS

Before reviewing therapeutic options for hypocalcemia, we would be remiss to fail to highlight the importance of prevention above therapy. Although a detailed discussion on preventive strategies is beyond the scope of this article, our job as veterinarians, in addition to diagnosing and treating illness, is to suggest and make improvements with other members of farm management teams that improve cow nutrition and comfort. Correctly applied preventive measures will drastically decrease the need for therapy.

Clinical hypocalcemia—individual cow treatment. Calcium solutions infused intravenously have been used to remedy clinical hypocalcemia for almost 100 years. In the United States, intravenous calcium often comes in the form of a 500 mL bottle of 23% calcium borogluconate, which provides approximately 10.5 g elemental calcium to the cow. When treating clinical hypocalcemia, administer a single bottle of 500 mL 23% calcium borogluconate intravenously over a period of approximately 5 to 10 minutes, which usually is the time it takes the fluid to flow into the cow when the bottle is held at the level of the cow's withers. Administering the bottle too quickly can cause cardiac arrhythmias. Visualizing and monitoring heartbeat reverberations at the thoracic inlet while administering intravenous calcium is an easy method to assess cardiac rhythm, and administration should be stopped if an abnormal rhythm is detected.

Blood calcium concentration peaks rapidly following intravenous administration, with peak blood calcium concentrations occurring in under 15 minutes.[46] For a 750 kg cow with a blood total calcium concentration of 1.0 mmol/L, a single bottle will increase calcium concentrations to approximately 4.5 mmol/L.[46,47] A second bottle is not necessary and even contraindicated because (1) the immediate calcium deficit has been resolved by the first bottle, (2) a second bottle can increase blood calcium concentration near a cardiotoxic concentration (~7.5 mmol/L), and (3) has been shown to offer no benefit over administration of a single bottle in a randomized trial.[47–49] For situations in which a vein is not accessible, or in which clients are untrained for intravenous calcium administration, a 500 mL bottle can be deposited subcutaneously; however, the time to peak calcium concentration is subsequently extended to 4 hours.[50,51]

Many cows first presenting with clinical hypocalcemia have hypocalcemic relapses and repeat recumbency following successful intravenous calcium administration. This occurs for two main reasons. First, cows treated with intravenous calcium often experience a rebound hypocalcemia 12 to 18 hours after administration (**Fig. 3**).[47,52] Second, the milk volume being produced by these cows continues the immense calcium pull from their systems. For these reasons, and to reduce the risk of relapse, continued calcium administration is warranted, and it is important for practitioners to understand when to administer additional calcium and what type of calcium is needed.

Unfortunately, given the low incidence of clinical hypocalcemia in many dairy herds, no trials have assessed the effects of multi-modal calcium therapy on recovery. Repeated administration of multiple bottles of intravenous or subcutaneous calcium is not the correct answer, as this creates a swinging pendulum of parathyroid hormone and calcitonin activity which impedes calcium homeostasis. Given the data presented

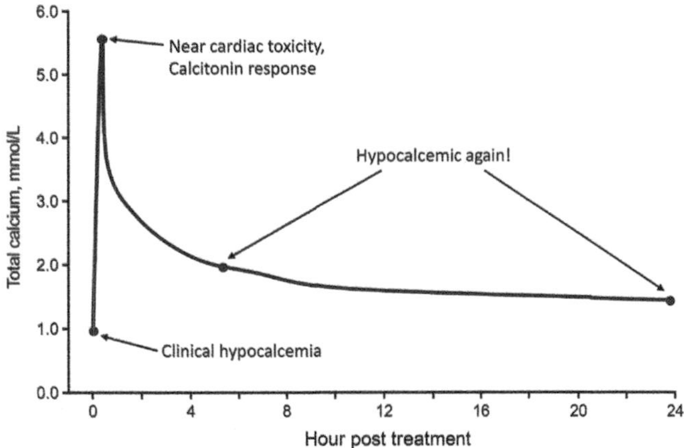

Fig. 3. The effect of intravenous administration of a 500 mL bottle of 23% calcium borogluconate to a cow with clinical hypocalcemia. Even in cows with very low blood calcium concentrations, rapid administration of intravenous calcium produces subsequent hypocalcemia due to (1) elevation of blood calcium concentration above physiologically normal thresholds resulting in negative feedback to parathyroid hormone secretion, (2) stimulation of calcitonin release from the hypercalcemic state, (3) the decrease of renal calcium absorption following calcitonin release, and (4) the calcitonin-mediated inhibition of bone calcium resorption.[47] The result is a reduction in blood calcium concentration approximately 24 hours following intravenous calcium administration. This rebound hypocalcemia encourages provision of additional and more moderate calcium supplementation to cows with clinical hypocalcemia after intravenous calcium administration and highlights the adverse effects of repetitive iatrogenic creation of a hypercalcemic state. This figure was adapted from Goff, 1999[47] by the authors.

below regarding blood calcium concentrations following subcutaneous or oral calcium administration for non-recumbent immediate postpartum cows, it is logical to either follow-up the initial administration of intravenous calcium with a single bottle of calcium administered subcutaneously approximately 8 hours after the initial treatment or to provide oral calcium supplementation via a bolus after the initial treatment once the cow is alert and able to swallow with a second oral calcium supplementation approximately 12 hours later. As subcutaneous calcium administration can also cause a rebound hypocalcemia, albeit to a lesser extent than intravenous administration, we recommend the use of oral calcium boluses after intravenous calcium administration in clinical hypocalcemia treatment protocols.

Clinical hypocalcemia—outbreak management. One of the more frustrating calls a bovine practitioner receives is one reporting multiple cows down with suspected clinical hypocalcemia. On the therapy side, it is important to put an incidence threshold in place, for example, more than 5% of fresh cows down within 48 hours of calving over the course of a week, in which a management change, most commonly immediate postparturient calcium supplementation, is put in place.

In an outbreak situation in which older multiparous cows are developing clinical hypocalcemia at an increased incidence, blanket administration of a single 500 mL bottle of 23% calcium borogluconate administered subcutaneously might be the most practical means of keeping cows on their feet while preventing too severe of a rebound hypocalcemia. Blood calcium concentration dynamics following administration of different methods of supplementation are discussed below; however, the subsequent rebound hypocalcemia resulting from intravenous calcium prevents the use of this method as a blanket treatment. Thus, subcutaneous calcium administration, likely followed by oral calcium administration, is the most appropriate immediate band-aid to control clinical hypocalcemia outbreaks in the short term. No studies have been conducted to confirm this hypothesis, but clinical experience has shown this to be an effective means of limiting recumbency to provide time for management investigations. Importantly, once the veterinarian and farm management team have addressed and stabilized any upstream issues (ie, nutrition, comfort, or handling) that might have initiated the outbreak, the calcium supplementation band-aid should be removed.

Subclinical hypocalcemia. Postpartum calcium supplementation aimed at preventing subclinical hypocalcemia was developed with the idea that supplying additional calcium at and/or soon after calving reduced the calcium deficit experienced by a cow and thus aided calcium homeostasis. However, as described below, postpartum calcium supplementation is clearly not associated with improved calcium homeostasis, partially because a subset of cows responds by producing more milk. In addition, with the recent evolution of new definitions of subclinical hypocalcemia in multiparous cows, two large questions loom regarding postpartum calcium supplementation: (1) if transient hypocalcemia is associated with well-regulated, high-producing cows, does exogenous calcium interfere with the natural homeorhetic processes of these cows and impeded performance, and (2) if dyscalcemia at 4 DIM is associated with negative health, production, and reproduction, does calcium supplementation at calving affect blood calcium concentrations long enough to improve dyscalcemia? These questions are currently being investigated by multiple research groups, and knowledge of their findings as well as a further inquiry into the risk factors and causes of dyscalcemia will hopefully inform our postpartum calcium management.

Postpartum calcium supplementation is not a therapy for subclinical hypocalcemia. It is a prevention strategy, as we do not know if a cow has subclinical hypocalcemia until after we have administered exogenous calcium. There are three main prevention options using postpartum calcium supplementation: (1) intravenous calcium, (2) subcutaneous calcium, and (3) oral calcium boluses. Although there are commercially available oral calcium gels, the caustic nature of their contents and availability of more effective alternatives should limit their use; similarly, although many practitioners and farm employees orally drench cows with a large volume of water and calcium-containing solution, this is more of an individual cow treatment and not practical for blanket use on farms. What follows is our current understanding of the effect of each of these different types of postpartum calcium supplementation on blood calcium dynamics, health, and production.

Intravenous calcium: We discourage intravenous use of calcium for the prevention of subclinical hypocalcemia. Although it increases blood calcium concentration drastically in the short term, approximately 12 hours, the rebound hypocalcemia is sustained and severe (**Fig. 4**).[50,53] There is evidence that the increase in blood calcium concentration following intravenous calcium administration has a negative effect on parathyroid concentrations which subsequently impedes calcium regulation mechanisms for days.[46] As a rule of thumb, standing cows do not require intravenous calcium.

Subcutaneous calcium: The same bottle of 23% gluconate or borogluconate used for intravenous calcium administration can be used for subcutaneous injection. It is important that practitioners ensure their injectable calcium products do not contain calcium chloride as calcium salt or glucose as these can cause osmotic injury to the tissues surrounding the injection sites and sloughing of the skin.[47] It has also been reported that the amount of calcium injected into a single site should be limited to 50 to 75 mL, as more than 1.0 to 1.5 g of calcium can cause local necrosis.[47] However, repeated injections cause additional pain to the cow, and repeated injections without changing needles can increase the risk of abscess formation. One of us (JAAM) has

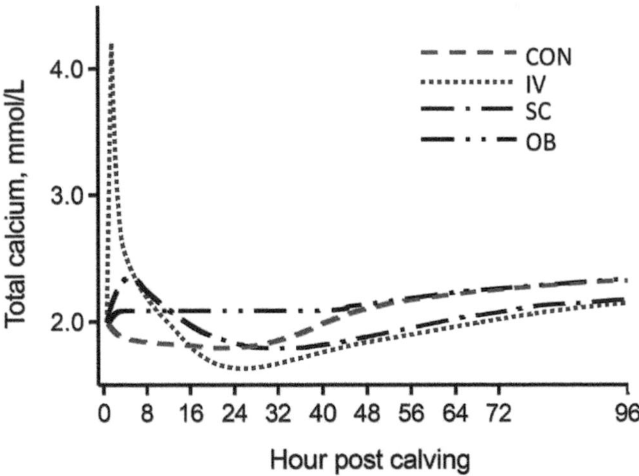

Fig. 4. The effect of various methods of postpartum calcium supplementation on blood calcium concentrations in non-recumbent multiparous cows. Demonstrated methods of administration include a 500 mL bottle of 23% calcium borogluconate administered intravenously (IV), a 500 mL bottle of 23% borogluconate administered subcutaneously across one or two locations (SC), and an oral calcium bolus containing 43 g of calcium administered at calving and again at 1 DIM (OB). Importantly, lines are intended to be schematic only and have been smoothed or imputed based on data from multiple studies.[50,51,54]

personally injected and trained many farm employees to inject cows in a single location with a new needle behind the shoulder, followed by massaging of the fluid under the skin post-administration, with apparent success. Although studies have not been conducted to assess the effect of multiple injection locations versus a single location on blood calcium concentrations, administration of a 500 mL bottle in a single location increases blood calcium drastically and has been performed in multiple studies without reports of adverse effects.[51,54]

Blood calcium concentrations peak approximately 4 hours following administration of subcutaneous calcium around 0.4 mmol/L above pre-treatment concentrations and 0.5 mmol/L above blood calcium concentrations of non-treated cows (see **Fig. 4**); blood calcium concentrations remain elevated for 12 hours post-administration.[51,55] Interestingly, in some studies, there is evidence of sustained rebound hypocalcemia following administration of subcutaneous calcium that can last up to 4 days following treatment.[54] Another study did not report this rebound hypocalcemia, although the product administered provided different grams of elemental calcium, and first lactation cows were included in the study, so results are difficult to compare.[56] Given the results in multiparous cows, if practitioners consider use of subcutaneous calcium in subclinical hypocalcemia prevention protocols, we suggest another calcium source, such as oral calcium boluses, be administered to prevent a rebound hypocalcemia at 12 hours post subcutaneous calcium administration and again the following day. Unfortunately, to date, there are no studies that provide evidence to support this recommendation.

The effect of subcutaneous calcium administration has been evaluated only for health and production outcomes. Across multiple studies, no effect of subcutaneous calcium administration has been reported on milk yield over multiple months postpartum.[51,56,57] In addition, there is little evidence to support administration of subcutaneous calcium reducing subsequent disease events, with most studies finding no difference in the incidence of metritis, displaced abomasum, or culling.[51,56,57] One study reported a benefit in the reduction of puerperal metritis following two repeat doses of subcutaneous administration, one at calving and the second 12 to 18 hours later.[56]

Given the negative effect of subcutaneous calcium infusion on blood calcium concentrations and the lack of substantial beneficial health and production outcomes reported in studies, the routine use of subcutaneous calcium administration on commercial dairies as a management strategy to prevent subclinical hypocalcemia cannot be supported.

Oral calcium boluses: Oral calcium boluses provide 40 to 100 g of calcium per bolus (or multiple boluses administered at the same time) via differing types of calcium salts and are intended to increase blood calcium concentrations through passive transport in the rumen and passive or active absorption in the small intestines.[47] However, not all calcium boluses are created equally, as different types of calcium salts have different solubility and absorption properties (**Box 2**). The effect of different types of calcium salts on blood calcium concentrations has been well described,[58] and many companies have used these results to formulate boluses with multiple different types of calcium salts that allow for an immediate absorption of calcium that increases blood calcium concentrations as well as a calcium salt that absorbs more slowly and thus sustains the increase in blood calcium concentrations. It is imperative that bovine practitioners understand the composition of calcium boluses used on their clients' farms and can recommend products based on their knowledge of absorption principles. For example, calcium carbonate is extremely insoluble in water. It is also inexpensive. This is an acceptable calcium source commonly used in diets as cows eat

Box 2
The solubility and absorption properties of different calcium salts commonly used in oral calcium boluses for dairy cows

Source	Solubility	Absorption
Calcium chloride	++++	++++
Calcium propionate	+++	+++
Calcium sulfate	++	+++
Calcium carbonate	+	+++
Calcium hydroxide	++	++

Solubility in water noted on a scale of + (minimally soluble) to ++++ (highly soluble). Absorption noted on a scale of + (minimally absorbed) to ++++ (highly absorbed).[58,68,69]

a large volume of calcium carbonate while often at calcium homeostasis. However, calcium carbonate in an oral calcium bolus is not present in enough quantity to positively affect blood calcium concentrations, and thus, has no place in a commercial product.

When administering oral calcium boluses, practitioners and trained farm employees should use safe handling techniques to avoid injury to the person administering the bolus as well as the cow receiving the bolus. A solid understanding of anatomy and the physiological process of swallowing is needed to ensure safe deposition of the bolus, or else they can end up in non-ideal locations.[59] Multiple dosing applicators are available commercially for this use, and boluses should be administered swiftly and correctly to the back of the throat. Incorrect handling can result in pharyngeal and retropharyngeal trauma and can be fatal. As calcium salts are irritating to the oral and esophageal mucosa,[47] some bolus products have fat or other coatings that assist in a rapid slide of the bolus down the esophagus into the rumen.

A summary of blood calcium concentrations following oral bolus administration, and their comparison to other methods of calcium supplementation methods, is in **Fig. 4**. Multiple studies have assessed blood calcium concentrations post oral bolus in a variety of combinations such as the number of boluses administered at one time, the timing of administration, and the length of time for which boluses are administered, and readers are encouraged to review the primary literature sources for more focused information.[30,50,51,54,60–63] When combining the results of these studies, the ability of oral calcium boluses to raise blood calcium concentrations is dose and frequency dependent. Administration of an oral calcium bolus at calving with a second dose given 12 to 24 hours later increases blood calcium concentrations; however, this increase is mild and each individual bolus time point does not sustain calcium concentrations for long periods, which is why repeat dosing is important. It is our opinion that administration of a single bolus or boluses at calving is not enough to have long-term beneficial effects on blood calcium concentrations.

Although a discussion on oral bolus administration and blood calcium concentration is necessary, the real question we should ask as practitioners is, "Do oral calcium boluses affect cow health or production?" Unfortunately, the answer is not unidirectional and depends on multiple factors. An excellent systematic review and meta-analysis have recently been published by Valldecabres and colleagues,[64] and readers are encouraged to access this review for further information. Multiple studies have found that blanket therapy of oral calcium boluses is not effective at increasing milk production or reducing subsequent disease events.[30,51,61,65–67] Interestingly, almost all of these same studies have found benefits of oral calcium supplementation in subgroups of cows, mainly older cows with greater milk production potential, and this demographic should be the focus of postpartum oral calcium bolus protocols. Although oral calcium benefits some cows, it has also been shown to reduce milk yield for cows with lower milk production potential and increase the risk of metritis and decrease reproductive success in primiparous cows.[30,61,63,66] Thus, great consideration must be given before adding routine administration of oral calcium boluses to protocols involving primiparous and perhaps even second parity cows.

Future therapy directions. Several research groups are conducting studies aimed at optimizing calcium dynamics in transiently hypocalcemic cows versus those with dyscalcemia. Postpartum calcium administration might affect each of these groups of cows differently, and future work on the method, timing, and frequency of administration is required. Unfortunately, until an accurate and economically reasonable on-farm test for blood calcium concentration is developed and commercialized, progress on the application of calcium supplementation in immediate postparturient cows will likely be stifled.

SUMMARY

Clinical hypocalcemia is one of the most historically relevant diseases of dairy cows, and although it occurs less commonly than in previous decades, the disease still requires veterinary intervention at individual cow therapy or herd prevention levels. Development or adjustment of effective treatment plans is essential, with special focus paid to the continual loss of calcium into milk by high-producing cows which requires continued therapeutic support. In addition, practitioners should identify a herd-level outbreak threshold at which blanket postpartum calcium supplementation is initiated while investigation into the cause of the increased disease incidence begins. This should be paired with a concerted effort to remove the blanket supplementation policy when positive management changes have been completed.

As the definition of subclinical hypocalcemia evolves, amassing evidence suggests that a reasonable proportion of cows, notably those with transient hypocalcemia, can balance high volumes of milk production and calcium homeorhesis without additional support. It is likely that the best approach for management of these cows is one in which we provide good cow comfort, adequate nutritional support, and allow them to thrive on their own. Our attention should primarily reside on dyscalcemic cows, the prevalence of which can be routinely monitored on farms by testing cows at 4 DIM at varying intervals. Future research into the causes of dyscalcemia will educate continued efforts at prevention and therapy. Until that time, bovine practitioners should develop hypocalcemia prevention strategies that assist with postpartum calcium dynamics rather than interfere with them.

Although well beyond the scope of this article, the importance of prepartum nutritional management of hypocalcemia, transition cow comfort and head abatement, handling, and management of maternity cows, and maximizing early lactation dry matter intake cannot be trivialized. The combination and successful management of these factors will do far more to reduce the incidence of clinical hypocalcemia and dyscalcemia than any postpartum prevention program. Veterinary involvement in these management aspects, along with other key farm personnel, is essential for successfully navigating calcium disturbances and improving cow health and farm productivity.

CLINICS CARE POINTS

- The best method of routine blood testing for monitoring hypocalcemia is by sampling multiparous cows at 4 DIM.
- Collect a blood sample from all cows with suspected clinical hypocalcemia before treatment and place it in a refrigerator; if a response to treatment is not seen, submit for total calcium analysis to confirm the diagnosis.
- Cows with clinical hypocalcemia are at high risk for hypocalcemic relapse. We recommend routine administration of an oral calcium supplement following an initial bottle of intravenous calcium.
- During a clinical hypocalcemia outbreak, we suggest blanket use of subcutaneous calcium followed by oral calcium supplementation for older cows.

DISCLOSURE

J. A. A. McArt has been provided compensation for speaking engagements related to cow health and research output from the McArt Dairy Cow Lab at Cornell University from Boehringer Ingelheim Animal Health and Phibro Animal Health, both companies with commercial products related to the prevention and/or treatment of hypocalcemia in dairy cows. G. R. Oetzel has been provided compensation for consulting, speaking engagements, and on-farm research from I.B Co., Ltd, which is developing an on-farm blood testing system. None of these companies were involved in the preparation of this article. The authors declare they have no additional conflicts of interest.

REFERENCES

1. Hutyra F, Marek J. Special pathology and therapeutics of the diseases of domestic animals, 1926, London.
2. Dryerre HG, Greig JR. The specific chemotherapy of milk fever by the parenteral administration of Ca-boro-gluconate. Vet Rec 1935;15:456–9.
3. USDA. Dairy 2014 - Trends in dairy health and management practices in the United States, 1991-2014. Fort Collins, CO: *USDA-APHIS-VS-CEAH-NAHMS*; 2021 (#711.0821).
4. Goff JP. Pathophysiology of calcium and phosphorus disorders. Vet Clin North Am Food Anim Pract 2000;16(2):319–37.
5. Wilkens MR, Nelson CD, Hernandez LL, et al. Symposium review: transition cow calcium homeostasis - health effects of hypocalcemia and strategies for prevention. J Dairy Sci 2020;103(3):2909–27.
6. Goff JP. Macromineral disorders of the transition cow. Vet Clin North Am Food Anim Pract 2004;20(3):471–94.
7. Goff JP. Calcium and magnesium disorders. Vet Clin North Am Food Anim Pract 2014;30(2):359–81.
8. DeGaris PJ, Lean IJ. Milk fever in dairy cows: a review of pathophysiology and control principles. Vet J 2008;176(1):58–69.
9. Santos JEP, Lean IJ, Golder H, et al. Meta-analysis of the effects of prepartum dietary cation-anion difference on performance and health of dairy cows. J Dairy Sci 2019;102(3):2134–54.
10. Lean IJ, DeGaris PJ, McNeil DM, et al. Hypocalcemia in dairy cows: meta-analysis and dietary cation anion difference theory revisited. J Dairy Sci 2006; 89(2):669–84.

11. Reinhardt TA, Lippolis JD, McCluskey BJ, et al. Prevalence of subclinical hypocalcemia in dairy herds. Vet J 2011;188(1):122–4.
12. Chapinal N, Carson M, Duffield TF, et al. The association of serum metabolites with clinical disease during the transition period. J Dairy Sci 2011;94(10): 4897–903.
13. McArt JAA, Neves RC. Association of transient, persistent, or delayed subclinical hypocalcemia with early lactation disease, removal, and milk yield in Holstein cows. J Dairy Sci 2020;103(1):690–701.
14. Mann S, McArt J, Abuelo A. Production-related metabolic disorders of cattle: ketosis, milk fever and grass staggers. Practice 2019;41(5):205–19.
15. Oetzel G.R. Parturient paresis in cows - metabolic disorders. Merck Veterinary Manual. 2022. Available at: https://www.merckvetmanual.com/metabolic-disorders/disorders-of-calcium-metabolism/parturient-paresis-in-cows. Accessed January 10, 2023.
16. Rajala-Schultz PJ, Grohn YT, McCulloch CE. Effects of milk fever, ketosis, and lameness on milk yield in dairy cows. J Dairy Sci 1999;82(2):288–94.
17. Markusfeld O. Periparturient traits in seven high dairy herds. Incidence rates, association with parity, and interrelationships among traits. J Dairy Sci 1987;70(1): 158–66.
18. Erb HN, Smith RD, Oltenacu PA, et al. Path model of reproductive disorders and performance, milk fever, mastitis, milk yield, and culling in Holstein cows. J Dairy Sci 1985;68(12):3337–49.
19. Oetzel GR. Effect of calcium chloride gel treatment in dairy cows on incidence of periparturient diseases. J Am Vet Med Assoc 1996;209(5):958–61.
20. Oetzel GR. Parturient paresis and hypocalcemia in ruminant livestock. Vet Clin North Am Food Anim Pract 1988;4(2):351–64.
21. Martinez N, Risco CA, Lima FS, et al. Evaluation of peripartal calcium status, energetic profile, and neutrophil function in dairy cows at low or high risk of developing uterine disease. J Dairy Sci 2012;95(12):7158–72.
22. Rodriguez EM, Aris A, Bach A. Associations between subclinical hypocalcemia and postparturient diseases in dairy cows. J Dairy Sci 2017;100(9):7427–34.
23. Wilhelm AL, Maquivar MG, Bas S, et al. Effect of serum calcium status at calving on survival, health, and performance of postpartum Holstein cows and calves under certified organic management. J Dairy Sci 2017;100(4):3059–67.
24. Venjakob PL, Pieper L, Heuwieser W, et al. Association of postpartum hypocalcemia with early-lactation milk yield, reproductive performance, and culling in dairy cows. J Dairy Sci 2018;101(10):9396–405.
25. Neves RC, Leno BM, Curler MD, et al. Association of immediate postpartum plasma calcium concentration with early-lactation clinical diseases, culling, reproduction, and milk production in Holstein cows. J Dairy Sci 2018;101(1): 547–55.
26. Neves RC, Leno BM, Bach KD, et al. Epidemiology of subclinical hypocalcemia in early-lactation Holstein dairy cows: The temporal associations of plasma calcium concentration in the first 4 days in milk with disease and milk production. J Dairy Sci 2018;101(10):9321–31.
27. Venjakob PL, Staufenbiel R, Heuwieser W, et al. Association between serum calcium dynamics around parturition and common postpartum diseases in dairy cows. J Dairy Sci 2021;104(2):2243–53.
28. Caixeta LS, Ospina PA, Capel MB, et al. Association between subclinical hypocalcemia in the first 3 days of lactation and reproductive performance of dairy cows. Theriogenology 2017;94:1–7.

29. Serrenho RC, DeVries TJ, Duffield TF, et al. Graduate Student Literature Review: What do we know about the effects of clinical and subclinical hypocalcemia on health and performance of dairy cows? J Dairy Sci 2021;104(5):6304–26.
30. Leno BM, Neves RC, Louge IM, et al. Differential effects of a single dose of oral calcium based on postpartum plasma calcium concentration in Holstein cows. J Dairy Sci 2018;101(4):3285–302.
31. Seely CR, Leno BM, Kerwin AL, et al. Association of subclinical hypocalcemia dynamics with dry matter intake, milk yield, and blood minerals during the periparturient period. J Dairy Sci 2021;104(4):4692–702.
32. Seely CR, McArt JAA. The association of subclinical hypocalcemia at 4 days in milk with reproductive outcomes in multiparous Holstein cows. JDS Communications 2023;4. https://doi.org/10.3168/jdsc.2022-0279.
33. Huzzey JM, Mann S, Nydam DV, et al. Associations of peripartum markers of stress and inflammation with milk yield and reproductive performance in Holstein dairy cows. Prev Vet Med 2015;120(3–4):291–7.
34. Horst EA, Kvidera SK, Baumgard LH. Invited review: The influence of immune activation on transition cow health and performance-A critical evaluation of traditional dogmas. J Dairy Sci 2021;104(8):8380–410.
35. Neves RC, Leno BM, Stokol T, et al. Risk factors associated with postpartum subclinical hypocalcemia in dairy cows. J Dairy Sci 2017;100(5):3796–804.
36. Neves RC, Stokol T, Bach KD, et al. Method comparison and validation of a prototype device for measurement of ionized calcium concentrations cow-side against a point-of-care instrument and a benchtop blood-gas analyzer reference method. J Dairy Sci 2018;101(2):1334–43.
37. Neves RC, Stokol T. Calcium. Available at: https://eclinpath.com/chemistry/minerals/calcium/
38. Bach KD, Neves RC, Stokol T, et al. Technical note: Effect of storage time and temperature on total calcium concentrations in bovine blood. J Dairy Sci 2020;103(1):922–8.
39. Fu Y, Colazo MG, De Buck J. Development of a blood calcium test for hypocalcemia diagnosis in dairy cows. Res Vet Sci 2022;147:60–7.
40. Serrenho RC, Bruinjé TC, Morrison EI, et al. Validation of a point-of-care handheld blood total calcium analyzer in postpartum dairy cows. JDS Communications 2021;2(1):41–5.
41. Seely CR, McArt JAA. The association of prepartum urine pH and periparturient activity and rumination time on postpartum subclinical hypocalcemia dynamics in Holstein cows. J Dairy Sci 2021;104(Suppl. 1):73.
42. Seminara JA, Callero KR, Frost IR, et al. Calcium dynamics and associated patterns of milk constituents in early lactation multiparous Holsteins. J Dairy Sci 2022;105(Suppl. 1):379–80.
43. Ospina PA, McArt JA, Overton TR, et al. Using nonesterified fatty acids and beta-hydroxybutyrate concentrations during the transition period for herd-level monitoring of increased risk of disease and decreased reproductive and milking performance. Vet Clin North Am Food Anim Pract 2013;29(2):387–412.
44. McArt JAA, Abuelo A, Mann S. Metabolic disease diagnosis on farm: epidemiological principles. Practice 2020;42(7):405–14.
45. Oetzel GR. Monitoring and testing dairy herds for metabolic disease. Vet Clin North Am Food Anim Pract 2004;20(3):651–74.
46. Braun U, Zulliger P, Liesegang A, et al. Effect of intravenous calcium borogluconate and sodium phosphate in cows with parturient paresis. Vet Rec 2009;164(10):296–9.

47. Goff JP. Treatment of Calcium, Phosphorus, and Magnesium Balance Disorders. Vet Clin North Am Food Anim Pract 1999;15(3):619–39.
48. Doze JG, Donders R, van der Kolk JH. Effects of intravenous administration of two volumes of calcium solution on plasma ionized calcium concentration and recovery from naturally occurring hypocalcemia in lactating dairy cows. Am J Vet Res 2008;69(10):1346–50.
49. Littledike ET, Glazier D, Cook HM. Electrocardiographic changes after induced hypercalcemia and hypocalcemia in cattle: reversal of the induced arrhythmia with atropine. Am J Vet Res 1976;37(4):383–8.
50. Blanc CD, Van der List M, Aly SS, et al. Blood calcium dynamics after prophylactic treatment of subclinical hypocalcemia with oral or intravenous calcium. J Dairy Sci 2014;97(11):6901–6.
51. Domino AR, Korzec HC, McArt JAA. Field trial of 2 calcium supplements on early lactation health and production in multiparous Holstein cows. J Dairy Sci 2017;100(12):9681–90.
52. Curtis RA, Cote JF, McLennan MC, et al. Relationship of methods of treatment of relapse rate and serum levels of calcium and phosphorous in parturient hypocalcaemia. Can Vet J 1978;19(6):155–8.
53. Wilms J, Wang G, Doelman J, et al. Intravenous calcium infusion in a calving protocol disrupts calcium homeostasis compared with an oral calcium supplement. J Dairy Sci 2019;102(7):6056–64.
54. Frost IR, Seely CR, Callero KR, et al. Effect of prophylactic calcium supplementation on regulators of calcium homeostasis in multiparous Holstein cows. J Dairy Sci 2022;105(Suppl. 1):228.
55. Jahani-Moghadam M, Yansari AT, Chashnidel Y, et al. Short- and long-term effects of postpartum oral bolus v. subcutaneous Ca supplements on blood metabolites and productivity of Holstein cows fed a prepartum anionic diet. Animal 2020;14(5):983–90.
56. Amanlou H, Akbari AP, Farsuni NE, et al. Effects of subcutaneous calcium administration at calving on mineral status, health, and production of Holstein cows. J Dairy Sci 2016;99(11):9199–210.
57. Miltenburg CL, Duffield TF, Bienzle D, et al. Randomized clinical trial of a calcium supplement for improvement of health in dairy cows in early lactation. J Dairy Sci 2016;99(8):6550–62.
58. Goff JP, Horst RL. Oral administration of calcium salts for treatment of hypocalcemia in cattle. J Dairy Sci 1993;76(1):101–8.
59. Mann S, Nuss KA, Feist M, et al. Balling gun-induced trauma in cattle: clinical presentation, diagnosis and prevention. Vet Rec 2013;172(26):685.
60. Valldecabres A, Pires JAA, Silva-Del-Río N. Effect of prophylactic oral calcium supplementation on postpartum mineral status and markers of energy balance of multiparous Jersey cows. J Dairy Sci 2018;101(5):4460–72.
61. Martinez N, Sinedino LDP, Bisinotto RS, et al. Effects of oral calcium supplementation on mineral and acid-base status, energy metabolites, and health of postpartum dairy cows. J Dairy Sci 2016;99(10):8397–416.
62. Jahani-Moghadam M, Chashnidel Y, Teimouri-Yansari A, et al. Effect of oral calcium bolus administration on milk production, concentrations of minerals and metabolites in serum, early-lactation health status, and reproductive performance of Holstein dairy cows. N Z Vet J 2018;66(3):132–7.
63. Melendez P, Bartolome J, Roeschmann C, et al. The association of prepartum urine pH, plasma total calcium concentration at calving and postpartum diseases in Holstein dairy cattle. Animal 2021;15(3):100148.

64. Valldecabres A, Branco-Lopes R, Bernal-Cordoba C, et al. Production and reproduction responses for dairy cattle supplemented with oral calcium bolus after calving: Systematic review and meta-analysis. JDS Communications 2023; 4:9–13.
65. Oetzel GR, Miller BE. Effect of oral calcium bolus supplementation on early-lactation health and milk yield in commercial dairy herds. J Dairy Sci 2012; 95(12):7051–65.
66. Martinez N, Sinedino LDP, Bisinotto RS, et al. Effects of oral calcium supplementation on productive and reproductive performance in Holstein cows. J Dairy Sci 2016;99(10):8417–30.
67. Menta PR, Fernandes L, Poit D, et al. A randomized clinical trial evaluating the effect of an oral calcium bolus supplementation strategy in postpartum jersey cows on mastitis, culling, milk production, and reproductive performance. Animals (Basel) 2021;11(12). https://doi.org/10.3390/ani11123361.
68. National Research Council. US subcommittee on dairy cattle nutrition. Nutrient requirements of dairy cattle. Washington: National Academy Press; 2001.
69. National center for biotechnology information (NCBI) 2023. Bethesda (MD): National Library of Medicine (US), National Center for Biotechnology Information. 2023. Available at: www.ncbi.nlm.nih.gov/.

Phosphorus Metabolism During Transition

Walter Grünberg, Dr. med. vet, MS, PhD, Dipl. ECBHM, Dipl. ECAR, assoc. Dipl. ACVIM large animal

KEYWORDS

- Hypophosphatemia • Deprivation • Dry matter intake • Hemolysis • Homeostasis
- Regulation • Muscle function • Dry cow

KEY POINTS

- Phosphorus (P) in ruminant nutrition is under scrutiny because of concerns with P in animal waste presenting an environmental concern.
- Progress was made in the understanding of the P regulation in cattle. P-deprivation results in bone mobilization independently of the calcium homeostasis, and independently of the activity of parathyroid hormone.
- Assessing the P status of an individual animal remains a challenge. The concentration of inorganic P in serum or plasma is unreliable to identify animals in negative P balance.
- Several clinical signs and conditions most commonly observed in dairy cows during early lactation have been associated to P balance disorders. The role of P in the cause of many of these conditions remains obscure.
- In particular, during the dry period, cows should not be fed P in excess of requirements. Risks for health and productivity mainly result from overfeeding P, not from deficient P supply during the dry period.

INTRODUCTION

Phosphorus (P) in ruminant nutrition has received increased attention in the last decades. In particular, environmental concerns with P from animal waste reaching surface waters and resulting in eutrophication of lakes and ponds, and the continuously shrinking reserves of phosphate rock, that is the primary and nonrenewable resource of P, dictate a need for more restrictive use of the mineral in animal production. However, P that is required for the body's structural integrity and metabolic activity is also essential to sustain health and productivity in high-yielding dairy cows. Concerns of producers and veterinarians with reducing the dietary P supply in dairy herds with continuously increasing productivity thus remain.

Considerable progress was made during the last years in unraveling the regulation of the P balance and pathophysiology of P balance disorders that primarily affect the

Clinic for Ruminants and Herd Health, Justus-Liebig University, Frankfurter Strasse 104, Giessen, D-35392, Germany
E-mail address: waltergruenberg@yahoo.com

Vet Clin Food Anim 39 (2023) 261–274
https://doi.org/10.1016/j.cvfa.2023.02.002 vetfood.theclinics.com

transition cow. Many questions around the metabolic and (sub-) clinical effects of P-balance disturbances in cattle, however, remain unresolved. Similarly, knowledge gaps persist in the understanding of the regulation of the P homeostasis in ruminants. This article aims at reviewing our current knowledge and recent updates on P metabolism in transition cows.

BACKGROUND

Use of fertilizers but also the application of P-laden manure onto farmland are major contributors the pollution of surface waters with P. The amount of manure applied onto fields increased considerably during the second half of the last century, particularly in countries with intensive livestock farming. Dairy farms that typically have high yearly surpluses in their P balance contributed considerably to this development.[1] To address this environmental concern with P of animal origin governmental authorities in different parts of the world adopted a variety of strategies. In some countries authorities aimed at limiting the amount of manure applicable to agricultural land, while others implemented measures to reduce livestock density, and still other countries implemented taxes to penalize the supplementation of P in feed.[1] Depending on how strictly they are enforced, these measures can provide compelling incentives to keep the dietary P content in diets for farm animals at lowest possible level. Another reason to aim for a more sustainable use of P in animal production is that the availability of phosphate rock, the primary source of P, is worldwide in rapid decline. Scarcity of this nonrenewable resource has the potential to jeopardize the future capacity of the agriculture worldwide to produce sufficient food for a rapidly growing population.[2]

In the last decades of the previous, and the first decade of this century official estimates of daily P requirements of cattle underwent thorough reappraisal. Research at the time indicated that previous studies on which earlier recommendations were based, considerably underestimated true absorption of dietary P in cattle.[3,4] As a result, authorities responsible to publish official recommendations for dietary requirements lowered their estimates for daily P requirements in cattle. This reduction of officially advised dietary P supply to cattle was received with skepticism by veterinarians and the dairy industry, particularly in view of continuously increasing productivity of the dairy herds. P is an element that historically has been associated with productivity, fertility, and clinical disease in cattle and other ruminant species.[5,6] Concerns associated with P deficiency or hypophosphatemia in cattle include hampered productivity, decreased dry matter (DM) intake, impaired fertility but also clinical signs and symptoms such as muscle weakness, the downer cow syndrome, or intravascular hemolysis occurring during early lactation.[7] The link between the aforementioned disturbances and low P supply or hypophosphatemia is in most cases solely based on empirical grounds, and without good understanding of underlying pathophysiological mechanisms.[7] Before rules to mitigate environmental pollution with P originating from animal waste were implemented, there was less incentive to adhere to these new official recommendations, and feeding P in excess of these requirements was commonplace in particular in the dairy industry.[3,8]

Controversy and uncertainties around the P balance of dairy cows primarily concern the dairy cow during the transition period that is the period from approximately 1 month before to 1 month after calving. Outside this high-risk period for the dairy cow P metabolism does not seem a matter of concern or debate for producers and veterinarians. In recent years, advances in the understanding of the regulation of the P homeostasis in cattle as well as on implications of P balance disorders in cattle were made that will be discussed below.

REGULATION OF PHOSPHORUS HOMEOSTASIS IN CATTLE

Historically the P homeostasis of cattle and other species was thought to be regulated indirectly through the regulation of the extracellular calcium (Ca) balance.[9] According to this understanding, the key hormones responsible for regulating the P homeostasis were parathyroid hormone (PTH), a peptide hormone synthetized and excreted from the parathyroid glands, and calcitriol ($1,25(OH)_2$-D_3), that is the bioactive form of vitamin D_3.[10] The concept of a combined regulation of Ca and P seems to be biologically meaningful, particularly in young and growing animals, as both minerals are accrued in bone as hydroxyapatite in a precise Ca: P ratio. Accordingly, in growing animals the availability of these macrominerals in the extracellular pool of the body in a specific ratio to each other is essential to ensure adequate bone mineralization.[11] To a certain extent, this also applies to lactating dairy cows, which excrete Ca and P through the mammary gland at a relatively constant ratio as well.[12]

Beyond bone mineralization and milk production, however, Ca and P have only limited common ground metabolically that would support the concept of common regulatory circuits.

One major differences between these minerals is that P is a predominantly intracellular mineral, whereas soluble Ca prevails in the extracellular space.[7] The extracellular Ca concentration is regulated tightly through well-defined regulatory circuits, and even moderate drops of the extracellular Ca balance are associated specific signs and symptoms.[10] In contrast to Ca, the regulation of the extracellular P-balance seems to be less responsive to sudden drops of the concentration of inorganic P (Pi) in blood as they commonly occur in early lactation (**Fig. 1**). Clinical signs associated with disturbances of the extracellular P balance are ill defined and are frequently not consistently reproducible.[7] Furthermore, the sensing mechanism through which the body identifies P balance disturbances and regulates the P homeostasis remain enigmatic.

Ca presents an example of a mineral with tightly regulated extracellular concentration (imbalances around calving are rapidly corrected) and P represents a mineral of which the extracellular concentration is only loosely regulated.

Recent studies conducted in dairy cattle with the objective to identify the effect of restricted dietary P supply on the bovine organism found that the extracellular P balance, characterized by the blood [Pi] is easily disturbed, while in contrast the

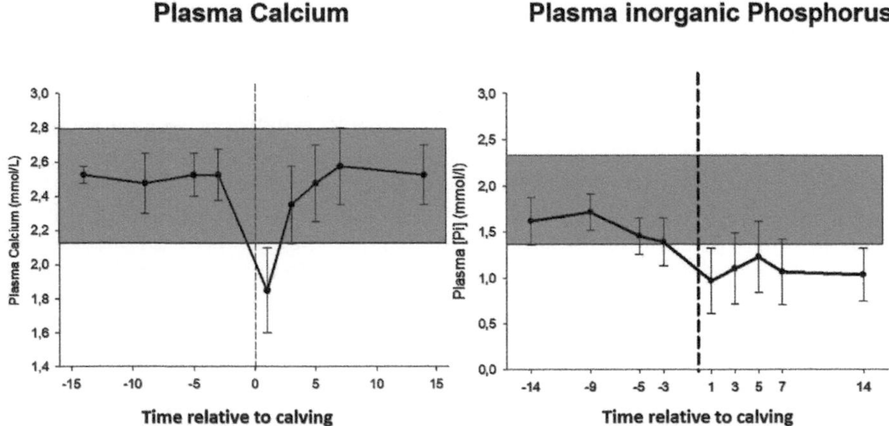

Fig. 1. Concentration time curves for Ca and Pi in plasma of healthy high-yielding dairy cows from 2 weeks before to 2 weeks after calving.

intracellular P homeostasis could not be disrupted in these experiments. One study aiming at inducing a negative P balance in midlactating dairy cows by feeding an approximately 50% P-deficient diet over a course of 5 weeks reported rapidly developing pronounced hypophosphatemia, with blood [Pi] less than detection limit (<0.2 mmol/L) for several days in some instances.[13] Study animals remained clinically unapparent, and the P content in muscle tissue or in red blood cells remained unaffected throughout the 5-week study period.[13,14] Similar results were obtained in dairy cows P depleted during transition.[15] The authors proposed that the emphasis of P regulation in the body is on maintaining a stable intracellular rather than extracellular P balance.

As mentioned above the question of how the body precisely senses a deregulation of the P balance either at intracellular or extracellular level remains unresolved. A series of recent studies conducted in cattle and small ruminants, however, provide compelling evidence that the ruminant organism can efficiently respond to P deprivation in the absence of Ca balance disturbances, which refutes the concept of a Ca-dependent P regulation.[13,16,17]

Primary pathways through which P deficiency is counterregulated seem to be activation of osteoclasts, resulting in release of P together with Ca from bone, and enhanced intestinal P absorption that may be upregulated through activation of vitamin D_3. Studies conducted on dairy cows in midlactation but also in transition cows showed that restricted P supply resulted in pronounced bone mobilization that was associated with marked increases of bone biomarkers such as pyridinoline and deoxypyridinoline in urine or crosslaps in plasma.[13,18] The precise mechanism through which P deprivation triggers activation of osteoclasts again has not yet been unraveled. In states of negative Ca balance bone mobilization is triggered by increased secretion of PTH in response to a signal from Ca-sensing receptors.[10] A similar peak in PTH secretion was not observed in P-deprived cattle with unaltered Ca balance in various stages of lactation.[18–20] These results led to the current understanding that although PTH affects P homeostasis, for example, by activating osteoclast activity, or increasing salivary P excretion, it should not be considered a hormone regulating the P homeostasis because it does not seem to respond to alterations of the P balance in ruminants.[7]

Controversy still exists about the role of vitamin D_3 as regulatory hormone of P homeostasis. One study reported a similar increase in $1,25(OH)_2D_3$, the active form of vitamin D_3 around parturition in cows on dry cow diets with adequate Ca, and in cows on diets with deficient dietary P content.[18] In this study, P-deprived cows had higher blood Ca concentrations and lacked the characteristic PTH-peak associated with periparturient hypocalcemia. This led the authors to hypothesize that the activation of vitamin D_3 may also occur in response to negative P balance and independently of PTH.[18] A negative association of $1,25(OH)_2D_3$ with blood [Pi] was observed in P deprived sheep but not in sheep on a diet with adequate P content, which corroborates the hypothesis of vitamin D contributing to the regulation of P balance in ruminants.[17] Other studies in contrast did not observe an increase of $1,25(OH)_2D_3$ in P-deprived cattle, which is consistent with earlier studies in small ruminants, and suggests that vitamin D_3 is not a primary regulatory hormone of P homeostasis in ruminants.[19–21]

At the beginning of this century, a new endocrine substance, fibroblast growth factor 23 (FGF23), which is thought to be a key player in the regulation of the P balance, at least in monogastric species, was identified.[22] This hormone synthetized in osteocytes counterregulates hyperphosphatemia by increasing renal P excretion and by hampering the synthesis of 1α-hydroxylase, the enzyme responsible of converting vitamin D_3 from its inactive form 25(OH)D_3 to its active form 1,25$(OH)_2$-D_3.[23] In ruminants, the role of FGF23 could not yet been clarified in detail due to lacking validated diagnostic tests allowing to measure FGF23 in ruminant species. One study investigating the effect of dietary P deprivation in sheep reported a marked reduction of the transcription rate of FGF23 in bone tissue of P-deprived sheep compared with sheep on adequate dietary P supply.[17] These results indicate FGF23 may not only be involved in the correction of hyperphosphatemia in ruminants as in other species but potentially also contributes to the counterregulation of P deprivation or hypophosphatemia. Downregulation of FGF23 synthesis in osteocytes in states of negative P balance would result in an enhanced activation of vitamin D_3, reduced renal P excretion, and possibly also to enhanced bone mobilization.[17]

In conclusion, recent advances in the understanding of P homeostasis regulation in cattle led to the awareness that earlier concepts of regulation of P homeostasis cannot be sustained. Novel regulatory circuits have been identified; the overall understanding of how the ruminant regulates the P homeostasis however remains incomplete.

PHOSPHORUS BALANCE DISTURBANCES IN TRANSITION COWS

Several clinical signs occurring in cattle have been associated with P balance disturbances, primarily affecting the transition cow. In veterinary practice the diagnosis of P balance disorders in cattle is based on blood biochemical analysis yielding concentrations of inorganic P ([Pi]) in serum or plasma outside the reference range for cattle (1.4–2.6 mmol/L).[7] Recurrent observation of a specific clinical sign such as recumbency or hemoglobinuria in combination with subnormal blood [Pi] will reasonably lead the veterinarian to suspect a causative relation between hypophosphatemia and the observed presentation. In the hierarchy of evidence, this corresponds either to empirical evidence or to the evidence level of observational studies, case series, or case reports.[24] Upgrading the level of evidence on the pyramid of evidence-based medicine requires to be able to reproduce this association in controlled and randomized prospective studies.[24] Despite of numerous attempts this step has not yet been achieved for several of the conditions discussed below. Another unresolved matter of debate is the metabolic and clinical relevance of hypophosphatemia that is commonly observed in dairy cows shortly after calving.

Postparturient Hypophosphatemia

Disturbances of P homeostasis in dairy cows are a matter of concern primarily when occurring in the first weeks of lactation. It is mainly for reasons of practicality that [Pi] in serum or plasma is the best-established parameter to assess P status of an animal.[7] Measuring [Pi] in serum or plasma (incorrectly often referred to as blood [Pi]) as integral part of a chemistry panel is common in farm animal practice. Hypophosphatemia is commonly diagnosed in sick periparturient dairy cows, for example, suffering of periparturient recumbency, abomasal displacement, ketosis, or hepatic lipidosis.[25–27] Metabolic profiling studies, however, revealed a larger number of clinically healthy cattle in the first days after calving show subnormal blood [Pi].[28–30] A German study that is based on laboratory study of more than 7000 clinical healthy dairy cows identified 93%, 53%, and 44% of studied animals with serum [Pi] of less than 1.6 mmol/L on days 1, 3, and 5, respectively. Using a cutoff value of 1.25 mmol/L, the authors identified 71%, 21% and 10% of cows on days 1, 3, and 5 of lactation as hypophosphatemic.[31]

The metabolic or even clinical relevance of hypophosphatemia in sick but also in healthy periparturient cows remains under contentious debate.[7] Although some may consider hypophosphatemia in a sick cow to cause or at least contribute to morbidity, others may interpret the drop in blood [Pi] in sick and feed depressed cows as a consequence rather than the cause of illness. Still others may consider hypophosphatemia in fresh cows to be a physiologic sign of adaptation of the metabolism from the dry period to lactation. Specifically the question whether transient postparturient hypophosphatemia that is devoid of any clinical signs is a physiologic development after calving, or if rather is a harbinger of a subclinical metabolic disturbance potentially affecting health or productivity of a high-yielding dairy cow remains unresolved.

The cause of postparturient hypophosphatemia has not been entirely elucidated. Common wisdom states that, the drop in plasma [Pi] is primarily the result of the sudden increase of P loss through the mammary gland at the onset of lactation in combination with low feed intake around calving, as it is the case for Ca. Pronounced declines in blood [Pi] around calving were also shown to occur in mastectomized cows not producing any milk.[32] Furthermore, a similar decline in blood [Pi] could be induced in nonpregnant and nonlactating dairy cows infused with adrenocorticotropic hormone (ACTH) to induce an increase in blood cortisol as it occurs around parturition.[33] These findings indicate the cause of the periparturient drop of blood Pi is more complex than is the case for Ca. Compartmental shifts of P from the extracellular to the intracellular space that are not associated with P losses from the body considerably contribute this periparturient extracellular P imbalance.[7]

A question that is distinct from the debate over the relevance of hypophosphatemia for health and productivity is the question about the suitability of [Pi] in serum or plasma to identify animals with negative P balance. There is general consensus that the plasma/serum [Pi] only characterizes the extracellular P pool of the body, equivalent to less than 1% of the P available in the body.[7] The [Pi] in serum or plasma thus at best can crudely reflect the short-term P supply through feed. The result of a single blood sample must be interpreted with caution as sudden and pronounced compartmental shifts, resulting in short-lived fluctuations in concentrations of [Pi] in serum or plasma that can exceed 30%, may mislead the interpretation of the biochemical analysis.[31] The [Pi] in serum or plasma is in particular not suited to identify chronically P-deficient animals or to assess severity of P deprivation. Counterregulation in the form of bone mobilization and enhanced P absorption from the gut that vary depending on severity and duration of P deprivation will confound the blood [Pi].[17,20,34,35] Hypophosphatemia thus cannot be considered as unambiguous sign for P deprivation.

Hypophosphatemic Recumbency

One condition that is widely believed to be associated with P deficiency or hypophosphatemia in cattle in particular during the periparturient period is the so-called downer cow syndrome, or what is sometimes referred as atypical milk fever.[36,37] Affected cows are commonly in early lactation, mentally alert with posture suggesting hind limb paresis, and typically do not respond to intravenous treatment with Ca salts. Laboratory study most consistently reveals subnormal blood [Pi] with or without subnormal blood [Ca].[37–39] The role of P in the etiology of downer cow syndrome, however, remains obscure. Despite various attempts reported in the literature, there is to this day not one single report of experimentally induced hypophosphatemic recumbency in cattle. Studies conducted in midlactating and in transition cows, feeding rations approximately 50% P deficient for periods of 5 to 9 weeks reported the development of pronounced hypophosphatemia without any concomitant clinical signs of muscle weakness.[13,15] Muscle biopsies conducted in these cows revealed unaltered contents of total P, creatine phosphate, and adenosine phosphates in muscle tissue throughout the study period. Electromyographs conducted throughout these studies determined muscle function disturbances at a subclinical level after several weeks of P deprivation. These were not pronounced enough to become clinically apparent.[13,15] In summary, currently available evidence suggests hypophosphatemia or P deprivation per se, at a level it may occur in practice without using P binders, does not result in clinically apparent muscle function disturbances in cattle. It is however conceivable that hypophosphatemia or P deprivation may contribute to the downer cow syndrome and cause recumbency when occurring in combination with another thus far undetermined contributing factor.

Postparturient Hemoglobinuria (PPH)

Another condition thought to be associated with hypophosphatemia or P deprivation and primarily occurring in dairy cows in the first weeks of lactation is postparturient hemoglobinuria (PPH). Affected animals develop sudden intravascular hemolysis severe enough to result in hemoglobinuria and that may lead to potentially life-threatening anemia within a matter of days.[40] Typically, PPH occurs as a sporadic disease, only affecting one or few cows of a herd, although a large number of fresh cows in the same herd can be diagnosed with subnormal [Pi] in serum or plasma. Blood biochemical analysis from samples obtained in the acute phase of the disease reveals pronounced hypophosphatemia as the most consistent finding, which led to the empirical association of PPH with hypophosphatemia or P deprivation.[41,42] The proposed underlying mechanism is intracellular P depletion, and ensuing ATP shortage in red blood cells of P-deficient cows. The lack of ATP in erythrocytes is thought to result in an increase of red blood cell volume, development of spherocytosis, increased osmotic fragility, and finally erythrolysis.[43] It is noteworthy; however, that P deprivation and hypophosphatemia is not routinely associated with P depletion in erythrocytes, and that P deprivation was found to induce hemolysis only when occurring in early lactation but not during the dry period or later in lactation.[14,44]

A recent study reported experimentally induced PPH consistently occurring in the second week of lactation in a subset of dairy cows subject to dietary P deprivation during late gestation and early lactation.[44] The authors, however, also reported several milder cases of hemolysis that were not associated with hemoglobinuria in this study, suggesting the existence of a subclinical form of PPH that is not yet acknowledged in the current literature.[44] In contrast, cows fed a control diet with adequate P content, and cows fed a P-deficient diet during the last 4 weeks of gestation only did not develop hemolysis. The authors furthermore provide anecdotal reports of PPH cases aggressively supplemented with P-salts, which rapidly corrected hypophosphatemia but did not interrupt hemolysis. In other instances, hemolysis resolved while cows remained on a deficient diet and without P supplementation.[44] The underlying mechanism causing PPH thus remain obscure, as does the role of P in the etiology.

Feed Intake Depression

Feed intake depression and altered eating behavior are among the oldest concerns associated with P deficiency and hypophosphatemia in cattle.[5,6] Anorexia and feed intake depression are the most consistent signs associated with P deficiency across species.[6,45–47] In cattle, pica has been reported to occur particularly in states of chronic and severe P deficiency.[48] The mechanism through which P deficiency may affect voluntary feed intake and eating behavior remains obscure. In ruminants, altered rumen fermentation in P-deprived animals has been suggested as possible cause for anorexia. This would however not explain identical clinical signs observed in other non-ruminant species in states of P deprivation.[35] An alternative mechanism of action proposed more recently is through metabolic disturbances of the central nervous system that may occur in states of P deprivation.[49] Neurologic symptoms such as altered demeanor or disorientation are consistently reported in hypophopshatemic human patients.[50] In rodents, experimental P depletion was found to significantly impair neurotransmitter synthesis in various regions of the central nervous system.[51]

Altered eating behavior in cattle is reported to occur after prolonged periods of P deprivation. The type of eating behavior disturbance is presumably associated with severity and duration of P deprivation. Pica is observed in more severe and pronounced states of P deficiency, whereas anorexia is more commonly seen with moderate P deprivation.[3,52,53] The matter of inadequate dietary P supply in dairy cows, in particular during the transition period, and its potential effect on DM intake was the subject of several studies. Feed intake depression in adult cattle, previously fed adequate amounts of P, developed after feeding P-deficient lactating cow diets with a content in the range of 0.26% P in DM during weeks to months.[6,52] Shorter episodes of restricted dietary P supply of 5 weeks in midlactating cows were, in contrast, not associated with feed intake depression.[13] Feed intake depression was also not observed during the dry period when P restriction (diets with 0.16% P in DM) was initiated 4 weeks before expected calving.[53,54] When P restriction was extended into early lactation, with rations containing between 0.20% and 0.23% P in DM, cows on restricted P supply showed smaller increases in DM intake in early lactation compared with control cows on adequate P supply.[13,49,53] Another recent study in which fresh cows were fed a diet with 0.29% P in DM for the first 8 weeks of lactation reported a trend toward lower increases in DM intake in the second and third week of lactation when compared with cows on a diet with a P content 0.38% in DM.[55] A difference between treatments was not perceptible later during the study.[55] In summary, the results presented here leave the question unresolved whether prolonged restricted access to P during the transition period, or rather restricted P supply from the time of calving on and into early lactating may cause feed intake depression in fresh cows. Based on the presented data, P restriction from the moment after calving and during the first weeks of lactation is strongly discouraged.

For decades, P deprivation has also been linked to impaired growth, poor fertility, and hampered productivity in ruminants.[56,57] In most reports, where such an association was apparent, P deprivation persisted for prolonged periods and was associated with marked feed intake depression or insufficient availability of feed.[6,52,54] Current wisdom states that negative effects on milk production, fertility, or weight gain are not caused by insufficient availability of P but are rather the consequence of inadequate energy and nutrient intake resulting from feed intake depression.[7] It is this widely held association between productivity, fertility, and P supply that is thought to have encouraged the still common practice in the field the feed rations with P contents well above current recommendations.[3] In the meantime, numerous studies have unequivocally documented that there is no benefit on productivity or fertility of feeding P in excess of current recommendations.[58,59]

PHOSPHORUS REQUIREMENTS OF DAIRY COWS IN TRANSITION

Estimates of daily cattle P requirements underwent a thorough reappraisal during the last decades of the previous century. Official recommendations for P supply to ruminants were lowered in many countries in the late 1990s and early 2000s, based on evidence indicating P absorption rates in ruminants were grossly underestimated in the past.[3,60] Current estimates of daily P requirements for cattle handled in various countries differ within a reasonable range (**Table 1**). The differences are primarily

Table 1
Official recommendations for dietary P supply to dairy cows in different countries

Milk Yield (kg/d)	DMI[a] (kg/d)	United Kingdom[b] (% in DM)	Germany[c] (% in DM)	United States[d] (% in DM)	The Netherlands[e] (% in DM)
Dry cow			0.25	0.23	0.20
15	17	0.33	0.28	0.30	0.24
25	20.3	0.38	0.33	0.32	0.27
35	23.6	0.42	0.37	0.35	0.29
45	26.9	0.45	0.40	0.36	0.31
55	30.9	0.47	0.42	0.38	0.32

[a] Assumed daily DM intake.
[b] AFRC, 1991.[4]
[c] GfE, 2001.[64]
[d] NASEM,2021.[61]
[e] CVB, 2018.[62]

attributable to different estimates of dietary P true absorption rate. The Netherlands handles the lowest values for recommended dietary P supply to ruminants and is furthermore among the countries with the strictest regulations to limit environmental pollution from farm animal waste. The Dutch recommendations are based on an estimated true absorption rate for P of 75%, compared with values between 64% and 70% handled in the United Kingdom and United States.[4,61,62] Overall, these are thought to be conservative estimates of the true P absorption in cattle.[4] Real absorption rates for P in cattle are assumed to exceed 80%.[3,63] These conservative estimates are considered to provide a safety margin for current recommendations and may furthermore provide scope for fine-tuning of current recommendation in the future.[63]

As it was the case for lactating cow rations, recommendations for dietary P supply to dry cows were revisited and revised over the past years. Estimating the P requirements of the dry cow presents several challenges. The limited duration of the dry period, the impossibility to include parameters related to production and reproduction, and the lack of unambiguous signs suggestive of mild-to-moderate P deficiency all complicate the objective assessment of P balance in the dry period. In the recent past attempts were made to identify the dietary P level in dry cow rations at which the body activates bone mobilization as response to insufficient dietary P supply.[13] Bone biomarkers determined in blood were suggested as potentially useful diagnostic tools for this purpose, and preliminary data suggest that bone mobilization in dry cows is not consistently activated with dry cow ration containing a dietary P content above 0.20% in DM.[31]

Effect of Dietary Phosphorus Content in Dry Cow Diets on the Calcium Homeostasis of the Periparturient Cow

Current knowledge indicates that a dietary P content in the range of 0.20% to 0.25% in DM covers dairy cow requirements in the dry period.[61,63,65] In the past century, feeding P well in excess of requirements was often advised not only to mitigate the risk of periparturient hypocalcemia and periparturient hypophosphatemia but also to prevent fertility issues in the following lactation.[3,5,66] More recent studies; however, provide compelling evidence that feeding P in excess of requirements not only does not improve health and productivity but is rather counterproductive in that it increases the risk for periparturient hypocalcemia.[55,67] A meta-analysis revealed an increase in the incidence of clinical hypocalcemia in the range of 18% when feeding dry cow rations with a dietary P content of 0.4% instead of 0.3% P in DM.[67] A recent case control study reported 4% higher blood Ca concentrations after calving in cows fed a dry cow diet with 0.22% P in DM when compared with cows fed a diet with 0.36% P in DM.[55] The same study reports more stable blood [Pi] in cows that were fed the ration with 0.22% when compared with the ration containing 0.36% P in DM.[55]

Studies exploring effects of dietary P deprivation during the dry period in dairy cows found that inducing a negative P balance in late gestation resulted in the activation of bone mobilization.[18,19] The result was significantly increased blood [Ca] during the first week of lactation when compared with cows on a diet with high P content.[16,19] Although extending P deprivation into early lactation seriously impacted health and productivity, no deleterious effects were observed when P deprivation was discontinued at the time of calving.[49,54] The same study showed that P restricting dairy cows during the dry period did not exacerbate but rather tended to mitigate the occurrence of postparturient hypophosphatemia.[54]

Feeding P-deficient diets during the last weeks of gestation has been discussed as a strategy to mitigate occurrence of periparturient hypocalcemia.[16,19,54] Before low P diets for dry cows can be recommended to prevent hypocalcemia large-scale studies confirming that P depriving cows during the dry period is innocuous for health and productivity in the following lactation must be performed. In this context it should be noted that formulating dry cow rations with a P content sufficiently low to drive the dry cow into negative balance (ie, well below 0.20% P in DM) is at least as challenging as formulating a dry cow ration with Ca content low enough to induce a negative Ca balance.

FUTURE DIRECTIONS FOR RESEARCH

Although important progress in understanding P homeostasis in ruminants was made in the recent past, many important questions remain unresolved. It remains an endeavor for veterinarians and nutritionists to provide substantiated advice on P requirements without in-depth understanding of P balance regulation. Important knowledge gaps remain in the understanding of P homeostasis regulation, including the question of how the body senses P balance disturbances, how FGF23 functions in ruminants, or how P recycling in ruminants is regulated. For disease prevention and improvement of treatment modalities, a better understanding of the pathophysiology and underlying mechanisms through which P balance disorders may affect health and productivity of the fresh cow in particular are urgently needed. This includes altered feeding behavior, altered red blood cell integrity, or muscle function disturbances.

CLINICS CARE POINTS

- Postparturient hypophosphatemia is commonly observed in cows shortly after calving. The metabolic and clinical relevance of it remains uncertain
- Hypophosphatemia is not a reliable indication for a negative P balance
- Feeding P in excess of requirements during the dry period must be avoided because this increases the risk of periparturient hypocalcemia
- P deprivation in cattle is of particular concern during the first weeks of lactation

DECLARATION OF INTERESTS

The author had several consultancy agreements and speaker appointments with Boehringer Ingelheim Vetmedica, Zoetis and Elanco.

REFERENCES

1. Bomans E, Fransen K, Gobin A, et al. Addressing phosphorus related problems in farm practice. *Final report to the, . European Commission.* Leuven-Heverlee, Belgium: Soild service of Belgium; 2005. p. 9–21.
2. Schroder J, Cordell D, Smit A, et al. Sustainable use of phosphorus: EU tender ENV. B1/ETU/2009/0025. Wageningen UR; 2010.
3. NRC. Nutrient Requirements of dairy cattle. 7th revised edition. Washington, D.C.: Nat. Acad. Sci; 2001.
4. AFRC. Reappraisal of the calcium and phosphorus requirements of sheep and cattle. Swindon wiltshire. Wallingford Oxon UK: CAB International; 1991.
5. Morrow DA. Phosphorus deficiency and infertility in dairy heifers. J Am Vet Med Assoc 1969;154:761.
6. Call JW, Butcher JE, Shupe JL, et al. Clinical effects of low dietary phosphorus concentration in feed given to lactating dairy-cows. American journal of veterinary research 1987;48:133–6.
7. Grunberg W. Treatment of Phosphorus Balance Disorders. Vet Clin Food Anim Pract 2014;30:383–408.
8. Plaizier J, Garner T, Droppo T, et al. Nutritional practices on Manitoba dairy farms. Can J Anim Sci 2004;84:501–9.
9. Goff JP. Pathophysiology of calcium and phosphorus disorders. Vet Clin Food Anim Pract 2000;16:319–38.
10. Horst RL. Regulation of calcium and phosphorus homeostasis in the dairy cow. J Dairy Sci 1986;69:604–16.
11. Chen Y-H, Goff JP, Horst RL. Restoring normal blood phosphorus concentrations in hypophosphatemic cattle with sodium phosphate. Vet Med 1998;93:4.
12. Cerbulis J, Farrell H Jr. Composition of the milks of dairy cattle. II. Ash, calcium, magnesium, and phosphorus. J Dairy Sci 1976;59:589–93.
13. Grunberg W, Scherpenisse P, Dobbelaar P, et al. The effect of transient, moderate dietary phosphorus deprivation on phosphorus metabolism, muscle content of different phosphorus-containing compounds, and muscle function in dairy cows. J Dairy Sci 2015;98:5385–400.
14. Grunberg W, Mol JA, Teske E. Red Blood Cell Phosphate Concentration and Osmotic Resistance During Dietary Phosphate Depletion in Dairy Cows. J Vet Intern Med 2015;29:395–9.
15. Grünberg W, Scherpenisse P, Cohrs I, et al. Phosphorus content of muscle tissue and muscle function in dairy cows fed a phosphorus-deficient diet during the transition period. J Dairy Sci 2019;102:4072–93.
16. Cohrs I, Wilkens MR, Grunberg W. Short communication: Effect of dietary phosphorus deprivation in late gestation and early lactation on the calcium homeostasis of periparturient dairy cows. J Dairy Sci 2018;101:9591–8.
17. Köhler OM, Grünberg W, Schnepel N, et al. Dietary phosphorus restriction affects bone metabolism, vitamin D metabolism and rumen fermentation traits in sheep. J Anim Physiol Anim Nutr 2021;105:35–50.
18. Cohrs I, Grunberg W. Suitability of oral administration of monosodium phosphate, disodium phosphate, and magnesium phosphate for the rapid correction of hypophosphatemia in cattle. J Vet Intern Med 2018;32:1253–8.
19. Wächter S, Cohrs I, Golbeck L, et al. Effects of restricted dietary phosphorus supply to dry cows on periparturient calcium status. J Dairy Sci 2021;105(1):748–60.
20. Keanthao P, Reappraisal of the phosphorus requirement of lactating dairy cows, 2022, Utrecht University; Utrecht, The Netherlands.

21. Schröder B, Käppner H, Failing K, et al. Mechanisms of intestinal phosphate transport in small ruminants. Br J Nutr 1995;74:635–48.
22. Razzaque MS. The FGF23–Klotho axis: endocrine regulation of phosphate homeostasis. Nat Rev Endocrinol 2009;5:611–9.
23. Kuro-o M. Overview of the FGF23-Klotho axis. Pediatr Nephrol 2010;25:583–90.
24. Holmes MA, Ramey DW. An Introduction to Evidence-Based Veterinary Medicine. Vet Clin N Am Equine Pract 2007;23:191–200.
25. Blum J, JW B, KG J, et al. Calcium (ionized and total), magnesium, phosphorus, and glucose in plasma from parturient cows. Am J Vet Res 1972;33(1):51–6.
26. Kalaitzakis E, Panousis N, Roubies N, et al. Macromineral status of dairy cows with concurrent left abomasal displacement and fatty liver. N Z Vet J 2010;58: 307–11.
27. Kalaitzakis E, Panousis N, Roubies N, et al. Clinicopathological evaluation of downer dairy cows with fatty liver. Canadian Veterinary Journal-Revue Veterinaire Canadienne 2010;51:615 +.
28. Macrae AI, Whitaker DA, Burrough E, et al. Use of metabolic profiles for the assessment of dietary adequacy in UK dairy herds. Vet Rec 2006;159:655–61.
29. Macrae AI, Burrough E, Forrest J. Assessment of nutrition in dairy herds: Use of metabolic profiles. Cattle Pract 2012;20:120–7.
30. Hansen K. Untersuchungen zur postpartalen Hypophosphatämie bei Holstein Friesian Kühen, 2018. Doctoral Thesis, Free University Berlin, Germany.
31. Cohrs I, Wächter S, Hansen K, et al. A potential new biomarker to monitor the phosphorus balance in dry dairy cows. Anim Feed Sci Technol 2022;287:115281.
32. Goff JP, Kimura K, Horst RL. Effect of mastectomy on milk fever, energy, and vitamins A, E, and beta-carotene status at parturition. J Dairy Sci 2002;85:1427–36.
33. Kim D, Yamagishi N, Devkota B, et al. Effects of cortisol secreted via a 12-h infusion of adrenocorticotropic hormone on mineral homeostasis and bone metabolism in ovariectomized cows. Domest Anim Endocrinol 2012;43:264–9.
34. Antoniucci DM, Yamashita T, Portale AA. Dietary phosphorus regulates serum fibroblast growth factor-23 concentrations in healthy men. The Journal of clinical endocrinology and metabolism 2006;91:3144–9.
35. Breves G, Schröder B. Comparative Aspects of Gastrointestinal Phosphorus Metabolism. Nutr Res Rev 1991;4:125–40.
36. Gerloff B, Swensen E. Acute recumbency and marginal phosphorus deficiency in dairy cattle. J Am Vet Med Assoc 1996;208:716–9.
37. Menard L, Thompson A. Milk fever and alert downer cows: Does hypophosphatemia affect the treatment response? Canadian Veterinary Journal-Revue Veterinaire Canadienne 2007;48:487–91.
38. Hofmann W, el-Amrousi S. Studies on bovine paresis. 5. Experiments on the medicamentous therapy of hypophosphoremia and paresis in atypical parturient paresis. DTW Deutsche tierarztliche Wochenschrift 1971;78:156–9.
39. Stolla R, Schulz H, Martin R. Changes in the clinical picture of parturient paresis. Tierärztliche Umsch 2000;55:295–9.
40. Macwilliams PS, Searcy GP, Bellamy JE. Bovine postparturient hemoglobinuria: a review of the literature. The Canadian veterinary journal = La revue veterinaire canadienne 1982;23:309–12.
41. Jubb TF, Jerrett IV, Browning JW, et al. Haemoglobinuria and hypophosphataemia in postparturient dairy cows without dietary deficiency of phosphorus. Aust Vet J 1990;67:86–9.
42. Stockdale CR, Moyes TE, Dyson R. Acute post-parturient haemoglobinuria in dairy cows and phosphorus status. Aust Vet J 2005;83:362–6.

43. Ogawa E, Kobayashi K, Yoshiura N, et al. Hemolytic anemia and red blood-cell metabolic disorder attributable to low phosphorus intake in cows. American journal of veterinary research 1989;50:388–92.
44. van den Brink L, Cohrs I, Golbeck L, et al. Effect of Dietary Phosphate Deprivation on Red Blood Cell Parameters of Periparturient Dairy Cows. Animals (Basel) 2023;13(3):404.
45. Knochel JP. Pathophysiology and clinical characteristics of severe hypophosphatemia *Archives of Internal Medicine* 1977;137:203–20.
46. Fuller TJ, Carter NW, Barcenas C, et al. Reversible changes of muscle-cell in experimental phosphorus deficiency. J Clin Invest 1976;57:1019–24.
47. Ternouth J, Sevilla C. The effects of low levels of dietary phosphorus upon the dry matter intake and metabolism of lambs. Aust J Agric Res 1990;41:175–84.
48. Dixon R, Fletcher M, Goodwin KL, et al. Learned behaviours lead to bone ingestion by phosphorus-deficient cattle. Anim Prod Sci 2018;59:921–32.
49. Grünberg W, Witte S, Cohrs I, et al. Liver phosphorus content and liver function in states of phosphorus deficiency in transition dairy cows. PLoS One 2019;14:e0219546.
50. Knochel JP. Hypophosphatemia. West J Med 1981;134:15–26.
51. Bhaskaran D, Massry SG, Campese VM. Effect of hypophosphatemia on brain catecholamines content in the rat. Mineral and electrolyte metabolism 1987;13:469–72.
52. Valk H, Sebek LBJ. Influence of long-term feeding of limited amounts of phosphorus on dry matter intake, milk production, and body weight of dairy cows. J Dairy Sci 1999;82:2157–63.
53. Puggaard L, Lund P, Liesegang A, et al. Long term effect of reduced dietary phosphorus on feed intake and milk yield in dry and lactating dairy cows. Livest Sci 2014;159:18–28.
54. Wächter S, Cohrs I, Golbeck L, et al. Effects of restricted dietary phosphorus supply during the dry period on productivity and metabolism in dairy cows. J Dairy Sci 2022;105:4370–92.
55. Keanthao P, Goselink R, Dijkstra J, et al. Effects of dietary phosphorus concentration during the transition period on plasma calcium concentrations, feed intake, and milk production in dairy cows. J Dairy Sci 2021;104(11):11646–59.
56. Gartner BJW, Murphy GM, Hoey WA. Effects of induced, subclinical phosphorus deficiency on feed intake and growth of beef heifers. J Agric Sci 1982;98:23–9.
57. Milton J, Ternouth J. Phosphorus metabolism in ruminants. 2. Effects of inorganic phosphorus concentration upon food intake and digestibility. Aust J Agric Res 1985;36:647–54.
58. Wu Z, Satter LD, Sojo R. Milk production, reproductive performance, and fecal excretion of phosphorus by dairy cows fed three amounts of phosphorus. J Dairy Sci 2000;83:1028–41.
59. Bach KD, Neves RC, Stokol T, et al. Technical note: Effect of storage time and temperature on total calcium concentrations in bovine blood. J Dairy Sci 2020;103:922–8.
60. Ernährungsphysiologie Gf. Ausschuss für Bedarfsnormen der Gesellschaft für Ernährungsphysiologie: empfehlung zur Energie-und Nährstoffversorgung der Milchkühe und Aufzuchtrinder. Main) Frankfurt: DLG-Verlag; 2001.
61. National Academies of Sciences E, Medicine. Nutrient requirements of dairy cattle. 8th Revised Edition. Washington, DC: The National Academies Press; 2021.

62. Table Booklet Feeding of uminants 2016. Nutrient requirements for cattle, sheep and goats and nutritional values of feeding ingredients for ruminants, Federatie Nederlandse Diervoederketen, 2018, The Hague, The Netherlands.
63. CVB. Handleiding Mineralenvoorzienin rundvee, schapen, geiten. The Hague, The Netherlands, 2005.
64. GfE. Empfehlungen Zur Energie- und Nährstoffversorgung der Milchkühe und Aufzuchtrinder. Frankfurt a.M.: DLG-Verlag; 2001.
65. Landwirtschaft BLf. Gruber Tabelle zur Fütterung der Milchkühe. 47 ed. Freising-Weihenstephan: bayerische Landesanstalt für Landwirtschaft (LfL, 2021.
66. Boda J, Cole H. The influence of dietary calcium and phosphorus on the incidence of milk fever in dairy cattle. J Dairy Sci 1954;37:360–72.
67. Lean IJ, DeGaris PJ, McNeil DM, et al. Hypocalcemia in dairy cows: Meta-analysis and dietary cation anion difference theory revisited. J Dairy Sci 2006; 89:669–84.

Pregnancy Toxemia in Sheep and Goats

Andrea Mongini, DVM, MS[a], Robert J. Van Saun, DVM, MS, PhD[b,*]

KEYWORDS

- Pregnancy toxemia • Small ruminants • Metabolic disease • Sheep • Goats

KEY POINTS

- Pregnancy toxemia is a metabolic disease associated with hypoglycemia and hyperketonemia in late gestation sheep and goats typically with multiple fetuses.
- Obesity or starvation during late pregnancy can predispose the ewe or doe to greater risk of pregnancy toxemia.
- Proper diagnosis and early detection of pregnancy toxemia are critical for favorable outcomes.
- Nutritional management of individuals and herds is an essential part of treatment of acute cases and prevention of future cases.

 **Video content accompanies this article at http://www.vetfood.theclinics.com.**

INTRODUCTION

Pregnancy toxemia is the most common and potentially disastrous metabolic disease of sheep and goats.[1,2] Pregnancy toxemia may occur with a limited number of individuals or present as a herd/flock outbreak depending upon prevailing farm circumstances (ie, management, feeding practices, environmental conditions). A survey of 10 goat dairies where pregnancy toxemia was identified based on presence of defined clinical signs reported an overall pregnancy toxemia prevalence of 10%, though the range was between 0% and 18% within herds.[3] In a case report of a pregnancy toxemia outbreak in a sheep flock, approximately 20% of early lambing ewes presented with some degree of pregnancy toxemia before nutritional intervention that reduced the disease prevalence.[4] Consequences of pregnancy toxemia are critical as often both dam and offspring can be lost resulting in significant economic losses. Proper diagnosis and care of these patients early in the disease course have a large

[a] M&M Veterinary Practice, Inc, Ewetopia Dairy, Inc, Denair, CA, USA; [b] Department of Veterinary and Biomedical Sciences, College of Agricultural Sciences, Pennsylvania State University, 108C Animal, Veterinary and Biomedical Sciences Building, University Park, PA 16802-3500, USA
* Corresponding author.
E-mail address: rjv10@psu.edu

Vet Clin Food Anim 39 (2023) 275–291
https://doi.org/10.1016/j.cvfa.2023.02.010

impact on case outcomes. This article will provide an overview of pregnancy toxemia in sheep and goats addressing underlying metabolic derangements, diagnostic methods, and preventive management strategies. An accompanying article in this issue will detail therapeutic intervention strategies for pregnancy toxemia.

DEFINING PREGNANCY TOXEMIA

Classically, pregnancy toxemia has been defined as a metabolic disease of energy deficiency often the result of reduced energy intake coupled with increased energy demand to support multiple fetuses in late gestation.[1,2,5] Often pregnancy toxemia is preceded or concurrent with hypocalcemia, which further exasperates energy deficiency through reduced intake.[1,4] Clinical signs most often are presented in the last 3 weeks of gestation but could occur earlier depending on maternal health and nutritional status. Any breed of sheep or goats can be affected by the disease. Boer goats were reported as having greater pregnancy toxemia susceptibility compared to other goat breeds in a veterinary hospital survey.[6] The syndrome is a consequence of combined mismanagement of animal, environment, and nutrition.[1,2,5]

Two maternal nutritional situations (very fat and very thin dams) occur commonly that lead to pregnancy toxemia. Due to differences in metabolism in the two scenarios, medical treatment and management approaches are not the same. Cases of pregnancy toxemia secondary to hepatic lipidosis tend to be sporadic and are associated more with pet goats, whereas starvation pregnancy toxemia can be a herd-wide problem.

- *Obesity-Related Pregnancy Toxemia*: Using a body condition scoring (BCS) scale from 1 (emaciated) to 5 (grossly obese),[7] ewes and does with BCS $\geq$ 4 are at greater risk for developing hepatic lipidosis, hypoglycemia, and ketosis most often related to reduced feed intake. Greater BCS is associated with reduced feed intake as well as having more available adipose tissue to be mobilized in the face of negative energy balance.[8]
- *Starvation Pregnancy Toxemia*: Occurs in ewes and does who did not receive adequate calories during pregnancy or became pregnant while under-conditioned, are carrying high multiples, or are geriatric. In these cases, hypocalcemia and hypoglycemia are the primary metabolic issues. These does can be adequately conditioned until the last month of pregnancy at which time, body condition drops dramatically and a rapid decline in health is observed. Starvation pregnancy toxemia usually occurs within 1 to 3 weeks of parturition and can be a cause of huge maternal death losses. Starvation pregnancy toxemia can be broken down into three stages (**Box 1**).

ETIOLOGY

The underpinning derangement of pregnancy toxemia is the loss of maternal glucose homeostatic control resulting in a state of negative energy balance characterized by hypoglycemia and adipose tissue mobilization.[9] The underlying pathogenesis of perturbed glucose homeostasis is not fully understood. Fetal growth is exponential with more than 70% occurring within the last 30 to 40 days of gestation accounting for greater glucose loss.[10,11] Elevation in nonesterified fatty acids (NEFA) from lipolysis in late gestation has been implicated in altering pancreatic insulin response and peripheral insulin resistance in the German black-headed mutton breed that is highly susceptible to pregnancy toxemia.[12] Neurologic consequences of clinical pregnancy toxemia may be related to reduced cerebral spinal fluid (CSF) glucose concentration

Box 1
Staging of starvation-induced pregnancy toxemia

Stage 1. The doe has a decreased appetite, swollen and painful distal extremities, and walks stiffly (**Fig. 1**). Timeline for when these clinical signs begin greatly determines case severity. Presenting with Stage 1 signs 3 to 4 weeks from estimated due date suggests this will likely become a severe case and the chances of a normal parturition are low unless medical intervention occurs. These does and ewes can be treated and isolated and will go on to normal parturition in some cases. If presenting within 2 weeks of expected parturition, then the chances of a normal birthing are likely with therapy.

Stage 2. Dam presents as anorexic and down but can stand for short periods with assistance, shows signs of polioencephalomalacia such as visual deficits possibly to the point of blindness, head pressing, and tremors (**Fig. 2**). These ewes or does tend to star-gaze also. At this stage, supportive care is necessary to save the dam and the pregnancy. With proper therapy these dams can be treated, and signs can be reversed. If the doe or ewe begins eating again, she can reverse the clinical signs and go on to birth normally. Ewes and does who do not begin eating must be supported until they give birth or have birthing induced.

Stage 3. Dam presents down, obtunded, and has labored breathing with very harsh lung sounds (**Fig. 3**). At this stage, the dam will have periods of 'somnolence' and fetuses are very close to death or already dead. The chance of saving the fetuses is essentially none, but the dam can be saved with a C-section. If finances are limited, some dams will survive the induction process, and many will be ready to birth in 24 hours. Supportive care with IV fluids is mandatory in these cases. Parturition induction may cause decompensation and the dam often goes into cardiac arrest when labor begins. A vaginal exam starting at 24 hours post-induction is usually indicated. If there is any cervical dilation, the cervix should be further dilated, and fetuses pulled. These dams will not deliver on their own and should be under close supervision during this time.

impacting brain function. Blood glucose concentration was highly correlated with CSF glucose concentration in ewes with pregnancy toxemia, undernourished and inappetent, and normal pregnant ewes.[13] Ewes affected by clinical pregnancy toxemia had significantly lower blood and CSF glucose concentrations compared to undernourished and healthy pregnant ewes suggesting hypoglycemic encephalopathy as an underlying pathology. Associated serum ß-hydroxybutyrate (BHB) concentrations were >30 mg/dL (3.0 mmol/L), 16 to 30 mg/dL (1.6–3.0 mmol/L), and < 7 mg/dL (0.7 mmol/L) for pregnancy toxic, undernourished, and normal ewes, respectively.[13] Recently, the role of a proinflammatory immune response has been related to pathogenesis of postpartum disease in dairy cattle.[14,15] Proinflammatory cytokines such as interleukin-1ß, tumor necrosis factor-α, and monocyte chemotactic protein-1 were

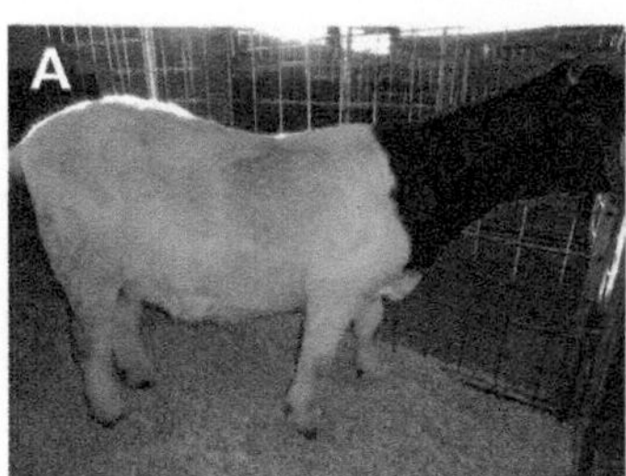

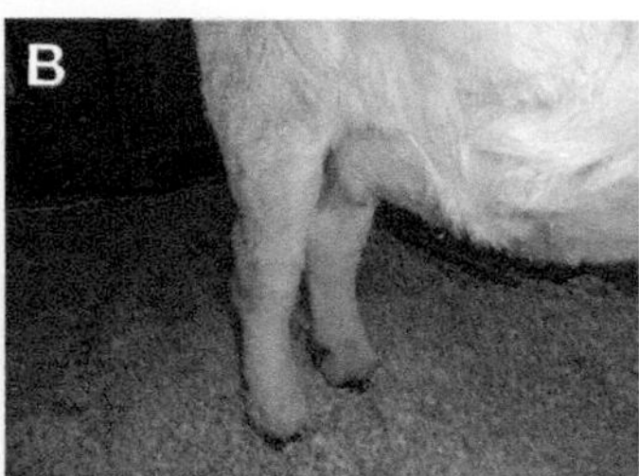

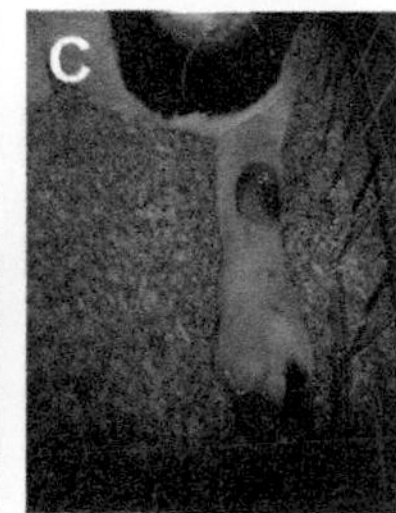

Fig. 1. Example of pregnant doe presenting in Stage 1 of pregnancy toxemia (*A*). Note the hind leg (*B*) and foreleg swelling (*C*) typically due to hypoproteinemia and hypoalbuminemia.

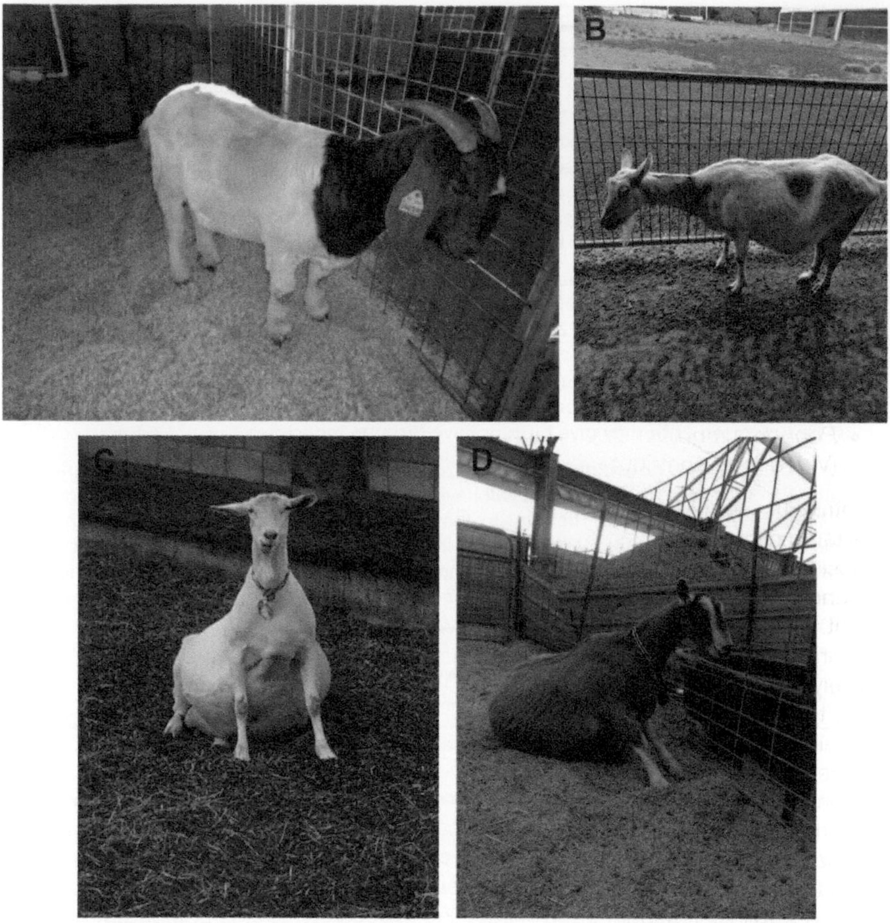

Fig. 2. Examples of pregnant does presenting in Stage 2 of pregnancy toxemia. Dams present as anorexic and may stand for limited times (*A, B*) or down (*C, D*).

found to be highly and moderately elevated in severe and mild pregnancy toxemic ewes compared to healthy pregnant ewes.[16] A proinflammatory immune response could redirect available nutrients in support of increased maintenance metabolism as well as inducing hypocalcemia and hypophagia.[14,15] Activated immune cells are

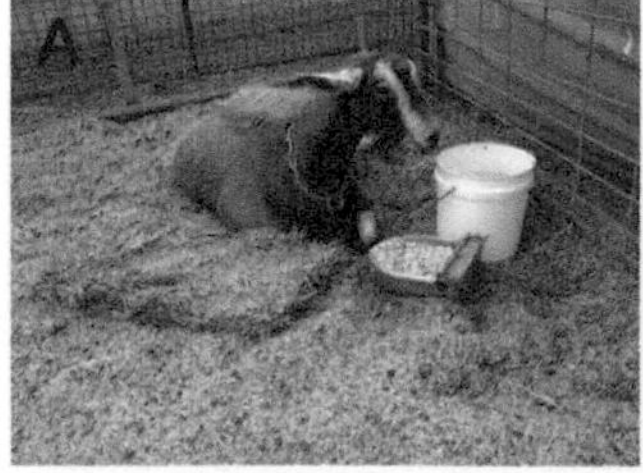

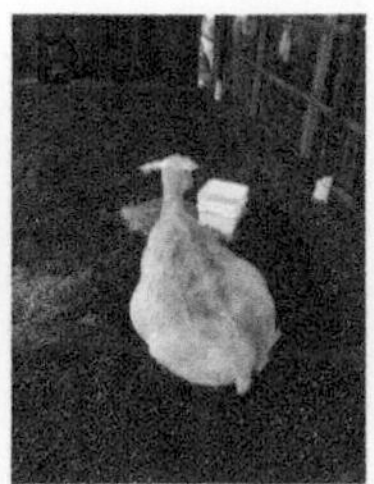

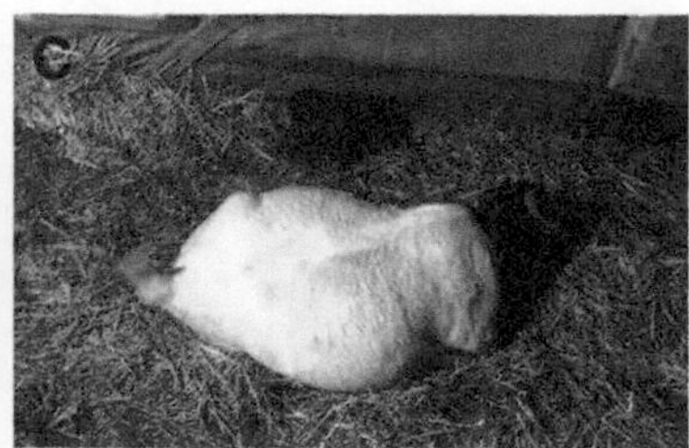

Fig. 3. Examples of pregnant does presenting in Stage 3 of pregnancy toxemia (*A–C*). Does are typically unable to rise, depressed, with labored breathing.

obligate consumers of glucose, and in the face of inflammation, are in a hypermetabolic state.[17]

Reasons for negative energy balance include the following.

- *Inadequate dietary caloric, protein, or both content.* Often due to inappropriate feed ingredients such as not providing a cereal grain or protein supplement to complement the forage or inadequate provision of sufficient feed.
- *Poor feed intake.* Result of providing poor quality, highly mature forages containing high neutral detergent fiber, limited bunk space, or inadequate feed amounts provided.
- *Hypocalcemia.* Primary form results from inadequate dietary calcium content or secondary to reduced feed intake.
- *Poor access to water.* Water consumption drives dry matter intake. Poorly maintained waterers, limited waterer space or numbers, and frozen waterers all will reduce intake.
- *Poor dam mobility.* Obesity, lameness due to various causes, and limb swelling (Video 1) all contribute to potential limited mobility of the pregnant ewe or doe.

Fetal glucose utilization is dependent upon maternal glucose availability given the facilitated diffusion across the placenta and inability of the fetus to perform gluconeogenesis.[18,19] In the face of maternal hypoglycemia, the fetus will become hypoglycemic and will shift metabolism to amino acid oxidation to make up the energy substrate deficit.[20] This situation may be reflected in the observation of increased urinary protein and uric acid in pregnancy toxic ewes.[16] In contrast to glucose, amino acids are actively transported across the placenta.[21] When confronted with nutritional limitations, the pregnant dam will mobilize labile body protein to support gluconeogenesis as well as amino acid supply to the conceptus.[22] As ketogenesis is resultant of reduced glucose and insulin status, hyperketonemia will suppress gluconeogenesis initiating a vicious cycle promoting lower blood glucose entry and exacerbating negative energy balance.[23] Fortunately, hyperketonemia also seems to reduce NEFA release from adipose, thus slowing ketogenesis.[24] Ewes presenting with more severe pregnancy toxemia leading to death had higher BHB and cortisol concentrations coupled with lower insulin concentration, all factors promoting excessive lipid mobilization and ketone production.[25] Ketones cannot be utilized for energy by the fetoplacental unit but most maternal tissues can oxidize ketones for energy.[21] Ewes with multiple fetuses in a state of hyperketonemia seemingly have a greater reduction in ketone body utilization by peripheral tissues compared to those with a single fetus, which may be a key component to pregnancy toxemia pathogenesis.[24] Multiparous does showed greater elevations in NEFA, BHB, and blood urea nitrogen concentrations in late pregnancy compared to primiparous does substantiating the greater risk of pregnancy toxemia in older dams.[26] Further research is needed to better understand the underlying metabolic pathogenesis of pregnancy toxemia and why the affected animal is often refractory to therapeutic interventions of glucose administration.

Diagnostic Methods

A preliminary diagnosis of pregnancy toxemia can be made based on presentation and a history of the ewe or doe being in late pregnancy with signs of decreased appetite or inappetence, poor mobility or non-ambulatory, and overall depressed demeanor. Confirmation of clinical pregnancy toxemia is based on identifying hypoglycemia, hyperketonemia, and ketonuria.[1,2,5] Similar to lactational ketosis in dairy cows, a subclinical state of pregnancy toxemia has been suggested based on slightly lower blood BHB concentrations (>0.86 mmol/L [8.6 mg/dL]).[27,28]

Physical examination

The common perception of the classic pregnancy toxemic ewe or doe is the obese dam in late pregnancy with multiple fetuses, an extrapolation from "fat cow syndrome" recognized with dairy cattle.[29] More often, the ewe or doe presents in poor body condition resultant of inadequate dietary supplementation. On physical examination, does or ewes will all show some degree of the following clinical signs. A combination of clinical signs and their severity will allow the practitioner to consider individual case prognosis.

1. *Decreased mobility or difficulty rising.* These animals will progress to being unable to rise as the case advances. Oftentimes, producers will comment the doe or ewe must rock back and forth before rising. Many cases will present with painful lower limbs on palpation with swelling in the pastern region as severity increases.
2. *Inappetence or decreased appetite.* In early stages of pregnancy toxemia, does or ewes will be noted to eat but for shorter periods. Inappetence progresses to complete anorexia in later disease stages. Anorexia can be attributed to multiple factors including difficulty or pain related to standing for periods, decreased rumen volume due to large uterine mass, and metabolic changes such as ketosis, which collectively suppress feed intake.
3. *Depression.* Does and ewes with pregnancy toxemia all exhibit some degree of depression. Owners will often notice behavioral changes first if not observant of feeding behavior or individual animals. Unfriendly does or ewes who become gentle in late-stage pregnancy should be examined or considered as potential pregnancy toxemia cases. With progression of the disease, a stuporous and eventually coma-like stage will develop. These cases are generally terminal, and in-utero fetal death is likely to have already occurred. Evaluation of fetal viability should be performed via trans-abdominal ultrasound in all advanced stages of pregnancy toxemia. Mild and moderate cases often can produce healthy full-term kids and lambs with appropriate interventions.

Clinical chemistry testing

The primary confirmatory diagnostic test for pregnancy toxemia is the presence of hyperketonemia as measured by elevated blood BHB concentration (>3 mmol/L [>30 mg/dL]) or moderate to heavy urinary ketone presence using nitroprusside-based urine dipstick testing for acetoacetate. Clinical signs of pregnancy toxemia may be associated with blood BHB concentrations > 1.6 mmol/L (16 mg/dL).[2] Blood BHB concentrations > 0.86 mmol/L (8.6 mg/dL) have been suggested to indicate a mild to moderate form of pregnancy toxemia that is often termed subclinical pregnancy toxemia.[27,28] This perspective is consistent with descriptions of subclinical and clinical lactational ketosis in dairy cattle and recognizes a progression in metabolic alterations leading to disease clinical signs rather than a dichotomous disease process. Hypoglycemia is the underpinning metabolic derangement in either subclinical or clinical pregnancy toxemia.[1,2,5,27,30] Hyperglycemia was reported to be common in pregnancy toxemic does.[6] Presence of hyperglycemia may represent a later stage of the disease process and reflect fetal viability.[31]

Historically, blood BHB concentration was determined by submitting a blood sample to a diagnostic laboratory for analysis resulting in a time delay for diagnostics. Hand-held glucometers used in monitoring human glucose have been validated for measuring whole blood BHB and glucose concentrations in sheep and goats.[32–35] Pichler and colleagues determined whole blood BHB concentrations>1.1 mmol/L (11 mg/dL) were significantly associated with greater risk for hyperketonemia in ewes.[36] Doré and colleagues determined whole blood BHB concentrations between

$\geq$ 0.4 mmol/L (4.0 mg/dL) and $\geq$ 0.9 mmol/L (9.0 mg/dL) during the final 5 weeks of gestation placed does at greater risk for pregnancy toxemia.[3] Whole blood BHB concentrations between $\geq$ 0.6 mmol/L (6 mg/dL) and $\geq$ 1.4 mmol/L (14 mg/dL) during the last 4 weeks of gestation were at greater risk for mortality.[3]

Other consistent blood metabolite changes associated with pregnancy toxemia include hypokalemia, hypoproteinemia, hypoalbuminemia, and indicators of metabolic acidosis (eg, reduced bicarbonate, base excess, and total carbon dioxide).[2,5,27,30] Reduced intake can be reflected in presence of hypokalemia, hypocalcemia, hypoazotemia (low urea nitrogen), and hypocholesteremia. With advancing disease severity comes a state of dehydration resulting in hyperazotemia and elevated creatinine. Serum creatine kinase and aspartate aminotransferase (AST) may be elevated due to muscle breakdown or damage from prolonged recumbency. Liver enzymes may be elevated with concurrent hepatic lipidosis. **Table 1** compares clinical chemistry profiles from two ewes showing these differences in early versus late-stage pregnancy toxemia.[4]

Nutritional management evaluation

Once a diagnosis has been made, it will be important to determine the underlying cause of negative energy balance, which will involve assessment of the feeding program. Collection of information related to all feeds and supplements being fed and feed amounts should be obtained. Accurate assessment of the actual number of does or ewes in the group and actual observation of feed delivery is critical. Proper evaluation of the diet requires both an understanding of the ingredients fed, and an accurate assessment of the actual feed amount presented to the doe or ewe.

Forages should be sampled appropriately and submitted to a feed analysis laboratory for nutritional analysis. Representative forage samples are best collected using a coring probe device. The American Forage Testing Association (www.foragetesting.org) provides information on hay sampling probes as well as certified laboratories by geographic region. Grain mixes and mineral supplements should have a basic nutrient analysis (ie, guaranteed analysis) on the associated feed tag that can provide

Table 1
Clinical chemistry values for late pregnant ewes with early (ewe 1) and late-stage (ewe 2) pregnancy toxemia

Parameter	Ewe 1	Ewe 2	Reference Range	Parameter	Ewe 1	Ewe 2	Reference Range
BUN	8	48	10–35 mg/dL	Sodium	149	146	145–155 mEq/L
Creatinine	0.7	3.7	0.9–2 mg/dL	Potassium	4.0	3.9	4.5–6.0 mEq/L
Glucose	24	17	50–85 mg/dL	Calcium	7.2	7.0	8.5–12 mg/dL
Total protein	6.6	6.1	5.5–7.5 g/dL	Phosphorus	6.7	6.6	5–7.5 mg/dL
Bilirubin, total	0.4	0.3	0–0.5 mg/dL	Magnesium	2.2	2.4	2.2–2.8 mg/dL
Creatine kinase (CK)	357	1,824	50–150 U/L	Triglycerides	27	13	< 100 mg/dL
Alkaline phosphatase	74	24	10–70 U/L	Cholesterol	59	38	> 70 mg/dL
GGT	39	45	30–94 IU/L	BHB	11.0	25.0	< 8.5 mg/dL
AST (SGOT)	84	1,243	60–280 IU/L	NEFA	1.43	0.29	< 0.4 mmol/L

Abbreviations: BHB, β-hydroxybutyrate; BUN, blood urea nitrogen; GGT, gamma-glutamyltransferase; NEFA, nonesterified fatty acids.

some information, though sending a representative sample to the forage lab would be appropriate. The guaranteed analysis is provided on an "as fed" basis, though this should not be a significant issue given the low moisture content of these feed sources. Guaranteed analysis values are presented as either "maximum", "minimum", or both depending upon the nutrient and state feed labeling regulations. This means the feed may have less or more than what is stated in the analysis. Review of the ingredient listing from the feed label will be useful in appreciating the potential for additional nutrient content relative to the analysis. Ingredients are required to be listed from highest to lowest incorporation rate based on as-fed composition.

Case Management Considerations

When pregnancy toxemia occurs in a fat ewe or doe, the remaining pregnant animals should be sorted according to BCS and stage of gestation. Any ewes or does who are borderline risk cases should be moved into pens where feed and water intake can be closely monitored. Ideally, a thorough evaluation of all diet ingredients with wet chemistry analysis should be performed with a nutrient analysis to create a balanced diet for the does or ewes based on breed, age, average body weight, and production class. In small farm or individual animal settings, this is often not achievable, and these general recommendations can be used for adult, full-sized goats and sheep. Does should be fed 1 to 1.5 lb of grain per day along with 4 to 5 pounds of alfalfa hay. If alfalfa hay is not available, highly palatable grass hay can be substituted, but grain supplementation will need to be increased to 1.5 to 2 lb to compensate for the lower energy density in the grass hay. It is critical that does and ewes in the last month of gestation be allowed free choice access to high-quality roughage. The goal should be 5% to 10% orts (ie, refused feed). Limit feeding close-up does and ewes will cause pregnancy toxemia in the animals within the group who are carrying larger litters or are less mobile. In settings where grain feeding is difficult, feeding molasses lick tubs can provide a glucose source, especially in grazing setting with non-dairy breed goats. It is preferable to use multiple tubs in groups as guarding can occur and subordinate does or ewes will not have access to the supplement. The mineral formulation in the tub should be evaluated as most tubs are made for cattle and sheep cannot handle the added copper in the mineral mixes commonly added to these tubs.

Herds and flocks with subclinical pregnancy toxemia often present to veterinarians as a situation where does and ewes are freshening without udder development or with inadequate colostrum production. The owner should be advised to be on close watch for signs of labor in the absence of any udder development. Frozen colostrum or colostrum replacer should be on hand in these situations. Although some does and ewes will recover after parturition and begin lactating, it is not uncommon for some cases to fail to lactate. This appears to be linked to both the severity of the pregnancy toxemia and the length of time during the pregnancy that the animal was affected.

Removal of environmental stressors is another factor in managing pregnancy toxemia. Goats are very social animals and social stress is a major factor in metabolic and infectious diseases. Important areas to consider and evaluate are feed bunk space and spatial layout. Feeders should be arranged so that all does and ewes can eat without being bullied. Dominant does will guard and protect feeders from subordinates. Goats with horns can cause serious trauma and injury to heavily pregnant female goats. Housing bucks with pregnant does is also not advised. Many bucks will take advantage of less mobile, heavily pregnant does, and continually try to breed them. This can lead to both injury and reluctance to eat at the manger where they are more likely to be harassed. Avoiding all types of stress is an extremely important part of preventing periparturient diseases in sheep and goats.

Observing sheep and goats at feeding time can help producers find bottlenecks in a feeder layout and is a very important step in the management of close-up does and ewes for prevention of pregnancy toxemia. If does or ewes eat along a manger, make sure that all animals can eat at the same time. The same evaluation should be done for shelter and water troughs. Shelters should be open enough that a dominant doe cannot block the doorway. If small 'hut' type shelters are used, then enough should be available that all does or ewes can access them in inclement weather. Regarding water troughs, multiple water troughs should always be available unless the trough is away from a fence line and there are only a few does in the pen. In cold climates, heated water troughs are very beneficial to maintaining pregnant doe and ewe health. Avoiding all types of stress is an extremely important part of preventing periparturient diseases in sheep and goats.

Preventive Management Considerations

In certain cases, does or ewes are highly likely to repeat a pregnancy toxemia event the following year or pregnancy. There are three main categories for repeat offenders: Older or geriatric does and ewes, structurally unsound does and ewes, and does or ewes with high total fetal kid weight. Old does and ewes who have arthritis, often related to caprine arthritis encephalitis virus (CAEV) infection, or broken down ligaments will struggle more with consecutive pregnancies. They are less competitive at the feed rack and do not graze as well. "Percentage" Boer does carry Nubian genetics, Dorpers and Katahdins have genetics for high milk production. If these does do not go into late pregnancy with adequate body condition, even a slight negative energy balance in the diet will start the process of starvation pregnancy toxemia. Does and ewes who are predisposed to this type of pregnancy toxemia are much worse in the following years. Finally, does who tend to carry high multiples (triplets and above) and have a high total fetal kid weight are predisposed to pregnancy toxemia. The high-energy demand along with a large uterus, which severely minimizes rumen volume, is the perfect combination for this syndrome.[8,37] Ultrasound pregnancy examinations are critical in these does or ewes to count fetuses and better prepare the client. Exams should be performed between 35 and 60 days for optimal fetal visualization and counting.

Proper ration balancing and body condition maintenance can prevent future problems in herds with widespread pregnancy toxemia secondary to inadequate nutrition. In these herds, the ration energy should be raised for the last 4 weeks of gestation. Does and ewes should be sorted on BCS into two groups. On a scale of 1 to 5, all does and ewes three or more months pregnant should be separated at a cut-off of <2.75 or >3. Thinner does and ewes require extra nutrition supplementation for adequate fetal and udder development. It is very important that clients be advised not to restrict calories or 'diet' does or ewes in the last 2 months of gestation. If breeding dates with ultrasound confirmation have not been performed in the herd or flock, then no dietary restrictions should occur at any time during the gestation. Over conditioned does and ewes are much easier to manage than under-conditioned ones. With adequate nutrition and avoidance of a negative energy balance, fat does and ewes can gestate with minimal issues. In addition, first-time kidders and lambers should not be grouped with mature does or ewes regardless of body weight, frame size, or body condition.

Preventive Nutritional Practices

Described issues of increasing fetal nutrient demand associated with rapid fetal growth in late gestation (**Fig. 4**) require appropriate modifications in the feeding

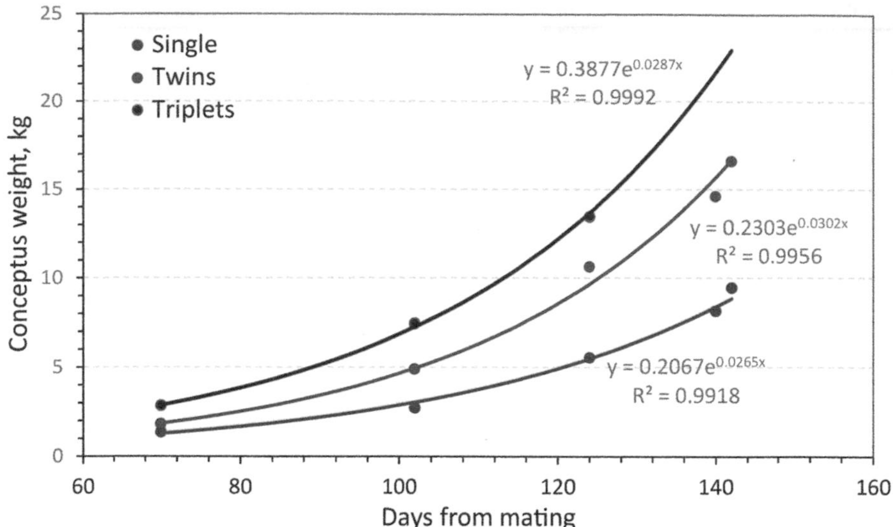

Fig. 4. Modeled growth of the ovine conceptus (ie, fetus, membranes, fluids) based on gestational age and number of fetuses. (Models based on data from Rattray and colleagues, 1974.[11])

program that complement maternal metabolic alterations to adequately support late gestation and minimize pregnancy toxemia risk. In dairy cattle, four critical control points have been identified relative to preventing periparturient problems,[38] of which (1) minimizing dry matter intake decline; (2) minimizing negative energy and protein balance; and (3) maintaining calcium homeostasis would be appropriate nutrition issues to address relative to pregnancy toxemia prevention.

Optimizing dry matter intake

Dietary recommendations for energy, crude protein, calcium, and phosphorus for the late gestation ewe or doe are 1.5 to 2.0 times greater compared to early gestation with an even larger increase to support lactation.[39] Of concern in reviewing dietary nutrient intakes recommended by NRC publications, one notices an expectation for dry matter intake to increase throughout these transitions. This is a point of concern in late pregnancy where physical fill limitation and other metabolic or endocrine factors may decrease intake capacity, thus resulting in greater potential for pregnancy toxemia and hypocalcemia metabolic problems.[37]

The neutral detergent fiber (NDF) content of forages or total diet has been shown to be a primary mediator of intake in dairy cattle. Research in cattle and sheep has shown an optimal limit of NDF intake as 1.2% of body weight. Other work has shown a lesser ability of pregnant cows to consume NDF. Expected NDF intakes for pregnant cows range from 0.8% of body weight at the end of pregnancy up to approximately 1.0% of body weight during the early dry period. Younger animals (first parity) have lower NDF capacity (0.1–0.2 units lower) compared to mature animals. Other issues such as forage quality and environmental factors will further influence intake capacity. As forage (or total dietary) NDF increases, maximal intake capacity is reduced. For example, if forage (or total diet) NDF is 50% and NDF intake capacity is 1% of body weight, then the animal could consume 2% of body weight (eg, 1/0.5 = 2.0) as forage or total diet. If NDF intake capacity is reduced to 0.8% of body weight, then intake would be only 1.6% of body weight (eg, 0.8/0.5 = 1.6) for this same NDF level. The reason NDF is a convenient measure of forage quality is because NDF levels in any forage increase with increasing maturity of the plant. A coarse stemmy grass hay will have a higher NDF than a younger, less mature plant. When selecting forages for close-up does and ewes, choosing the finer-stemmed, less mature hay will allow for greater intake of the roughage, better energy utilization, and more optimal rumen health.

Limitation of intake by NDF physical fill can be applied to other ruminant species, including small ruminants. However, selective feeding behaviors typical of goats may overcome dietary limitations from NDF content. This is assuming the animal is capable of separating digestible feed components from fibrous components. Legume forages facilitate this process as the stems are separate from the leaves; however, grass forages do not have this distinction. Data from the literature suggest sheep have similar NDF capacities during pregnancy as cattle.[40,41]

In the McNeil study, twin pregnant ewes were fed isocaloric diets with differing protein content (8%, 11%, and 15% crude protein).[22] Diets contained similar NDF content ranging from 39.3% to 42.9%. Calculated NDF intake as a percent of body weight was 0.71, 0.78, and 0.89 for 8%, 11% and 15% crude protein diets, respectively. These diets were fed between 110 and 140 days of gestation and are consistent with the observed lower NDF intake capacity of late pregnant cows. Of interest is the dietary protein effect, which may be the result of improved fiber digestibility with increasing dietary protein. Another study monitoring intake with silage-based diets calculated NDF intake as a percent of body weight decreased with the increasing week of gestation and fetal numbers (**Table 2**).[41] Neutral detergent fiber intake was below 0.8% of body weight in late pregnancy similar to what is observed in dairy cattle. In this same study, forage quality effects on NDF intake at different weeks of gestation and

Table 2
Calculated neutral detergent fiber intake as a percent of body weight in ewes fed differing quality silages over weeks of gestation and pregnancy status

	NDF Intake as % of Body Weight		
Pregnancy Week[a]	Singles	Twins	Triplets
15	0.83	0.81	0.74
16	0.81	0.73	0.71
17	0.81	0.65	0.68
18	0.74	0.65	0.64
19	0.69	0.62	0.59
20	0.70	0.60	0.55
Mean	0.76	0.68	0.65

		NDF Intake as %BW		
Forage NDF%	Week	Singles	Twins	Triplets
48.5	15–17	0.82	0.74	0.71
63.8	15–17	0.78	0.70	0.70
44.9	18–20	0.83	0.70	0.70
48.5	18–20	0.71	0.62	0.59

[a] Silage (48.5% NDF) fed at 25% of dietary dry matter.

From Orr R, Newton J, Jackson CA. The intake and performance of ewes offered concentrates and grass silage in late pregnancy. Animal Science 1983;36:21-27.

pregnancy status were evaluated and showed higher fetal numbers and later gestational status resulted in lower NDF intake capacity.[41]

Based on NRC recommendations, a late pregnant ewe (154 lb body weight) with twins should consume 4.0 lb dry matter (2.6% of body weight).[39] Using an NDF intake capacity of 0.7% of body weight, maximal dietary NDF content would be 27% (0.7/2.6*100). Extending this example further, if one assumes a 65% forage ration suggested by NRC, this suggests forage NDF could not exceed 41%. Forage quality may be the most limiting factor in maintaining transition intake for small ruminants. To maintain high intake potential, late pregnant animals should receive higher quality forages (<40% NDF), have feed available at least 21 hour/day, and should be managed to minimize excess body condition. Based on an author's (AM) experience, close-up dairy does and ewes consume 60% of the feed weight they will consume during lactation. During the last week before parturition, it appears this level drops closer to 50%.

Minimizing negative energy and protein balance

Nutrient balance is a function of dry matter intake and dietary nutrient composition. If dry matter intake declines in late gestation, appropriate modifications to nutrient density will be necessary to ensure adequate nutrient intake. Otherwise, the pregnant dam will experience negative energy balance, which could lead to rapid mobilization of fat reserves and body protein leading to hepatic lipidosis and pregnancy toxemia. Increasing grain amount in the diet (1.0–2.0 lb/d) can help compensate for low dietary energy availability, and more importantly, stimulate microbial growth and consequently microbial protein. In some situations, especially where diets are grass-based, grain supplement may approach 2.5 lb per day to mature does and ewes. It is very important to factor in the herd demographics and to consider what feed ingredients are regionally available.

Gestation diet protein content needs to be considered when one increases grain to accommodate intake. The authors, based on their experience in feeding sheep and goats, consider dietary protein to be a critical factor in preventing pregnancy toxemia. Severe or prolonged maternal inadequate protein feeding can result in intrauterine growth retardation of the fetus.[42] Feeding higher dietary protein content (~15% crude protein), which is above current recommendations for ewes with twins, has shown improved ewe and lamb performance, colostrum quality, and lamb growth via greater milk yield.[22,43–45] Feeding higher dietary protein to singleton-carrying ewes resulted in reduced colostrum yield and great lamb losses due to dystocia.[46] Limited studies have been performed in pregnant does. Using data from multiple goat feeding studies new equations were developed for goat nutrient requirements; however, pregnancy requirements were not addressed.[47] Sahlou and colleagues[48] determined a 9% crude protein diet was insufficient to meet the pregnant does needs and recommended 11% crude protein (9.8 g/kg $BW^{.75}$), which was 40% higher than the previous NRC recommendation; however, does fed the 14.5% crude protein diet performed as well and had better metabolic status relative to protein.[49]

If the diet cannot meet protein needs, due to reduced dry matter intake, inadequate protein content, or some combination, then the dam will mobilize body protein to meet fetal amino acid needs. Mobilization of maternal skeletal protein (termed "labile protein") can explain why birth weight is not dramatically affected within reasonable variation in maternal nutritional status, at the expense of maternal protein mass. Twin pregnant ewes needed to consume a 15% CP diet to provide required protein amount as a result of reduced intake and increase body protein.[22] Data defining protein needs of highly prolific ewes and does are limited, but suggest that higher litter size with

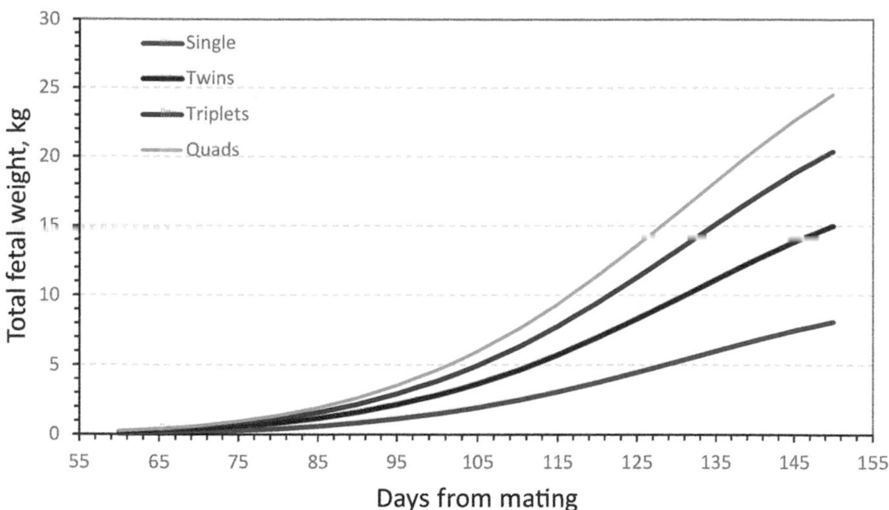

Fig. 5. Modeled growth of the ovine fetus based on gestational age and number of fetuses. (Models adapted from data presented by Koong and colleagues, 1975 and Rattray and colleagues, 1974 using Targhee x Suffolk ewes.[10,11] Predicted individual birth weights for single, twin, triplet, and quadruple lambs were 8.1, 7.5, 6.8, and 6.1 kg (18, 16.6, 15, and 13.5 lb).)

subsequent smaller rumen volume and dry matter intake would require a dietary protein content greater than 15%. **Fig. 5** shows modeled fetal growth in ewes with single, twin, triplet, and quadruplet lambs based on data from Rattray and colleagues where the fetus accounted for 70% of conceptus weight across fetal numbers between 1 and 3.[11] Other comparative slaughter data of ewes with one to five fetuses suggested a decline in fetal birth weight by 11% for every increase in fetal number.[50] As fetal numbers increase, there is greater reduction in intake capacity resulting from limited abdominal space.[37] Current NRC recommendations do not account for this greater fetal mass, intake reduction, and greater nutrient requirements for these prolific ewes who would be more susceptible to pregnancy toxemia.[39] Based on these issues, prolific ewes and does (≥3 fetuses) should be fed a minimum of 15% crude protein diets to meet increased needs and prevent pregnancy toxemia. Yearling ewes or does who are also pregnant have a higher protein requirement (suggest 16.5% in a close-up diet) to support both fetal growth and structural growth of the dam. Limiting protein to first-time fresheners will result in poor lactation performance, poor growth rates in kids and lambs, and structurally smaller mature body weights.

Maintaining calcium homeostasis

Ewes and does can experience prepartum hypocalcemia because of insufficient calcium intake to meet fetal calcium demands, often due to inappetence from some other disease process. A primary initiator of hypocalcemia in small ruminants is inadequate dietary calcium to meet needs for fetal bone development and inappropriate dietary calcium-to-phosphorus ratio. Excess phosphorus in the diet can inhibit dietary calcium uptake and potentially suppress parathormone activity that promotes vitamin D activation and increased efficiency of intestinal calcium absorption. Milk fever can be prevented by ensuring sufficient calcium and phosphorus are available in the diet, accounting for the observed level of intake. A common cause of hypocalcemia in close-up does and ewes is decreased feed intake. Similar to dairy heifers, first-freshening does and ewes do not develop hypocalcemia and seldom develop fulminant pregnancy toxemia. This may be related to the general tendency to produce small litters and have kids or lambs with smaller birth weights than mature dams.

CLINICS CARE POINTS

- Any late pregnant doe or ewe, irrespective of body condition, showing inappetence, separation behaviors, and appendage edema should be further evaluated for the potential of pregnancy toxemia
- Hand-held glucometers can be used to determine glucose and BHB concentrations to aid in pregnancy toxemia diagnostics where BHB concentration >0.85 mmol/L (8.5 mg/dL) would warrant further intervention
- Forage maturity, recognized as increased NDF content, is an important regulator of DMI. Forages exceeding 55% NDF should not be fed to late pregnant ewes or does and an NDF intake of 0.65% to 0.8% of live body weight is targeted for the late gestation diet.
- Essential nutrient content, especially energy and protein, need to be adjusted relative to intake rate. A minimum dietary crude protein of 12% and 65% total digestible nutrients is recommended for prevention.

DISCLOSURE

Grant funding received from the Pennsylvania Department of Agriculture, United States, American Dairy Goat Association, United States, Zoetis, United States.

SUPPLEMENTARY DATA

Supplementary data related to this article can be found online at https://doi.org/10.1016/j.cvfa.2023.02.010.

REFERENCES

1. Brozos C, Mavrogianni VS, Fthenakis GC. Treatment and control of peri-parturient metabolic diseases: pregnancy toxemia, hypocalcemia, hypomagnesemia. Vet Clin North Am Food Anim Pract 2011;27:105–13.
2. Rook JS. Pregnancy Toxemia of Ewes, Does, and Beef Cows. *Vet Clin North Am.* Food Animal Practice 2000;16:293–317.
3. Dore V, Dubuc J, Belanger AM, et al. Definition of prepartum hyperketonemia in dairy goats. J Dairy Sci 2015;98:4535–43.
4. Van Saun RJ. Pregnancy toxemia in a flock of sheep. *JAVMA* 2000;217:1536–9.
5. Cal-Pereyra L, Acosta-Dibarrat J, Benech A, et al. Toxemia de la gestación en ovejas: Revisión. Revista mexicana de ciencias pecuarias 2012;3:247–64.
6. Simpson KM, Taylor JD, Streeter RN. Evaluation of prognostic indicators for goats with pregnancy toxemia, *JAVMA* 2019;254:859–67.
7. Thompson J., Meyer H., Body condition scoring of sheep. Technical Report EC 1433, Oregon State University, Corvallis (OR): Oregon State University Extension Service, 1994, 4.
8. Forbes JM. The effect of pregnancy and fatness on the volume of rumen contents in the ewe. J Agric Sci 1969;72:119–21.
9. Fthenakis GC, Arsenos G, Brozos C, et al. Health management of ewes during pregnancy. Anim Reprod Sci 2012;130:198–212.

10. Koong LJ, Garrett WN, Rattray PV. A description of the dynamics of fetal growth in sheep. J Anim Sci 1875;41:1065–8.
11. Rattray PV, Garrett WN, East NE, et al. Growth, development and composition of the ovine conceptus and mammary gland during pregnancy. J Anim Sci 1974;38: 613–26.
12. Duehlmeier R, Noldt S, Ganter M. Pancreatic insulin release and peripheral insulin sensitivity in German black headed mutton and Finish Landrace ewes: evaluation of the role of insulin resistance in the susceptibility to ovine pregnancy toxemia. Domest Anim Endocrinol 2013;44:213–21.
13. Scott P, Sargison N, Penny C, et al. Cerebrospinal fluid and plasma glucose concentrations of ovine pregnancy toxaemia cases, inappetant ewes and normal ewes during late gestation. Br Vet J 1995;151:39–44.
14. Horst EA, Kvidera SK, Baumgard LH. Invited review: The influence of immune activation on transition cow health and performance-A critical evaluation of traditional dogmas. J Dairy Sci 2021;104:8380–410.
15. Bradford BJ, Swartz TH. Review: Following the smoke signals: inflammatory signaling in metabolic homeostasis and homeorhesis in dairy cattle. Animal 2020;14:s144–54.
16. Yarım G, Karahan S, Nisbet C. Elevated Plasma Levels of Interleukin 1β, Tumour Necrosis Factor α and Monocyte Chemotactic Protein 1 Are Associated with Pregnancy Toxaemia in Ewes. Vet Res Commun 2007;31:565–73.
17. Lochmiller RL, Deerenberg C. Trade-offs in evolutionary immunology: just what is the cost of immunity? Oikos 2000;88:87–98.
18. Bell AW, Ehrhardt RA. Regulation of placental nutrient transport and implications for fetal growth. Nutr Res Rev 2002;15:211–30.
19. Steinhoff-Wagner J, Gors S, Junghans P, et al. Maturation of endogenous glucose production in preterm and term calves. J Dairy Sci 2011;94:5111–23.
20. Faichney G, White G. Effects of maternal nutritional status on fetal and placental growth and on fetal urea synthesis in sheep. Aust J Biol Sci 1987;40:365–78.
21. Battaglia F, Meschia G. Principal substrates of fetal metabolism. Physiol Rev 1978;58:499–527.
22. McNeill D, Slepetis R, Ehrhardt R, et al. Protein requirements of sheep in late pregnancy: partitioning of nitrogen between gravid uterus and maternal tissues. J Anim Sci 1997;75:809–16.
23. Schlumbohm C, Harmeyer J. Hyperketonemia impairs glucose metabolism in pregnant and nonpregnant ewes. J Dairy Sci 2004;87:350–8.
24. Harmeyer J, Schlumbohm C. Pregnancy impairs ketone body disposal in late gestating ewes: Implications for onset of pregnancy toxaemia. Res Vet Sci 2006;81:254–64.
25. Henze P, Bickhardt K, Fuhrmann H, et al. Spontaneous pregnancy toxaemia (ketosis) in sheep and the role of insulin. Zentralbl Veterinarmed A 1998;45: 255–66.
26. Zamuner F, DiGiacomo K, Cameron AWN, et al. Endocrine and metabolic status of commercial dairy goats during the transition period. J Dairy Sci 2020;103: 5616–28.
27. Ismail ZA, Al-Majali AM, Amireh F, et al. Metabolic profiles in goat does in late pregnancy with and without subclinical pregnancy toxemia. Vet Clin Pathol 2008;37:434–7.
28. Lacetera N, Bernabucci U, Ronchi B, et al. Effects of subclinical pregnancy toxemia on immune responses in sheep. Am J Vet Res 2001;62:1020–4.
29. Morrow DA. Fat cow syndrome. J Dairy Sci 1976;59:1625–9.

30. Lima MS, Pascoal RA, Stilwell GT, et al. Clinical findings, blood chemistry values, and epidemiologic data from dairy goats with pregnancy toxemia. Bov Pract 2012;46:102–10.
31. Lima MS, Pascoal RA, Stilwell GT. Glycaemia as a sign of the viability of the foetuses in the last days of gestation in dairy goats with pregnancy toxaemia. Ir Vet J 2012;65:1.
32. Dore V, Dubuc J, Belanger AM, et al. Short communication: evaluation of the accuracy of an electronic on-farm test to quantify blood beta-hydroxybutyrate concentration in dairy goats. J Dairy Sci 2013;96:4505–7.
33. Pichler M, Damberger A, Arnholdt T, et al. Evaluation of 2 electronic handheld devices for diagnosis of ketonemia and glycemia in dairy goats. J Dairy Sci 2014;97: 7538–46.
34. Katsoulos PD, Minas A, Karatzia MA, et al. Evaluation of a portable glucose meter for use in cattle and sheep. Vet Clin Pathol 2011;40:245–7.
35. Panousis N, Brozos C, Karagiannis I, et al. Evaluation of Precision Xceed(R) meter for on-site monitoring of blood beta-hydroxybutyric acid and glucose concentrations in dairy sheep. Res Vet Sci 2012;93:435–9.
36. Pichler M, Damberger A, Schwendenwein I, et al. Thresholds of whole-blood beta-hydroxybutyrate and glucose concentrations measured with an electronic hand-held device to identify ovine hyperketonemia. J Dairy Sci 2014;97:1388–99.
37. Forbes JM. The physical relationships of the abdominal organs in the pregnant ewe. J Agric Sci 1968;70:171–7.
38. Goff J, Horst R. Physiological changes at parturition and their relationship to metabolic disorders. J Dairy Sci 1997;80:1260–8.
39. Council NR. Nutrient requirements of small ruminants: sheep, goats, cervids, and new world camelids. Washington, DC: The National Academies Press; 2007.
40. Newton J, Orr R. The intake of silage and grazed herbage by Masham ewes with single or twin lambs and its repeatability during pregnancy, lactation and after weaning. Anim Sci 1981;33:121–7.
41. Orr R, Newton J, Jackson CA. The intake and performance of ewes offered concentrates and grass silage in late pregnancy. Anim Sci 1983;36:21–7.
42. Mellor D, Matheson I. Daily changes in the curved crown-rump length of individual sheep fetuses during the last 60 days of pregnancy and effects of different levels of maternal nutrition. Q J Exp Physiol Cogn Med Sci: Translation and Integration 1979;64:119–31.
43. Ahmed MH, Salem AZM, Olafadehan OA, et al. Effect of pre- and post-partum dietary crude protein level on the performance of ewes and their lambs. Small Rumin Res 2016;136:221–6.
44. Dawson L, Carson A, Kilpatrick D. The effect of the digestible undegradable protein concentration of concentrates and protein source offered to ewes in late pregnancy on colostrum production and lamb performance. Anim Feed Sci Technol 1999;82:21–36.
45. Hashemi M, Zamiri MJ, Safdarian M. Effects of nutritional level during late pregnancy on colostral production and blood immunoglobulin levels of Karakul ewes and their lambs. Small Rumin Res 2008;75:204–9.
46. Ocak N, Cam MA, Kuran M. The effect of high dietary protein levels during late gestation on colostrum yield and lamb survival rate in singleton-bearing ewes. Small Rumin Res 2005;56:89–94.
47. Sahlu T, Goetsch AL, Luo J, et al. Nutrient requirements of goats: developed equations, other considerations and future research to improve them. Small Rumin Res 2004;53:191–219.

48. Sahlu T, Fernandez JM, Lu CD, et al. Influence of dietary protein on performance of dairy goats during pregnancy. J Dairy Science 1992;75:220–7.
49. National Research Council. Nutrient requirements of goats: angora, dairy, and meat goats in temperate and tropical countries. National Academies Press: Washington, DC; 1981.
50. Robinson J, McDonald I, Fraser C, et al. Studies on reproduction in prolific ewes: I. Growth of the products of conception. J Agric Sci 1977;88:539–52.

Pregnancy Toxemia Therapeutic Options

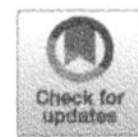

Jenna E. Bayne, DVM, PhD, DACVIM-LA

KEYWORDS

- Pregnancy toxemia • Therapy • Propylene glycol • Dextrose infusion • Insulin
- Induction • C-section

KEY POINTS

- Stabilization and correction of metabolic and electrolyte derangements is critical.
- Treatment goals need to reflect producer priorities of survival of dam or offspring.
- Current knowledge of prognostic indicators to guide evidence-based decisions is limited.
- Survival of dams and offspring is highly variable, but intensive care can achieve successful outcomes.

CASE DEFINITION

Pregnancy toxemia (PT) is a life-threatening metabolic disease of late gestation sheep and goats carrying multiple fetuses. Dysregulation of intermediary energy metabolism and failure of homeostasis results in the worsening of a negative energy balance and clinical disease. Untreated cases almost always result in death.[1] Clinical signs of PT and stages of disease progression depression, anorexia, increased respiratory rate, reduced to absent rumen motility, weakness, and incoordination leading to recumbency are described in detail elsewhere in this issue. Neurologic signs may include impaired vision, reduced pupillary light responses, stargazing, opisthotonos, and convulsions. Other signs may include teeth grinding, clamping of the jaw, abnormal vocalization, and edema of the limbs.[1–4] Limb edema has been observed in PT cases with and without albumin abnormalities and the pathogenesis is unknown.[5,6] The development of neurologic signs is thought to be a negative prognostic indicator[1] though reports of the association between neurologic manifestations and prognosis are inconsistent.[5–8] Progression to recumbency has also been associated with a poor prognosis[2,5,8] but was not negatively associated with survival in one report.[6] The course of the disease is only a few to several days, with death occurring within a week in most untreated cases.[2] Spontaneous recovery in untreated cases is rare, with a case fatality rate exceeding 80% in untreated cases.[5,9]

Department of Clinical Sciences, Auburn University College of Veterinary Medicine, 1500 Wire Road, Auburn, AL, USA
E-mail address: jeb0036@auburn.edu

Vet Clin Food Anim 39 (2023) 293–305
https://doi.org/10.1016/j.cvfa.2023.02.003
vetfood.theclinics.com
0749-0720/23/

Evaluation and Additional Testing

Many therapies have been attempted to treat PT. Failure to identify underlying pathophysiologic conditions, including dehydration, renal and liver dysfunction, and acid-base and electrolyte derangements, may contribute to variable and erratic responses to therapy and often lead to high case fatality rates.[2] To identify underlying imbalances, the minimal clinicopathological dataset should include a thorough physical examination, packed cell volume, total solids, blood glucose concentration, a serum biochemistry panel, and a complete blood cell count.[2] Validated point-of-care (POC) meters to determine blood glucose and beta-hydroxybutyrate concentrations aid in the establishment of a diagnosis of PT and provide the ability to serially monitor these parameters to assess response to therapy.[10,11] Transabdominal ultrasound can provide information on the fetal number and fetal viability. Estimating of degree of fetal maturation would be useful to guide the timing of parturition induction or C-section but has proven difficult.[12,13] Improved treatment recommendations and survival of PT cases will require well-designed, randomized control trials to determine if certain biochemical indices are of prognostic value.

Given the pathophysiology of PT, hyperketonemia and ketonuria are expectant findings. The degree of ketonemia varies considerably, with plasma concentrations of beta-hydroxybutyrate above 3 mmol/L in most clinical cases.[2] Although it would be expected that increased ketone concentrations would accompany worsening disease states, this relationship is inconsistent and not predictive of treatment response or survival.[6,14] Ketone bodies (beta-hydroxybutyrate and acetoacetate) are strong acids, and accumulation in the blood contributes to metabolic acidosis (ketoacidosis) observed in PT.[15] Mild to severe decreases in pH, HCO3-, and base excess are frequently present in both experimental and naturally occurring cases.[5,6,16] The contribution of L-lactate in acid-base derangements in PT has not been extensively evaluated but it was found to be increased in approximately 50% of small ruminant PT cases.[17] In dairy goats with PT, the probability of survival decreased with decreasing pH and HCO3 concentration.[5,8] In meat goats with PT, death was significantly more likely in does with severely low bicarbonate concentrations.[6] The condition of the patient can deteriorate quickly with rapid decreases in pH.[5,8] Lima and colleagues also indicate that blood pH is a useful prognostic indicator and should be used to direct therapy decisions concerning induction of parturition versus immediate C-section delivery.[8] However, the study design precludes drawing these conclusions, given pH determined treatment allocation (ie, all does with pH <7.15 underwent C-section) rather than a determined correlate of the outcome. Plausibly, a worse prognosis is to be expected in cases more profoundly acidotic and perhaps, as suggested by Lima and colleagues, a point of no return exists in severe cases.[5]

Hydration status will reflect ongoing acid-base and electrolyte derangements, and dehydration may be severe with evidence of shock. Recognizing renal impairment is crucial prognostically as well as in developing a treatment plan that avoids potentially nephrotoxic medications. Increases in blood urea nitrogen and decreases in serum potassium concentration may be poor prognostic indicators.[5,6] Depending on the degree of dehydration and electrolyte imbalances, resuscitative efforts may require oral or intravenous (IV) isotonic fluids or a combination.

The development of PT in late gestation is intricately linked to energy metabolism and glucose utilization. In early literature, low blood glucose was purported to be a consistent feature of the condition,[1,18] but glucose concentrations can vary, and the onset of clinical signs does not necessarily correlate well with deviations in glucose concentrations.[6,14,19,20] In the late stages of the disease, hyperglycemia has often been thought to signal fetal demise.[1] In contrast, Simpson and colleagues[6] reported that 90% of PT does as either normoglycemic or hyperglycemic at admission, and the presence of hyperglycemia was not predictive of fetal death, but rather these kids had an increased survival rate. Souto and colleagues[20] suggest that survival rates are higher in hypoglycemic dams and that the unnecessary administration of parenteral glucose can lead to hyperglycemic shock and death.

Individual and breed-dependent predisposition to insulin resistance should be considered especially in cases where normoglycemia or hyperglycemia are present. The possibility of low endogenous insulin concentrations may impact treatment responses in other cases.[9] Glucose intolerance has been shown in obese dairy goats with naturally occurring PT,[14] and PT-susceptible breeds of sheep show alterations in insulin secretion and altered peripheral ketone utilization.[21–23] In cases where blood glucose is demonstrably low, particularly when showing clinical signs of hypoglycemic encephalopathy, glucose treatment should be administered during initial resuscitative efforts. A bolus of 0.5 to 1 mL per kg body weight of 50% dextrose (0.25 to 0.5 g/kg) can be administered intravenously over several minutes.[24]

An estimated 20% of PT cases have concurrent clinical hypocalcemia.[19] In late gestation there is an increasing demand for calcium due to fetal skeletal development and most small ruminants are in a negative calcium balance during late gestation.[25] Approximately 50% of pregnant ewes have total calcium concentrations below 2.1 mmol/L in late gestation.[9] A link between the effects of hypocalcemia and hyperketonemia on the impairment of endogenous glucose metabolism has been described in dairy cattle and sheep and may contribute to insulin insufficiency.[25,26] Recommended dosages of 20% calcium borogluconate range from 30 to 60 mL (up to 100 mL).[3,27] Commercially available products contain 23% calcium borogluconate alone or its equivalence in calcium-magnesium–phosphite–potassium combination products contain approximately 10 g of calcium per 500 mL. This equates to a crude dose of 0.5 mL per pound body weight (1 mL per kg body weight). IV calcium must be delivered slowly over 7 to 10 min to avoid the development of arrhythmias and cardiac toxicity.[3] Products without dextrose can be administered subcutaneously to achieve a more prolonged absorption and be repeated at 24 h in high-yielding dairy does and ewes.[3] Dividing the total dose into several smaller volumes minimizes the risk of tissue irritation and sloughing. In hospitalized cases receiving long-term IV fluid infusions, supplementation with calcium, magnesium, and potassium can be provided, with adjustments made depending on serial biochemistry findings and feed intake levels. In states where subclinical hypocalcemia is expected to persist, continuous rate infusions of elemental calcium can be delivered at 1 to 3 mg/kg/h[28] When rumen motility is present, oral calcium gels may be used to provide more sustained calcium elevation profiles.[29,30]

Therapeutic Options

Treatment of PT involves correcting metabolic derangements and improvement of dysregulated metabolic processes that are furthering the negative energy balance. Recognition of concurrent acid-base and electrolyte imbalances plays a vital role in treatment response. Resuscitation efforts should correct dehydration, metabolic acidosis, and electrolyte derangements, reestablish glycemic control and curtail ketone body production. General principles include the administration of energy sources and the removal of factors that increase energy requirements. Individual case specifics and goals of the producer, including financial considerations, dictate choice of treatment options. Broad goals may include (1) survival of the dam with minimal regard for offspring viability or (2) prolonging gestation and directed intervention to maximize fetal viability and survival of the dam. In the former, induction of parturition and supportive care to address comorbidities of the dam are often elected. Depending on the gestational age of the offspring and the systemic state of the dam, management of PT cases to deliver healthy, viable offspring and survive the dam can be complicated, requiring intensive monitoring and therapy, often in a hospital setting. These cases are financially costly, and even with intensive supportive care, outcomes are variable.

Treatment Approach

The intensity level of treatment protocols implemented on-farm by the veterinarian depends on the producer's knowledge, skills, and resources and should be a collaborative effort in their development. Depending on the resources available, intensive on-farm therapy may include oral drenching or frequent IV administration of solutions in affected dams. In the early stages, when the animal is not completely anorexic and rumen motility is present, increasing the ration's availability, palatability, energy density, and starch content may be all that is needed.[2] These animals should be individually penned and provided easy access to highly palatable and energy-dense feed. Calcium supplementation may be warranted.[4]

Oral Drenches-Glucogenic Precursors

Early cases often benefit from oral drenching with glucogenic precursors, largely propylene glycol, and oral electrolyte solutions. Other substances, including sodium propionate, liquid molasses, sodium lactate, or ammonium lactate, have been used as glucose precursors.[3,9] Overzealous drenching with any glucogenic precursor can lead to disruption of rumen flora and predispose to ruminal acidosis.[3] Oral drenching of glucose is of little direct benefit, as it is rapidly fermented by rumen flora.[4]

Definitive studies evaluating different dosing volumes and frequencies of propylene glycol (or glycerol) treatments in terms of optimizing outcomes and financial considerations are lacking[4] but provision of glucogenic precursors (eg, propylene glycol, glycerol) remains a mainstay of therapy in on-farm settings, and has been useful in experimentally induced subclinical and clinical PT and mild cases of naturally occurring PT.[31–34] Many review articles[1–4] cite a study by Buswell and colleagues,[35] and a description is provided here, as modified drenching doses often stem from the study's findings. In a pilot study, Buswell and colleagues[35] compared the ability of an oral rehydration product, Liquid Lectade (c) (44.6 g glucose, 8.55 g sodium chloride, 6.17 g glycine, 4.084 g potassium dihydrogen phosphate, 0.12 g potassium citrate, and 0.525 g citric acid) to raise blood glucose concentrations in non-pregnant, healthy ewes to other drenches, including glucose alone (44.6 g in 160 mL), 120 mL of glycerol, or 120 mL of a propylene glycol based drench (Ketol; Intervet) containing 92 mg propylene glycol, 2.3 g choline chloride, and 204.7 mg potassium iodide). Findings included significant increases in blood glucose following Liquid Lectade dosing compared with oral drenches containing glucose or glycerol. Oral glucose and glycerol drenching significantly increased blood glucose concentrations from baseline, whereas propylene glycol drenching had little effect on blood glucose concentrations.[35] A follow-up field study was undertaken by the same researchers on 11 farms in naturally occurring PT cases. The Liquid Lectade drench was administered every 4 to 8 h until recovery was observed. Mild cases and severe cases (eg, neurologic signs present) showed 90% and 55% recovery rates, respectively, with an overall recovery rate of 68% with the delivery of live lambs and survival of the ewe.[35] Use of the same product drenched at 160 mL three times daily resulted in a survival rate of 34.8% and 24.7% in ewes and lambs, respectively.[36]

Oral drenching of propylene glycol or glycerol two to three times daily has been advocated as a sole treatment in mild cases and as a supplement to more aggressive therapy in more advanced cases.[2,19] The daily volume of propylene glycol ranges from 100 to 200 mL.[1,3] Others recommend 60 to 100 mL per dose of propylene glycol administered twice daily to minimize side effects.[2,19] which can include disruption of rumen flora. Duration of therapy is variable, often continuing until the return of normal appetite but seldom beyond a week to minimize complications. A tapered dosing regimen of 120 mL, PO, q12 h on the first day of therapy, followed by 60 mL, PO, q12 h thereafter, is also recommended.[6] Alternatively, glycerol can be administered at 60 mL, PO, q12 h for 3 to 6 days.[3] Commercially available products containing combinations of propylene glycol and glycerol (eg, Acetolena, Santa Elena, Uruguay) have been evaluated under experimental conditions.[31] Although propylene glycol and glycerol could be administered as IV solutions,[32] there is limited evidence to suggest this route of administration is superior to oral drenching, and it carries the risk of intravascular hemolysis.

INTRAVENOUS DEXTROSE

Parenteral injection of hypertonic glucose solutions as a single treatment has generally yielded poor results in the management of PT in the field.[2] There is limited evidence suggesting that frequent IV dextrose solution infusion is more effective than oral drenching of glucogenic precursors in mild to moderate PT cases under production settings.[4] Frequent infusions of hypertonic glucose solutions on farm are labor intensive, require maintenance of an IV catheter, and are therefore limited in practicality. However, it can be of value, and the injection of 5 to 7 g of glucose every 3 to 4 h, delivered as a 50% dextrose solution was reportedly successful in the treatment of PT in dairy goats.[2]

In a hospital setting, it is more feasible for clinicians to deliver continuous rate infusions of IV fluids supplemented with dextrose, in conjunction with the drenching of oral glucogenic precursors and insulin therapy. IV hypertonic dextrose infusion is cited as a therapy for hospitalized cases.[1,3] Many clinicians prefer less concentrated dextrose solutions supplemented with calcium and B vitamins for example, 500 mL and 250 mL boluses of 10% to 20% dextrose solutions, respectively.[1]

In the author's experience, use of continuous rate infusions of IV dextrose solutions is common for intensively managed cases in tertiary referral settings when the survival of both dam and offspring is the end goal. A dedicated high-quality, long-term venous jugular catheter is required for delivery of (partial) parenteral nutrition. Dextrose solution concentrations are typically between 5% and 10% to minimize the risk of thrombophlebitis. The total grams of glucose delivered per day are matched to the estimated energy requirements of the patient. When prolonged extensive parenteral nutritional support is necessary, use of commercial parenteral amino acids in dextrose solutions (eg, Clinimix, Baxter) should be considered. Serial measurement of blood glucose concentrations four to six times daily is necessary to guide treatment. BHB concentrations are monitored approximately once or twice daily, depending on the stability of metabolic regulation in individual cases. Depending on rumen motility and appetite, IV fluids are frequently combined in combination with twice-daily oral drenching of propylene glycol (60 mL, PO, q12 h) and rumen transfaunation (1 to 4 L/d). IV fluids are supplemented with electrolytes, including potassium and calcium, to correct deficits and anticipated ongoing losses in anorexic patients. Vitamin B complex or thiamine (10 mg/kg, IV, q6-12h) is recommended, given that rumen function and production of B vitamins are compromised. Supplementation of vitamin B12 has been advocated,[1,19] but has not consistently been shown to be of benefit in the treatment of PT.[20,37]

Insulin

The inclusion of insulin in PT treatment protocols to reduce ketogenesis and fatty acid mobilization is logical and has shown reasonably strong evidence of efficacy when used in conjunction with other treatments.[2–4,38] On-farm, when used in conjunction with oral propylene glycol (or other glucogenic precursor drenches), long-acting protamine zinc insulin, administered at 20 to 40 IU/animal once every 48 h for 3 days (or until recovery) has improved recovery rates in severely affected cases.[9,38] In naturally occurring cases of PT in ewes, the inclusion of Depot insulin at 0.4 mg/kg, SC, q24 h (Depot-insulin) in conjunction with twice-daily oral drench with glucogenic substrates significantly reduced the time to treatment response—typically within 2 days, and inclusion of insulin significantly improved survival rates to 86.7% compared with drenching alone (62.7%) or daily IV infusion of glucose and fructose (53.6%).[9] The benefit of including insulin as part of a standard treatment protocol for moderate to severe PT cases managed in the hospital setting is less clear. As reported by Simpson and colleagues, PT goats treated with insulin were at an increased risk of non-survival, which likely reflects the inclusion of insulin in more severely affected cases[6] as well as other inherent biases of retrospective studies. Alternatively, a short-acting formulation (regular insulin) can be used, at an initial dose of 0.1 to 0.2 U/kg, IM, followed by an additional dose of 0.05 to 0.1 U/kg, IM 60 to 90 min later, if necessary. If further doses are required to achieve normoglycemia, an insulin continuous infusion should be considered, as it is easier to titrate to effect than with repeated intramuscular doses. Based on infusion rates recommended in children and small animals, a continuous rate infusion (CRI) dosage of 0.025 to 0.05 U/kg/h should be initiated.[39] Glucose concentrations should decrease by no more than 50 to 75 mg/dl/h, monitored hourly during CRI implementation and frequently (q3-4h) once glycemic control is achieved.[39] Importantly, insulin administration should only be used in conjunction with either oral glucogenic precursors or IV dextrose supplementation to ensure hypoglycemia does not result.

Other Therapies

Previous reports suggest that low-dose corticosteroids may stimulate appetite, although most cases of PT show high concentrations of endogenous corticosteroids, and further supplementation is unlikely to alter the course of the disease short of inducing parturition.[4,9] The inclusion of nonsteroidal anti-inflammatory drugs, for example, flunixin meglumine, may be useful in controlling discomfort and potentially mitigate inflammatory cascades suggested to be present in PT.[4,40] Given the risk of renal insufficiency in PT cases, judicious use of nonsteroidal anti-inflammatory drugs (NSAIDs) and other nephrotoxic medication is prudent. In cases where significant gastrointestinal parasitism is present, anthelmintic treatment is justified.

Induction or C-Section

Termination of pregnancy eliminates the energy drain of the fetoplacental unit in the affected dam and has been advocated for decades to be a prudent approach in PT treatment.[1–4] In production settings, depending on the gestation stage and the dam's overall condition, induction of parturition is often carried out to survive the dam at the risk of delivery of weak or nonviable fetuses.[4] Induction protocols to maximize fetal viability are discussed later in this review.

It must be stressed that regardless of whether the dam, offspring, or both are the priority, ewes and does suffering from PT are systemically compromised and must continue to receive supportive care to correct dehydration, acid-base, and electrolyte imbalances, and ensure glycemic control until delivery of offspring.[2,3] The necessity of stabilization applies to all treatment goals, whether prolonging gestation, medical induction of parturition, or in the perioperative period for cases undergoing emergency or planned C-section delivery. Ewes and does with PT are at an increased risk of dystocia and post-partum complications, including retained fetal membranes and metritis, and should be monitored closely.[3,41,42] There are few studies evaluating treatment regimens that compare morbidity and mortality outcomes of dam and offspring following induction of parturition or C-section delivery of offspring (immediate or delayed) in naturally occurring PT. Given welfare and economic considerations, euthanasia should be considered in severely debilitated dams and scenarios where supportive care cannot be guaranteed or economics dictate.[4,5]

Parturition induction protocols using the combination of corticosteroids and a prostaglandin analog in both ewes and does is advocated, with potential benefits to both dam and offspring. The inclusion of corticosteroids may be advantageous for fetal lung maturation.[2,3] Because exact gestational age is generally unknown for most cases, and the dams are metabolically compromised, parturition following induction may be more protracted than induction in healthy ewes and does.[3,43] Corticosteroid choices include dexamethasone 15 to 20 mg (in does/ewes), 10 mg betamethasone (ewes), or 2.5 mg flumethazone (ewes/does). Addition of cloprostenol in ewes (0.375 mg) or prostaglandin F2 alpha in does (15 mg) increases the efficacy of the regime, with parturition at 40 to 45 ($\pm$ 10 to 15) h in ewes, and 48 to 72 h in does.[3]

Recently, some authors have called into question a once-held perception that an immediate C-section is the best option for saving the dam's life.[3] This recommendation lacks rigorous evidence and maybe the contrary.[4,5,14,44] In hopeless cases where euthanasia is indicated, a salvage C-section may be attempted to save the life of the offspring; however, the outcome remains guarded.[4] Extremely poor survival rates were reported by Lima and colleagues in dairy goats affected with PT, with case fatality rates of 64% to 86% and 88% to 100% in dams managed via induced parturition and C-section, respectively.[5,8] In a retrospective study evaluating risk factors in ewe and lamb survival in sheep undergoing emergency C-section, ewes with concurrent conditions, including PT, were at an increased risk of nonsurvival compared with simple dystocias, at 31.5% versus 3.8%, respectively.[45] Interestingly, dead and emphysematous fetuses were not found to increase the risk of postoperative complications or mortality in ewes that underwent C-sections.[45] Similarly, an 81% survival rate in non-complicated dystocias resolved via C-section was reported by Brounts and colleagues, whereas 100% of all PT cases that underwent C-section therein did not survive.[46] The authors criticized the previous recommendation of the necessity of C-section to save the dam; rather, doing so may put the dam's life at an increased risk compared with medical management, and the overall survival rates of dams with advanced PT may very well not be improved via prompt C-section.[46] In a recent retrospective study evaluating intensive management of PT in predominately Boer goats, does that underwent C-section delivery had a decreased survival rate of 43% compared with 86% survival in does that delivered kids naturally.[6] Offspring survival was also higher in vaginal delivery compared with C-sections at 72% and 15%, respectively.[6]

Future studies critically evaluating various treatment protocols for naturally occurring cases of PT and clinicopathological variables relevant to guide clinical decision-making are needed. Conclusions drawn from retrospective studies should be cautiously interpreted due to biases in case selection, data collection, and the inability to control for variation in treatment protocols used in case management. To the author's knowledge, no randomized controlled trials compare morbidity and mortality in dams and offspring treated with medical therapy, including induction of parturition, to surgical intervention. Clear evidence of either treatment as superior to the other for surviving the dam or offspring is largely empirical and requires further study in naturally occurring cases.

Maximizing Fetal Viability

The normal gestation length of sheep ranges from 138 to 152 days, with most breed averaging between 144 to 148 days. In goats, the average gestational length is approximately 150 days, varying from 147 to 155 days. Gestational ages of at least 140 and 143 days in lambs and kids, respectively, are reported ideal for delivery of uncompromised offspring,[3] with induction before day 138 of gestation advised against.[27,47] Perinatal mortality rises as prematurity increases, with lambs of less than 95% full gestational age without any medical induction showing mortality rates of 25% to greater than 90%.[48]

In studies using premature lambs as a research model, antenatal corticosteroid therapy is considered a standard of care for women at risk of preterm delivery to hasten lung maturation in the fetus.[49] Postnatal corticosteroid therapy is also used to minimize pulmonary inflammation and support continued lung development following birth.[50] Evaluation of induction protocols at gestational stages commonly encountered in small ruminants suffering from PT from the standpoint of fetal maturation and maximization of pulmonary function in a food animal practice setting is limited. Most studies involve healthy animals with a lack of field trials assessing different induction protocols in naturally occurring PT. In Zoller and colleagues, comparable lamb survival rates were shown between two induction protocols (parturition at day 137 to 139 of gestation) compared with C-section derived (day 147 to 148) and natural delivery at term (day 149) in healthy ewes.[51] Induction of parturition via a long-term protocol (LTP) entailed increasing daily doses of dexamethasone (administered intravenously) over 6 days, starting at 2 mg on days 130 to 133, followed by 4 mg on day 134 and 16 mg on day 135, which was repeated after that every 12 h until lambing occurred. The short-term protocol (STP) included 16 mg dexamethasone, IV, starting on day 135 of gestation, repeated every 12 h until lambing. Caesarian sections received 10 mg of dexamethasone 12 h before surgery. Vitality scores between the LTP and STP premature lambs were similar, and no lambs developed signs of respiratory distress syndrome (RDS).[51] Survival rates were 89%, 75%, 95%, and 96% for long-term protocol (LTP), short-term protocol (STP), C-section, and naturally delivered lambs, respectively, with no statistically significant differences found between treatment groups, although the study was limited in the number of animals in treatment groups.[51] Prolonged exposure to antenatal, low-dose corticosteroids appears to be beneficial for improving offspring vitality and survival; however, even in humans, response to antenatal corticosteroid therapy is variable, with only 40% of fetuses reported to respond favorably in its prevention of RDS.[52] In cases where it is not feasible for prolonged antenatal corticosteroid exposure before parturition, Regazzi and colleagues found that postnatal corticosteroids, therein long-acting betamethasone (0.5 mg/kg), had positive effects on vitality scores of preterm lambs (day 135) similar to antenatal betamethasone treatment as compared with controls during the first 72 h of life.[50] Postnatal steroid treatment had impacts on metabolic processes, including hyperglycemia and increases in lactate concentrations, the latter presumably reflecting increased cellular respiration and oxygen consumption.[50] Imprudent use of corticosteroids in neonates is cautioned against due to potential immunosuppression, potentially increasing the risk of sepsis.

Following medical induction of parturition, the effect of the delivery method, that is, vaginal delivery versus C-section, and its association with offspring survival in naturally occurring PT cases is currently limited to retrospective cohort studies. As reported by Lima and colleagues, management of PT on a large commercial goat dairy involves either induced parturition by injection of dexamethasone and dexcloprostenol or, if blood pH is less than 7.15, a C-section performed in PT cases. The case fatality rate of PT-does undergoing medically induced parturition was 64%, whereas 100% of does that underwent C-sections died.[5] Offspring survival was 96% and 77% in induced vaginal delivery and C-section, respectively.[5] In contrast, Simpson and colleagues report an overall PT doe survival rate of 70% in intensively managed, hospitalized cases in a predominately Boer meat goats referral population.[6] Offspring survival in these intensively managed PT cases was significantly higher in vaginal births compared with C-section delivery, at 72% and 15%, respectively.[6]

Clinicopathologically, offspring of PT-affected dams show variable degrees of hypoxemia and hypoventilation, significantly lower blood pH, and increased L-lactate concentrations.[42,53] Does with severely low bicarbonate concentrations had poorer offspring survival rates than does with values within or greater than reference ranges.[6] Similarly, Andrade and colleagues observed an association in C-section-born goat kids associated with decreased blood pH, base excess, increased L-lactate, and increased P_{CO_2} with poorer survival outcomes.[53] Offspring of dams with PT are at risk for increased short- and long-term morbidity and mortality, including reduced average daily gain and increased risk of nonsurvival to 3 months.[42]

Resuscitation of neonates from PT dams at the time of delivery is like other deliveries—clear airways of mucus and secretions, ensure normal respiration and response to stimuli, maintain sternal recumbency, and provide supplemental heat. Reversal agents for sedatives used in the dam for surgical delivery may be necessary if depression of respiratory or circulatory function is present. In cases of RDS, ideally, mechanical ventilation via endotracheal intubation is provided; however, this is very unlikely to be feasible in most scenarios. Although limited in its effect in the case of surfactant insufficiency, supplemental oxygen via nasal cannula can be used and may be of benefit. Maladapted respiratory function may persist for the first few days of life in offspring born to PT dams.[42] In premature neonates with underdeveloped respiratory center drive, respiratory stimulants (eg, doxapram hydrochloride) may be attempted, being mindful that potential cardiovascular side effects exist.[54] When possible, assessment of pulmonary function and characterization of the acid-base and electrolyte derangements should be used to direct therapy, including arterial blood gas analysis. Imprudent use of sodium bicarbonate to correct metabolic acidosis in the face of impaired pulmonary function (respiratory acidosis) will compound the metabolic derangements present.

Severely compromised dams may not be systemically stable enough to allow offspring to nurse colostrum. These animals should be milked out and colostrum bottle or tube fed to offspring. Colostrum production may also be severely decreased. Bovine colostrum replacement products can be used and fed to provide a minimum of 10% of body weight in volume. Weaver and colleagues found that kids born to dams suffering from PT are more likely to require tube feeding and should be monitored for appropriate nursing behavior and weight gain.[42]

CLINICS CARE POINTS

- Survival rates of dams and offspring in PT cases can be highly variable.
- Provision of gluogenic precursors - e.g., oral propylene glycol, is a mainstay of on-farm therapy.
- Nutritional support, e.g., parenteral nutrition, B vitamins, and when indicated, insulin, should be considered as part of the medical management in cases wherein prolonging gestation to maximize fetal viability is the goal.
- PT offspring are at risk for perinatal morbidity and mortality. Nursing care should include ensuring colostrum consumption and maximizing the maturation of lung development prior to delivery.

DISCLOSURE

The Author has nothing to disclose.

REFERENCES

1. Rook JS. Pregnancy toxemia of ewes, does, and beef cows. Vet Clin North Am Food Anim Pract 2000;16:293–317, vi-vii.
2. Marteniuk JV, Herdt TH. Pregnancy toxemia and ketosis of ewes and does. Vet Clin North Am Food Anim Pract 1988;4:307–15.
3. Brozos C, Mavrogianni VS, Fthenakis GC. Treatment and control of peri-parturient metabolic diseases: pregnancy toxemia, hypocalcemia, hypomagnesemia. Vet Clin North Am Food Anim Pract 2011;27:105–13.
4. Crilly J, Phythian C, Evans M. Advances in managing pregnancy toxaemia in sheep. Practice 2021;43:79–94.
5. Lima MS, Silveira JM, Carolino N, et al. Usefulness of clinical observations and blood chemistry values for predicting clinical outcomes in dairy goats with pregnancy toxaemia. Ir Vet J 2016;69:16.
6. Simpson KM, Taylor JD, Streeter RN. Evaluation of prognostic indicators for goats with pregnancy toxemia. J Am Vet Med Assoc 2019;254:859–67.
7. Vasava PR, Jani RG, Goswami HV, et al. Studies on clinical signs and biochemical alteration in pregnancy toxemic goats. Vet World 2016;9:869–74.
8. Lima MS, Pascoal RA, Stilwell GT, et al. Clinical findings, blood chemistry values, and epidemiologic data from dairy goats with pregnancy toxemia. Bov Pract 2012;46:102–10.
9. Henze P, Bickhardt K, Fuhrmann H, et al. Spontaneous pregnancy toxaemia (ketosis) in sheep and the role of insulin. Zentralbl Veterinarmed A 1998;45:255–66.
10. Doré V, Dubuc J, Bélanger AM, et al. Definition of prepartum hyperketonemia in dairy goats. J Dairy Sci 2015;98:4535–43.
11. Doré V, Dubuc J, Bélanger AM, et al. Short communication: evaluation of the accuracy of an electronic on-farm test to quantify blood β-hydroxybutyrate concentration in dairy goats. J Dairy Sci 2013;96:4505–7.
12. Doizé F, Vaillancourt D, Carabin H, et al. Determination of gestational age in sheep and goats using transrectal ultrasonographic measurement of placentomes. Theriogenology 1997;48:449–60.
13. Vannucchi CI, Veiga GAL, Silva LCG, et al. Relationship between fetal biometric assessment by ultrasonography and neonatal lamb vitality, birth weight and growth. Anim Reprod 2019;16:923–9.

14. Lima MS, Cota JB, Vaz YM, et al. Glucose intolerance in dairy goats with pregnancy toxemia: Lack of correlation between blood pH and beta hydroxybutyric acid values. Can Vet J 2016;57:635–40.
15. EE R. Dukes' Physiology of domestic animals. 13th edition. Ames Iowa USA: Wiley Blackwell; 2015.
16. González FH, Hernández F, Madrid J, et al. Acid-base and electrolyte status during early induced pregnancy toxaemia in goats. Vet J 2012;193:598–9.
17. Gomez DE, Bedford S, Darby S, et al. Acid-base disorders in sick goats and their association with mortality: A simplified strong ion difference approach. J Vet Intern Med 2020;34:2776–86.
18. Jeffrey M, Higgins RJ. Brain lesions of naturally occurring pregnancy toxemia of sheep. Vet Pathol 1992;29:301–7.
19. Andrews A. Pregnancy toxaemia in the ewe. Practice 1997;19:306–14.
20. Souto R, Afonso J, Mendonça C, et al. Biochemical, endocrine, and histopathological profile of liver and kidneys of sheep with pregnancy toxemia. Pesq Vet Bras 2019;39(10):780–8.
21. Duehlmeier R, Fluegge I, Schwert B, et al. Insulin sensitivity during late gestation in ewes affected by pregnancy toxemia and in ewes with high and low susceptibility to this disorder. J Vet Intern Med 2013;27:359–66.
22. Duehlmeier R, Noldt S, Ganter M. Pancreatic insulin release and peripheral insulin sensitivity in German black headed mutton and Finish Landrace ewes: evaluation of the role of insulin resistance in the susceptibility to ovine pregnancy toxemia. Domest Anim Endocrinol 2013;44:213–21.
23. Duehlmeier R, Fluegge I, Schwert B, et al. Post-glucose load changes of plasma key metabolite and insulin concentrations during pregnancy and lactation in ewes with different susceptibility to pregnancy toxaemia. J Anim Physiol Anim Nutr 2013;97:971–85.
24. Koenig A. Chapter 66 - Hypoglycemia. In: Silverstein DC, Hopper K, editors. Small animal critical care medicine. 2nd Edition. St. Louis: W.B. Saunders; 2015. p. 352–7.
25. Schlumbohm C, Sporleder HP, Gürtler H, et al. [Effect of insulin on glucose and and fat metabolism in ewes during various reproductive states in normal and hypocalcemia]. Dtsch Tierarztl Wochenschr 1997;104:359–65.
26. Harmeyer J, Schlumbohm C. Pregnancy impairs ketone body disposal in late gestating ewes: implications for onset of pregnancy toxaemia. Res Vet Sci 2006;81:254–64.
27. Edmondson MA, Shipley CF. 8 - Theriogenology of sheep, goats, and cervids. In: Pugh DG, Baird AN, Edmondson MA, et al, editors. Sheep, goat, and cervid medicine. 3rd Edition. St. Louis: Elsevier; 2021. p. 141–208.
28. Green TA, Chew DJ. Chapter 52 - Calcium Disorders. In: Silverstein DC, Hopper K, editors. Small animal critical care medicine. 2nd Edition. St. Louis: W.B. Saunders; 2015. p. 274–80.
29. Goff JP, Horst RL. Oral administration of calcium salts for treatment of hypocalcemia in cattle. J Dairy Sci 1993;76:101–8.
30. Blanc CD, Van der List M, Aly SS, et al. Blood calcium dynamics after prophylactic treatment of subclinical hypocalcemia with oral or intravenous calcium. J Dairy Sci 2014;97:6901–6.
31. Cal-Pereyra L, Benech A, González-Montaña JR, et al. Changes in the metabolic profile of pregnant ewes to an acute feed restriction in late gestation. N Z Vet J 2015;63:141–6.

32. Kalyesubula M, Rosov A, Alon T, et al. Intravenous infusions of glycerol versus propylene glycol for the regulation of negative energy balance in sheep: a randomized trial. Animals (Basel) 2019;9(10):731.
33. Wierda A, Verhoeff J, van Dijk S, et al. Effects of trenbolone acetate and propylene glycol on pregnancy toxaemia in ewes. Vet Rec 1985;116:284–7.
34. Alon T, Rosov A, Lifshitz L, et al. The distinctive short-term response of late-pregnant prolific ewes to propylene glycol or glycerol drenching. J Dairy Sci 2020;103:10245–57.
35. Buswell JF, Haddy JP, Bywater RJ. Treatment of pregnancy toxaemia in sheep using a concentrated oral rehydration solution. Vet Rec 1986;118:208–9.
36. Scott PR, Sargison ND, Penny CD. Evaluation of recombinant bovine somatotropin in the treatment of ovine pregnancy toxaemia. Vet J 1998;155:197–9.
37. Temizel EM, Batmaz H, Keskin A, et al. Butaphosphan and cyanocobalamin treatment of pregnant ewes: Metabolic effects and potential prophylactic effect for pregnancy toxaemia. Small Rumin Res 2015;125:163–72.
38. Burtis CA, Troutt HF, Goetsch GD, et al. Effects of glucagon, glycerol, and insulin on phlorizin-induced ketosis in fasted, nonpregnant ewes. Am J Vet Res 1968;29: 647–55.
39. Hess RS. Chapter 64 - Diabetic Ketoacidosis. In: Silverstein DC, Hopper K, editors. Small animal critical care medicine. 2nd Edition. St. Louis: W.B. Saunders; 2015. p. 343–6.
40. Zamir S, Rozov A, Gootwine E. Treatment of pregnancy toxaemia in sheep with flunixin meglumine. Vet Rec 2009;165:265–6.
41. Ioannidi KS, Vasileiou NGC, Barbagianni MS, et al. Clinical, ultrasonographic, bacteriological, cytological and histological findings during uterine involution in ewes with pregnancy toxaemia and subsequent reproductive efficiency. Anim Reprod Sci 2020;218:106460.
42. Weaver LF, Boileau MJ, Gilliam LL, et al. Characterization of short- and long-term morbidity and mortality of goat kids born to does with pregnancy toxemia. J Vet Intern Med 2021;35:1155–63.
43. Pollock JM, Miner K, Buzzell N, et al. Induction of parturition in a large number of pregnant dairy goats and its benefits as a management tool in a commercial scale goat operation. Theriogenology 2021;172:1–7.
44. Lima MS, Pascoal RA, Stilwell GT. Glycaemia as a sign of the viability of the foetuses in the last days of gestation in dairy goats with pregnancy toxaemia. Ir Vet J 2012;65:1.
45. Voigt K, Najm NA, Zablotski Y, et al. Factors associated with ewe and lamb survival, and subsequent reproductive performance of sheep undergoing emergency caesarean section. Reprod Domest Anim 2021;56:120–9.
46. Brounts SH, Hawkins JF, Baird AN, et al. Outcome and subsequent fertility of sheep and goats undergoing cesarean section because of dystocia: 110 cases (1981-2001). J Am Vet Med Assoc 2004;224:275–9.
47. Kastelic JP, Cook RB, McMahon LR, et al. Induction of parturition in ewes with dexamethasone or dexamethasone and cloprostenol. Can Vet J 1996;37:101–2.
48. Dawes GS, Parry HB. Premature delivery and survival in lambs. Nature 1965; 207:330.
49. Roberts D, Brown J, Medley N, et al. Antenatal corticosteroids for accelerating fetal lung maturation for women at risk of preterm birth. Cochrane Database Syst Rev 2017;3:Cd004454.
50. Regazzi FM, Justo BM, Vidal ABG, et al. Prenatal or postnatal corticosteroids favor clinical, respiratory, metabolic outcomes and oxidative balance of preterm

lambs corticotherapy for premature neonatal lambs. Theriogenology 2022;182: 129–37.
51. Zoller DK, Vassiliadis P, Voigt K, et al. Two treatment protocols for induction of preterm parturition in ewes—Evaluation of the effects on lung maturation and lamb survival. Small Rumin Res 2015;124:112–9.
52. Jobe AH, Schmidt AF. Chapter for antenatal steroids - Treatment drift for a potent therapy with unknown long-term safety seminars in fetal and neonatal medicine. Semin Fetal Neonatal Med 2021;26:101231.
53. Andrade IM, Simões PBA, Lamas LP, et al. Blood lactate, pH, base excess and pCO(2) as prognostic indicators in caesarean-born kids from goats with pregnancy toxaemia. Ir Vet J 2019;72:10.
54. Bleul U, Bircher B, Jud RS, et al. Respiratory and cardiovascular effects of doxapram and theophylline for the treatment of asphyxia in neonatal calves. Theriogenology 2010;73:612–9.

Hyperketonemia

A Marker of Disease, a Sign of a High-Producing Dairy Cow, or Both?

Sabine Mann, Dr. med. vet, PhD, Dip. ACVPM, Dip. ECBHM (Epidemiology),
Jessica A.A. McArt, DVM, PhD, DABVP (Dairy Practice)*

KEYWORDS

• Hyperketonemia • Ketone • β-Hydroxybutyrate • Transition • Epidemiology
• Treatment

KEY POINTS

- Focus hyperketonemia diagnosis at 3 to 9 days in milk.
- On-farm blood ß-hydroxybutyrate (BHB) meters offer the best balance of testing accuracy, convenience, and economics when used appropriately.
- Oral propylene glycol administered for 3 to 5 days remains the most evidence-based treatment of hyperketonemia.
- Hyperketonemic cows with concurrent hypoglycemia benefit more with treatment than cows with hyperketonemia alone.
- High-yielding cows will often have blood BHB greater than or equal to 1.2 mmol/L during the second and subsequent weeks of lactation, which is indicative of an appropriate adaptation to copious milk production.

BACKGROUND

Before the terminology used today, this disorder was described as acetonemia and reported as early as 1849 according to Udall.[1] In 1938, the Canadian veterinarian Legard[2] remarked that acetonemia was a recently recognized disease of cattle that practitioners had likely been presented with for a long time but that they lacked understanding of how to differentiate it from other postpartum disorders such as milk fever. The clinical signs of acetonemia were described by Fox[3] as diminished appetite, drop in milk production, nervousness, abnormal biting and licking behavior, refusal of grain, pica, and irritability. In the 1940s, this metabolic disorder became known as "ketosis" based on presence of these clinical signs. In the 1990s, Holtenius and Holtenius[4]

Department of Population Medicine and Diagnostic Sciences, College of Veterinary Medicine, Cornell University, 240 Farrier Road, Ithaca, NY 14853, USA
* Corresponding author.
E-mail address: jmcart@cornell.edu
Twitter: jmcartdvm (J.A.A.M.)

Vet Clin Food Anim 39 (2023) 307–324
https://doi.org/10.1016/j.cvfa.2023.02.004
vetfood.theclinics.com

differentiated this disorder into type I and II ketosis, proposing that the former occurred 3 to 6 weeks after calving and was associated with hypoglycemia and hypoinsulinemia, whereas the latter occurred immediately after calving with presence of hyperglycemia and hyperinsulinemia. These investigators ascribed the proposed type II ketosis to overfeeding in the dry period; however, the opposite has been found to be true in more recent work, that is, cows overfed in the dry period are at increased risk of elevated blood ketone concentrations, but they have concurrent lower glucose and insulin concentrations than controlled-energy fed cows.[5] The recent literature does not support the presence of hyperglycemia and hyperinsulinemia in early postpartum ketosis; therefore, we discourage the use of the terminology of type I and type II ketosis.

In the late 1990s, ketosis was further distinguished as clinical ketosis based either on presence or on absence of the typical clinical signs described earlier or as subclinical ketosis defined by severity of blood, urine, or milk ketone elevation greater than a certain threshold. In recent decades, direct testing for ketone concentrations in blood, or estimation of blood concentrations by testing urine or milk, has largely replaced reliance on clinical diagnosis; this is facilitated by the ready availability of cow-side blood ketone meters and other on-farm tests, including estimation of ketone bodies by Fourier-transform infrared spectroscopy (FTIR). Out of this quantitative measurement of ketone concentrations, the term "hyperketonemia" as a descriptor of this disorder has risen in popularity. Hyperketonemia is any increase in blood concentrations of ketone bodies (the parent compound acetoacetate and its derivatives ß-hydroxybutyrate [BHB] and acetone) greater than those considered physiologically normal.

It is important to note that hyperketonemia does not describe a clinical presentation. Hyperketonemia is not a disease per se, as it is not defined by distinguishing clinical signs, but exists rather as the elevated concentration of a metabolic marker, which is different from ketosis, a defined disorder that includes abnormal clinical signs; these should be clearly distinguished, as the former is associated with risk for diseases, but the latter is, itself, a disease. In our opinion, the use of the term hyperketonemia is the most appropriate and unbiased definition for the metabolic disorder of early lactation.

PHYSIOLOGY—THE SOURCE AND USE OF KETONES IN TRANSITION COWS

The cause of early lactation energy deficit leading to the production of ketone bodies and the development of hyperketonemia has been well described and will not be reviewed here.[6,7] Instead, we offer a short review of the source and use of ketones in transition cows.

Production of ketone bodies from 16 to 18 chain length fatty acids of adipose tissue origin, butyrate, and ketogenic amino acids (tyrosine, isoleucine, phenylalanine, and leucine) occurs primarily in the liver and is therefore called hepatic ketogenesis[8] (**Fig. 1**). Ketogenesis is one possible outcome of hepatic fatty acid utilization, the 2 other being esterification to triglycerides or complete oxidation. During times of energy deficit, ketone bodies play an important part in homeostasis, as they provide a form of energy to tissues, particularly when circulating glucose concentrations are low and hepatic gluconeogenesis capacity has reached its maximum.[9] In addition, alimentary ketogenesis from butyrate occurs in the rumen, especially when animals consume diets high in this fatty acid, but this plays a minor role during postpartum hyperketonemia,[8] especially when cows decline in intake.[10]

Concurrent with ketogenesis, hyperketonemic cows are often hypoglycemic.[8] Infusion of BHB stimulates insulin secretion and reduces gluconeogenesis in monogastric animals,[11,12] which is thought to represent a negative feedback loop on ketone

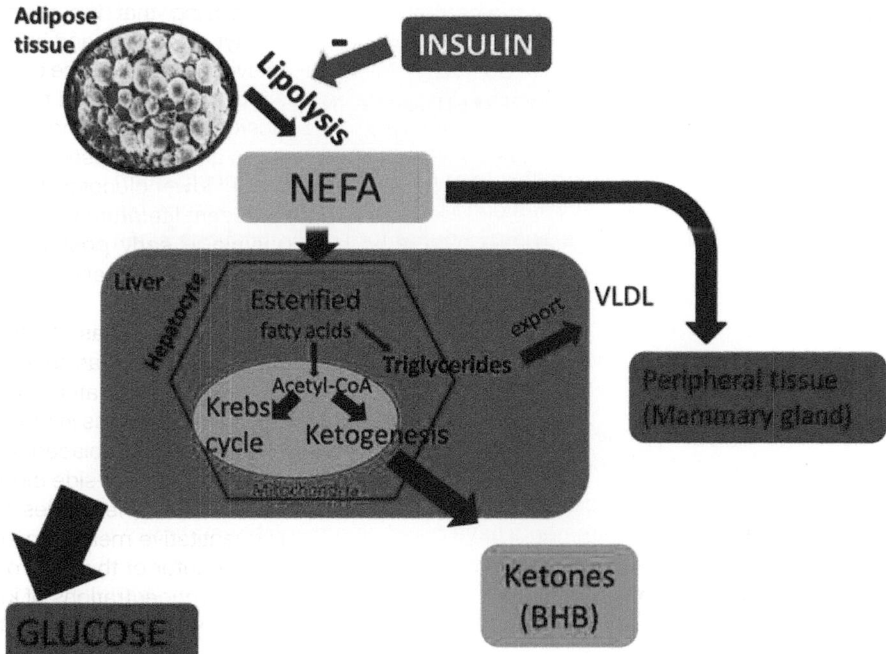

Fig. 1. Physiology of hepatic ketogenesis in cattle. Ketogenesis increases in magnitude due to an influx of fatty acids (NEFA) from lipolysis of adipose tissue during times of negative energy balance when circulating concentrations of insulin are low. Fatty acids in circulation are taken up by peripheral tissues, such as the mammary gland, as well as the liver. In the liver, NEFA can follow 3 different fates: (1) reesterification and export as triglycerides, (2) complete oxidation in the Krebs cycle to generate energy intermediates (eg, for gluconeogenesis), and (3) ketogenesis, particularly when Krebs cycle intermediates such as oxalacetate become limiting. Ketones enter the circulation and can be used by several tissues, including the mammary gland.

production.[13] The same reduction in glucose concentrations, albeit in absence of an increase in insulin concentrations, was seen in postpartum dairy cows infused for 4 hours with BHB to maintain concentrations between 1.5 and 2 mmol/L,[14] in mid-lactation cows at 1.7 mmol/L over 48 hours,[15] and in late-lactation cows at 1.8 mmol/L over 72 hours.[16] A promising explanation for the reduction in glucose concentrations in postpartum dairy cows was discussed by Zarrin and colleagues[14] as a possible consequence of reduced gluconeogenesis and use of BHB as an alternative energy substrate. It is likely that postpartum cows experiencing energy deficit with low circulating concentrations of insulin[5] are unable to make use of the regulatory feedback of insulin on ketogenesis, permitting the increase in ketone body concentrations in excess of their utilization.[13] There is also a possibility that ketone bodies, themselves, suppress gluconeogenesis even further.[14]

The mammary gland is a net user of ketones for milk fat production,[8,17] but other tissues such as the heart, kidney, and skeletal muscle can use ketone bodies as well.[9,17] The use of ketone bodies by the brain is still disputed for ruminants, but in other species seems compartmentalized and generally highest in areas without a blood-brain barrier, although it increases with starvation as reviewed by Laeger and colleagues.[18] The fact that severely hyperketonemic cows can develop nervous signs consistent with the concurrent hypoglycemia, and that signs resolve upon administration of intravenous glucose, suggests that the central nervous system in cows is dependent on glucose.

CONTROVERSIES—THE ROLE OF HYPERKETONEMIA IN HEALTH AND PRODUCTIVITY OF DAIRY COWS

As explained earlier, an elevation of ketone bodies in the early postpartum period is a hallmark of the physiological adaptation to lactation. Therefore, ketone bodies should be considered as an alternative energy source for bodily functions when gluconeogenic capacity is reached, and fatty acids are used in a complementary role to glucose in achieving "caloric homeostasis."[9] However, ketone bodies have been found to be harmful when produced in high quantities and have also been associated with several undesirable outcomes in observational studies. The most well studied of these ketone bodies is BHB.

Associations of Hyperketonemia with Reproduction and Health: ß-Hydroxybutyrate as a Marker

Studies of elevated BHB concentrations in terms of disease risk, reproductive parameters, and production measurements have relied on observational studies that cannot establish causal relationships of the direct effect of BHB on the measured outcome parameters. Therefore, we stress the importance of refraining from language when reporting these studies that would suggest otherwise, for example, discussing direct effects of BHB on outcomes.

Negative associations

Elevated BHB concentrations and their association with detrimental effects on health (displaced abomasum, mastitis, metritis, lameness, fatty liver) and reproduction (risk of pregnancy to first service, estrus expression and duration, number of services per pregnancy) as well as greater overall culling risk have been reported extensively[7,19–26] and summarized by McArt and colleagues[27] and Raboisson and colleagues.[28] Although the threshold for diagnosing hyperketonemia via elevated BHB concentrations and the magnitude of the point estimate and confidence for the association under investigation varied between studies, the negative association with undesirable events was shown consistently across studies. Of note, early hyperketonemia diagnosis (within the first week) has been found to be associated with higher risk for negative outcomes than diagnosis in the second week of lactation or later.[21,29]

Positive associations

BHB concentrations less than 1.2 mmol/L at the time of displaced abomasum diagnosis, before surgical correction, were associated with 2.5 times greater likelihood to be culled within 30 days of the surgery than cows with BHB greater than or equal to 1.2 mmol/L.[30] Similar associations (3 times greater odds) were shown by Reynen and colleagues[31] for the risk of culling within 60 days of surgery for cows with BHB concentrations less than 1.2 mmol/L. Both groups concluded, based on their observational studies, that hyperketonemia at time of surgery indicated a higher milk production level and the ability to return to full milking potential, whereas cows with lower BHB concentrations at time of diagnosis were thought to either have lower overall productivity or had dropped in productivity before the time of diagnosis.[30,31]

Evidence for Higher ß-Hydroxybutyrate in High-Producing Cows

As explained earlier, Krebs[9] differentiated physiological from pathological ketosis. He defined pathological ketosis as an increase in ketone bodies that exceeds possible needs under conditions of relative oxalacetate deficiency during times of increased gluconeogenesis and physiological ketosis as a complementary caloric contribution to glucose when the latter is in short supply. Because ketone bodies can be used by the mammary gland, an increase in blood ketone concentrations might play a role in supporting lactation.

Conflicting results in the literature abound regarding the association of hyperketonemia and milk production.[32] When considering studies from the last 25 years using blood BHB measurements to diagnose hyperketonemia with a diagnostic threshold of 1.2 to 1.4 mmol/L, some investigators find a positive association of hyperketonemia with milk production, that is, increased milk yield in cows with hyperketonemia,[33–35] whereas others find a negative association, that is, reduced milk yield in cows with hyperketonemia.[7,21,29,36] Some of this discrepancy might be explained by methodology and length of time considered for milk loss measurements. However, the timing of hyperketonemia diagnosis seems to play a role in these differences and is best demonstrated in studies that separated diagnosis by week relative to calving (**Fig. 2**).

In a large field trial including 1717 cows in 4 dairies in New York and Wisconsin, cows with blood BHB greater than or equal to 1.2 mmol/L first diagnosed between 3 and 7 days in milk (DIM) produced 2.2 kg/d less milk across the first 30 DIM than cows first diagnosed between 8 and 16 DIM, and hyperketonemic cows diagnosed at any point

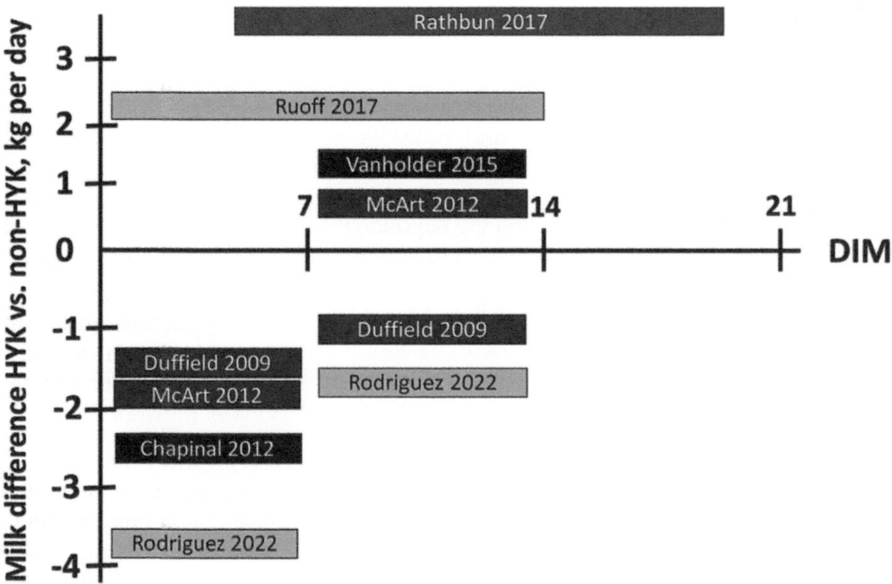

Fig. 2. Difference in kilogram milk per cow per day between cows diagnosed with hyperketonemia (HYK) and nonhyperketonemic cows based on blood BHB threshold definitions ranging from 1.2 to 1.4 mmol/L at varying days in milk (DIM). Studies include those published since 2009 included in a meta-analysis by Raboisson and colleagues[28] that measured BHB in blood, as well as recent publications meeting these criteria. The milk outcome is based on milk yield per cow per day across the first 30 DIM or at first test except for Rodriguez and colleagues,[29] which reported milk across the entire lactation. Data from McArt et al.[21] are reanalyzed from the original publication, which did not compare milk yield by week of hyperketonemia diagnosis with nonhyperketonemic cows. Readers are encouraged to read the primary literature sources to understand effect size and variance of these graphical outcomes and assess external validity.

between 3 and 16 DIM produced 1.2 kg/d less milk across the first 30 DIM than nonhyperketonemic cows.[21] In an unpublished reanalysis of this dataset, multiparous nonhyperketonemic cows across the first 30 DIM produced 0.8 kg/d less milk than cows first diagnosed with hyperketonemia between 8 and 16 DIM, whereas there was no difference between primiparous cows. This reanalysis was triggered by a recent study of multiparous cows in a single commercial dairy in Minnesota that cows diagnosed with hyperketonemia in week 1 of lactation produced 3.7 kg/d less milk across and entire lactation than nonhyperketonemic herd mates, whereas cows not diagnosed with hyperketonemia until week 2 were not different from herd mates not diagnosed with hyperketonemia at all.[29] Although not statistically different for both time points, a numerical difference was also shown by data from 1010 cows in 25 predominately tie-stall dairy farms in southwest Ontario,[7] with cows positive in the first week making 1.2 kg/d less milk at first DHI test and cows positive in week 2 making 1.0 kg/d less milk than cows with less than 1.2 mmol/L BHB threshold for hyperketonemia diagnosis. However, it was not reported if cows with elevated BHB in week 2 were also elevated in week 1, and thus the true effect of week of first diagnosis is unable to be determined from this study. Combined, these data suggest that the association with milk production differs in cows experiencing hyperketonemia in the first week postpartum compared with cows identified during or after the second week of lactation.

In addition to using caution in assuming all elevations of blood BHB are detrimental for productivity, it is important to note that the association of severity of BHB elevation and milk production may not follow a linear relationship. Although for most reported studies a linear regression line is fit for model predictions, examination of raw date for a possible nonlinear relationship is lacking. In summary, the relationship between hyperketonemia and milk production merits further investigation, particularly regarding the timing of diagnosis and possible nonlinear associations between severity of hyperketonemia and milk loss. We note the plausibility that an elevation of blood BHB during the first week of lactation is a marker of an underlying physiological issue, whereas an elevation during the second week of lactation is solely a marker of a high-producing dairy cow attempting to achieve "caloric homeostasis."

EPIDEMIOLOGY—PREVALENCE AND INCIDENCE

Evaluating 38 studies from 6 different continents, Loiklung and colleagues[37] calculated a pooled global hyperketonemia prevalence of 22.7% (95% confidence interval, 21.2%–24.3%), with an overall lower prevalence in Holstein cows compared with other breeds and a higher prevalence in confinement herds compared with pastured herds. However, care must be taken when interpreting these results, as information on breed and feeding system is often confounded by management differences between locations. In addition, although the association of hyperketonemia and negative consequences, defined as exceeding a BHB threshold of around 1.2 mmol/L, has been well reported in confinement herds as discussed earlier, the same threshold might not be appropriate for pasture-based herds.[38,39]

Peak incidence of hyperketonemia, that is, the first occurrence of a positive test defined as a concentration greater than a predefined threshold, occurs in the first week of lactation.[21,29,40] Given the expense and labor required to accurately determine hyperketonemia incidence, many studies underreport the true incidence, and thus this measure is not often used to discuss the epidemiology of hyperketonemia outside of research-based inquiries.

On the individual cow level, although hyperketonemia occurs in all lactations, the risk increases in older animals as demonstrated for Holstein cows.[33,41,42] In addition, high body condition score at calving has been associated with a greater risk of hyperketonemia.[41,43]

DIAGNOSIS—HOW TO TEST, WHEN TO TEST, AND HOW MANY COWS?

Testing individual cows and monitoring herd-level hyperketonemia can be done via direct tests for ketone bodies or more recent indirect testing methodology.

Direct Testing

Ketone bodies are most concentrated in urine, followed by blood, and lowest in milk.[8] The ketone body BHB is the predominant and most stable in blood,[8] and thus it is often the ketone body of choice in direct measurement, gold-standard laboratory tests as explained by Duffield.[32] Availability of handheld blood meters, in addition to presence of urine and milk dip strips and milk powder tests, have improved our ability to conduct accurate on-farm testing. Knowledge of the substrate tested, measured ketone body, and sensitivity and specificity of each test are required to fully understand the implications of results. For example, nitroprusside-based tests detect acetoacetate and acetone but not BHB.[32] In addition, users should read testing directions carefully, calibrate testing methods as recommended in the instructions, and understand how environmental conditions might change reported results. For example, instructions for milk dip strip tests specify use of room-temperature milk; however, on-farm and in research trials they are often used cow side on milk taken directly from the udder. From our experience, handheld meters should not be operated in cold temperatures often encountered in barns in the winter season, as they either do not work or they report erroneous results. Fortunately, many handheld meters can be left in warm rooms, and serum, plasma, or anticoagulated whole blood can be later tested to provide an accurate measurement.[44–46] Given the availability of multiple accurate and cost-effective on-farm testing methods, direct testing of ketone concentrations is relatively straightforward (**Box 1**).

Although urine tests are less expensive, only about 50% of cows can be induced to urinate on demand, which can create frustration when testing specific cows as part of a physical examination. There are multiple validated handheld blood ketone meters available for on-farm use.[46–49] Milk tests are a more expensive diagnostic test than either blood or urine and are often used incorrectly. Given these comments, and a recent study by Serrenho and colleagues[50] showing that milk and urine ketone tests detected cows with hyperketonemia after a delay of approximately 2 days after a blood BHB test, we recommend the use of on-farm blood BHB meters for diagnosis of hyperketonemia, rather than relying on diagnosis of hyperketonuria or hyperketolactia.

Indirect Testing

Indirect measurements of hyperketonemia mainly rely on associations with milk constituents, which are arguably an easier method of sample collection than via blood or urine testing, and include the fat-to-protein ratio of milk and estimated milk BHB concentrations. Hyperketonemia is often associated with an increase in milk fat concentration due to incorporation of preformed fatty acids originating from lipolysis, as well as a decrease in protein concentration due to energy deficit. However, use of milk fat-to-protein ratio for individual cow diagnosis of hyperketonemia is discouraged due to its low sensitivity and specificity.[51]

A review of measurement methods for hyperketonemia, including via milk-based FTIR, has been recently published.[52] Methods relying on FTIR do not allow direct measurement of analytes but rather predict milk constituents based on light spectra

Box 1

Pooled cow-level summary of sensitivity and specificity of direct ketone strip measurement strategies used for on-farm diagnosis of hyperketonemia reported by multiple studies

Matrix	Ketone	Diagnostic Threshold	Sn (%)	Sp (%)	Study
Blood	BHB	1.2 mmol/L	96	93	Sailer et al,[49] 2018 Bach et al,[48] 2016 Iwersen et al,[43] 2013 Iwersen et al,[47] 2009
Urine	AcAc	5 mg/dL (trace)	90	84	Reviewed by Oetzel, 2004
Urine	AcAc	15 mg/dL (small)	79	95	Reviewed by Oetzel, 2004
Urine	AcAc	40 mg/dL (moderate)	53	99	Reviewed by Oetzel, 2004
Milk	BHB	100 μmol/L	83	82	Reviewed by Oetzel, 2004
Milk	BHB	200 μmol/L	54	94	Reviewed by Oetzel, 2004

Milk and urine tests were compared with a gold standard of either handheld on-farm blood meters or laboratory-based β-hydroxybutyrate (BHB) measurement methods; handheld on-farm blood meters were compared with a gold standard of laboratory-based BHB measurement methods. The concentration of blood BHB used to diagnose hyperketonemia in the summarized studies ranges from 1.2 to 1.4 mmol/L. Given these on-farm results, and that milk and urine ketone tests detect cows with hyperketonemia approximately 2 d after a blood BHB test,[50] we recommend the use of on-farm blood BHB meters for diagnosis of hyperketonemia. However, we urge veterinarians to use caution when operating them in the cold and to read and follow the instruction manual regarding regular meter calibration.*Abbreviation:* AcAc, acetoacetic acid, Sn, sensitivity; Sp, specificity.

(**Fig. 3**). Estimated milk BHB concentrations have been associated with an increased risk of early lactation disease and herd removal but also increased milk yield.[53] This association needs to be further investigated within the context of timing of blood BHB elevations, further described later. In addition to estimation of milk BHB alone, use of FTIR predicted milk BHB and acetone as a component of a multivariable logistic regression model aimed to predict hyperketonemia, which also contained other individual animal parameters, was found to have high specificity (>95%) for both Holsteins and Jerseys, although sensitivity at the chosen thresholds was low (<60%).[42] To date, milk constituent estimation is conducted on proportional milk samples, which limits the utility of indirect measurement of hyperketonemia, as in-line FTIR testing systems do not yet exist. From a logistical standpoint, monthly DHI sampling conducted in smaller herds prevents timely identification of individual animals.[54] If herds are larger but also only sampled monthly, classification of herd hyperketonemia risk status is possible although individual identification is equally limited.

Testing Timeline and Sample Size

Traditionally, it has been recommended to test cows in the first 2 to 3 weeks of lactation. However, as discussed earlier, evidence is building that hyperketonemia identified in the first week of lactation has the strongest association with negative health and milk production outcomes.[7,21,29] Together with the fact that the highest incidence of hyperketonemia occurs in the first week of lactation, we recommend that sampling strategies should be adjusted to target the first week postpartum. Concentrations of blood BHB follow a diurnal pattern with highest concentrations reaching approximately 6 hours after a single total mixed ration feeding in the morning, and the amplitude of difference throughout a day is more pronounced in cows with hyperketonemia.[55] Therefore, the sampling time point in relation to feeding and diurnal patterns needs to be considered and standardized, especially when comparisons are

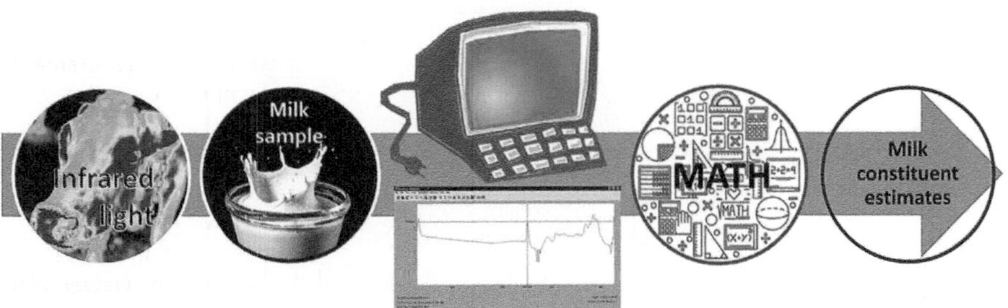

Fig. 3. Diagram simplifying the method of milk constituent estimation via Fourier transform infrared spectroscopy. This technique is used to create an infrared absorption or emission pattern of a solid, liquid, or gas by measuring how well a sample absorbs light at each wavelength. Simplifying the explanation of this methodology, infrared light is passed through a milk sample, an interferometer modifies the light to allow for data processing, and a computer uses Fourier transformation technology to create a spectra. Certain milk constituents such as fat, protein, and lactose are measured via specific chemical bonds present in the spectra, whereas partial least squares models are created to estimate additional milk constituents such as milk β-hydroxybutyrate and acetone. This figure was created with input from the authors, K D Bach, and D M Barbano.

made over time. Blood samples are often collected from the coccygeal vessels for which the BHB concentration is the same as from blood taken from the jugular vein or via an ear or vulvar skin prick.[56–59] Blood sampled from the milk vein, which in our opinion should not be conducted, will report BHB concentrations approximately 0.3 mmol/L lower than samples taken elsewhere,[56] likely due to uptake of BHB by the mammary gland.

Considerations for the number of cows required to estimate hyperketonemia prevalence within a herd have been thoroughly described and reviewed.[60,61] A ballpark estimate is to sample at least 12 cows, which will often provide sufficient confidence around the estimate for herd-level monitoring. Of course, the higher the proportion of at-risk cows sampled, the more precise the resulting hyperketonemia prevalence estimate. The required confidence in this estimate is a balance between the cost of sampling (test and labor) and possible actions resulting from the subsequent estimate.

THERAPEUTIC OPTIONS

Treatment of hyperketonemia should target the underlying metabolic derailment, not the reduction of ketone concentrations per se. Ketosis treatments, and the lack of appropriately conducted studies to understand the benefit of these treatment approaches, were comprehensively reviewed a decade ago.[62] An overview of evidence-based treatments follows and is summarized in **Box 2**.

Glucose

Administration of an intravenous glucose solution is the most historic treatment of ketosis. In 1938, Legard[2] recommended 250 g of dextrose administered intravenously for up to 8 consecutive days to greatly reduce mortality from the then newly recognized metabolic disorder, and this quantity of glucose has been typical for ketosis treatment over the last century. However, in a systematic review by Gordon and colleagues,[62] no studies at the time had been conducted on glucose treatment of ketosis, and they concluded that use of glucose should be considered as a second-line treatment in animals with concurrent hypoglycemia or those suffering from nervous signs. A small study comparing treatments of hyperketonemia (diagnosed in multiparous

Box 2

Summarized overview of evidence-based hyperketonemia treatments to reduce blood β-hydroxybutyrate concentrations one week following treatment, reduce postdiagnosis disease incidence, and increase production outcomes

Therapeutic vs Control	Dose & Route of Administration	Length of Administration	Blood [BHB]	Disease Incidence	Milk Yield
Glucose vs nontreatment	250 g IV glucose	3 d	.	N/A	N/A
PG[a] vs nontreatment	310 g oral PG	3 to 5 d	+	+++	+++
Glucose + PG vs PG	250 g IV glucose + 310 g oral PG vs. 310 g oral PG	1 to 3 d (glucose) 3 d (PG)	.	.	.
Glucocorticoids + PG vs PG	20 mg IM dexamethasone + 312 g oral PG vs. 312 g oral PG	1 d (dexamethasone) 4 d (PG)	–	.	.
B + C[b] + PG vs PG	25 mL SC B + C + 300 g oral PG vs 300 g oral PG	3 d (B + C) 3 d PG	+	N/A	+

[a] PG, propylene glycol.[b] B + C, butaphosphan + cyanocobalamin."+++", "++", and "+" represent strong, moderate, and weak evidence of positive benefit, respectively; "." Represents no evidence of benefit or detriment; "—", "–", and "–" represent evidence of strong, moderate, and weak evidence of detriment, respectively; and "N/A" represents the outcome has not been assessed compared with a nontreatment control group.*Abbreviations:* IM, intramuscular, IV, intravenous, SC, subcutaneous.

cows between 3 and 9 DIM with a blood BHB ≥1.2 mmol/L) showed that a single administration of 250 g of intravenous glucose to hyperketonemic cows reduced BHB concentrations for only 2 hours.[63] To date, no field trials assessing solely the use of glucose as a treatment of hyperketonemia have been conducted to assess health and production outcomes.

Propylene Glycol

The use of oral propylene glycol for its ketone-lowering effects began several decades after the use of intravenous glucose.[64] Antiketogenic benefits of propylene glycol have been shown,[65] although changes in circulating concentrations of insulin and glucose have been found to be moderate and short-lived[63]; this may be due to a slower plasma appearance and subsequent immediate use of glucose in tissues derived from the contribution of propylene glycol to the oxalacetate pool via the pyruvate or lactate-pyruvate routes.[66] Daily treatment with propylene glycol until resolution of hyperketonemia (BHB <1.2 mmol/L) resulted in increased milk production on 2 of 4 herds in a large field trial and greater pregnancy risk to first service, and cows were less likely to develop a displaced abomasum or leave the herd.[67] Extending the treatment duration of PG from 3 to 5 days has been found to aid in the improvement of ketosis of cows with higher blood BHB concentrations (>2.4 mmol/L).[68] In the prior described study by Mann and colleagues[63] comparing treatments in multiparous cows diagnosed with hyperketonemia between 3 and 9 DIM, administration of 300 mL of propylene glycol only reduced blood BHB concentrations at 2 hours postdosing compared with the nontreated control group. This small window of reduction in blood BHB concentrations, paired with field trials showing positive health and production benefits of propylene glycol administration to hyperketonemia cows, supports our goal of targeting the underlying metabolic derangement and not focusing on reducing blood BHB concentrations.

Combination of Glucose and Propylene Glycol

As early as 1971, Fox[3] described his standard ketosis treatment as 200 g intravenous dextrose followed with 171 to 342 g of oral propylene glycol. In a controlled study, the combination of both 300 mL of oral propylene glycol and 250 g of intravenous glucose given for 3 days to hyperketonemic multiparous cows diagnosed between 3 and 9 DIM led to the greatest degree and longest lasting decrease in BHB concentrations for the duration of the treatment; however, effects did not persist after treatment.[63] Accordingly, when 250 g of intravenous glucose was added for either 1 or 3 days to a 3-day course of 300 mL oral propylene glycol drench and tested in a multiherd field trial, no beneficial effects on the incidence of health disorders, milk production, or culling risk were found with the addition of glucose versus propylene glycol alone.[69] Given the lack of clinical benefit of intravenous glucose, paired with the invasive treatment method and labor needs, the routine use of intravenous glucose in the treatment of hyperketonemia should be questioned. Additional consideration around the use of intravenous glucose should be given to cows with severely elevated BHB concentrations showing clinical signs of ketosis, as the studies assessing the use of glucose were conducted based on the diagnosis of hyperketonemia and not of clinical ketosis.

Glucocorticoids

Glucocorticoids have long been used in the treatment of ketosis.[70] However, recently their use has been discouraged due to the lack of evidence for beneficial effects in the treatment of hyperketonemia.[62,70] A large multifarm trial subsequently conducted by the same research group randomized cows diagnosed with hyperketonemia between

3 and 16 DIM to receive 300 mL oral propylene glycol for 4 days and either a single intramuscular injection of 20 mg dexamethasone or a placebo on the day of hyperketonemia diagnosis. There was no difference between treatment groups in the odds of postpartum disease or milk production, and cows with high blood BHB concentrations (>3.2 mmol/L) had increased odds of remaining hyperketonemic a week following their first diagnosis. Given the lack of beneficial effects, the potential effect of administration of dexamethasone on immune function (which will not be reviewed here), and the detrimental effects on cows with high BHB concentrations, the use of glucocorticoids as a treatment of hyperketonemia cannot be supported.

Cyanocobalamin

Cyanocobalamin has often been used as an adjunct therapy for the treatment of hyperketonemia, although there are limited trials assessing the impact of vitamin B_{12} on hyperketonemic cows. Use of a combination butaphosphan-cyanocobalamin product in conjunction with oral propylene glycol in cows diagnosed with hyperketonemia between 3 and 16 DIM suggested subcutaneous administration of 25 mL of butaphosphan-cyanocobalamin might be beneficial in reducing the time to resolution of hyperketonemia and increasing milk yield, especially in cows with concurrent hypoglycemia.[68] To our knowledge, no studies have solely assessed the use of vitamin B_{12} in the treatment of hyperketonemia in a noncombination product. Given the suggested benefits and lack of evidence of negative effects, veterinarians should weigh the cost of treatment with the potential benefits when treating cows for hyperketonemia or creating treatment protocols for on-farm use.

Reduced Milking Frequency

Reduction of milking frequency from twice to once daily was tested as an adjunct treatment to oral propylene glycol drenching in a study of 104 hyperketonemic cows and led to rapidly declining BHB concentrations. However, it also reduced milk production during and after the intervention, particularly in parity more than or equal to 3 cows.[71] In addition, the welfare aspect of discomfort and pain due to udder engorgement after reducing milking frequency in early lactation has yet to be investigated.

Concurrent Hypoglycemia

Cows with concurrent hyperketonemia and hypoglycemia are more likely to benefit from treatment than cows with hyperketonemia alone. Treatment with 300 mL propylene glycol for 5 days increased 305-day mature equivalent milk production (305ME) compared with nontreated cows with blood BHB greater than or equal to 1.2 mmol/L and glucose less than or equal to 2.2 mmol/L diagnosed between 3 and 9 DIM, whereas this treatment did not affect 305ME in cows with only hyperketonemia at this time point of lactation.[72] Similarly, cows with hyperketonemia and hypoglycemia, diagnosed between 3 and 16 DIM, were more likely to resolve their hyperketonemia within 1 week following diagnosis and produce more milk when treated with 3 days of 300 g oral propylene glycol and 3 days of 25 mL subcutaneous butaphosphan-cyanocobalamin than cows only diagnosed with hyperketonemia.[73] Together, these studies suggest that hyperketonemic cows with concurrent hypoglycemia are more likely to be positively affected by treatment.

SUMMARY

Amassing evidence suggests that cows first diagnosed as hyperketonemic during week one of lactation are not adapting well to the initiation of lactation, whereas hyperketonemia appearing in cows during the second or subsequent week of lactation is indicative of high milk production. Given that numerous economically reasonable and accurate on-farm testing methods for hyperketonemia exist, veterinarians are encouraged to (1) include hyperketonemia testing as part of every early postpartum physical examination and (2) discuss routine monitoring for hyperketonemia with their clients to track herd-level prevalence over time, targeting testing to cows between 3 and 9 DIM. Although numerous concoctions and combinations of treatments exist and are commonly used for the treatment of hyperketonemia, propylene glycol remains the only therapeutic with positive evidence of subsequent production and health improvements. Unfortunately, no studies have been conducted that report on the effect of treatment by week of hyperketonemia diagnosis, so there is no evidence to support or refute the treatment of cows based on week of hyperketonemia development. Given the lack of detrimental evidence surrounding treatment of hyperketonemia (with the exception of glucocorticoids), it seems prudent to treat early lactation hyperketonemic cows regardless of their DIM at diagnosis until appropriate data have been generated.

Although this review does not cover prevention of hyperketonemia, which has been briefly summarized elsewhere,[74] we feel strongly that transition cow management, with particular emphasis on cow comfort,[75–77] heat abatement, calving management, and appropriate nutrition quality,[5,78,79] quantity, and timing, is likely more important and cost-effective for producers than the identification and treatment of individual cows for hyperketonemia. Hence the importance of veterinary involvement on farms regarding transition cow management and nutritional strategies in addition to developing on-farm testing and treatment protocols.

CLINICS CARE POINTS

- Focus hyperketonemia diagnosis at 3 to 9 DIM.
- On-farm blood BHB meters offer the best balance of testing accuracy and price when used appropriately.
- Oral propylene glycol administered for 3 to 5 days remains the most effective treatment of hyperketonemia.
- Hyperketonemic cows with concurrent hypoglycemia benefit more from treatment than cows with hyperketonemia alone.
- High-yielding cows will often have blood BHB greater than or equal to 1.2 mmol/L during the second week of lactation, which is indicative of an appropriate adaptation to copious milk production.

DISCLOSURE

The authors have nothing to disclose.

REFERENCES

1. Udall DH. The practice of veterinary medicine: with one hundred and two illustrations. Ithaca, NY: Published by the author; 1943.
2. Legard HM. Observations of acetonaemia of cattle. Can J Comp Med 1938;2(3):60.
3. Fox FH. Clinical diagnosis and treatment of ketosis. J Dairy Sci 1971;54(6):974–8.

4. Holtenius P, Holtenius K. New aspects of ketone bodies in energy metabolism of dairy cows: a review. Zentralbl Veterinarmed A 1996;43(10):579–87.
5. Mann S, Leal Yepes FA, Duplessis M, et al. Dry period plane of energy: effects on glucose tolerance in transition dairy cows. J Dairy Sci 2016;99(1):701–17.
6. Herdt TH. Ruminant adaptation to negative energy balance. Influences on the etiology of ketosis and fatty liver. Vet Clin North Am Food Anim Pract 2000; 16(2):215–30.
7. Duffield TF, Lissemore KD, McBride BW, et al. Impact of hyperketonemia in early lactation dairy cows on health and production. J Dairy Sci 2009;92(2):571–80.
8. Bergman EN. Hyperketonemia-ketogenesis and ketone body metabolism. J Dairy Sci 1971;54(6):936–48.
9. Krebs HA. Bovine ketosis. Vet Rec 1966;78(6):187–92.
10. Brockman RP. Roles for insulin and glucagon in the development of ruminant ketosis - a review. Can Vet J 1979;20(5):121–6.
11. Felts PW, Crofford OB, Park CR. Effect of infused ketone bodies on glucose utilization in the dog. J Clin Invest 1964;43(4):638–46.
12. Mebane D, Madison LL. Hypoglycemic action of ketones. I. Effects of ketones on hepatic glucose output and peripheral glucose utilization. J Lab Clin Med 1964; 63:177–92.
13. Herdt TH, Emery RS. Therapy of Diseases of Ruminant Intermediary Metabolism. Vet Clin North Am Food Anim Pract 1992;8(1):91–106.
14. Zarrin M, Grossen-Rösti L, Bruckmaier RM, et al. Elevation of blood β-hydroxybutyrate concentration affects glucose metabolism in dairy cows before and after parturition. J Dairy Sci 2017;100(3):2323–33.
15. Zarrin M, De Matteis L, Vernay MCMB, et al. Long-term elevation of β-hydroxybutyrate in dairy cows through infusion: Effects on feed intake, milk production, and metabolism. J Dairy Sci 2013;96(5):2960–72.
16. Swartz TH, Bradford BJ, Mamedova LK. Connecting metabolism to mastitis: Hyperketonemia impaired mammary gland defenses during a Streptococcus uberis challenge in dairy cattle. Front Immunol 2021;12:700278.
17. Heitmann RN, Dawes DJ, Sensenig SC. Hepatic ketogenesis and peripheral ketone body utilization in the ruminant. J Nutr 1987;117(6):1174–80.
18. Laeger T, Metges CC, Kuhla B. Role of β-hydroxybutyric acid in the central regulation of energy balance. Appetite 2010;54(3):450–5.
19. Ospina PA, Nydam DV, Stokol T, et al. Associations of elevated nonesterified fatty acids and beta-hydroxybutyrate concentrations with early lactation reproductive performance and milk production in transition dairy cattle in the northeastern United States. J Dairy Sci 2010;93(4):1596–603.
20. Chapinal N, Leblanc SJ, Carson ME, et al. Herd-level association of serum metabolites in the transition period with disease, milk production, and early lactation reproductive performance. J Dairy Sci 2012;95(10):5676–82.
21. McArt JA, Nydam DV, Oetzel GR. Epidemiology of subclinical ketosis in early lactation dairy cattle. J Dairy Sci 2012;95(9):5056–66.
22. LeBlanc SJ, Leslie KE, Duffield TF. Metabolic predictors of displaced abomasum in dairy cattle. J Dairy Sci 2005;88(1):159–70.
23. Kerwin AL, Burhans WS, Mann S, et al. Transition cow nutrition and management strategies of dairy herds in the northeastern United States: Part II-Associations of metabolic- and inflammation-related analytes with health, milk yield, and reproduction. J Dairy Sci 2022;105(6):5349–69.

24. Albaaj A, Jattiot M, Manciaux L, et al. Hyperketolactia occurrence before or after artificial insemination is associated with a decreased pregnancy per artificial insemination in dairy cows. J Dairy Sci 2019;102(9):8527–36.
25. Bogado Pascottini O, Probo M, LeBlanc SJ, et al. Assessment of associations between transition diseases and reproductive performance of dairy cows using survival analysis and decision tree algorithms. Prev Vet Med 2020;176:104908.
26. Rutherford AJ, Oikonomou G, Smith RF. The effect of subclinical ketosis on activity at estrus and reproductive performance in dairy cattle. J Dairy Sci 2016;99(6): 4000–15.
27. McArt JA, Nydam DV, Oetzel GR, et al. Elevated non-esterified fatty acids and β-hydroxybutyrate and their association with transition dairy cow performance. Vet J 2013;198(3):560–70.
28. Raboisson D, Mounié M, Maigné E. Diseases, reproductive performance, and changes in milk production associated with subclinical ketosis in dairy cows: a meta-analysis and review. J Dairy Sci 2014;97(12):7547–63.
29. Rodriguez Z, Shepley E, Endres MI, et al. Assessment of milk yield and composition, early reproductive performance, and herd removal in multiparous dairy cattle based on the week of diagnosis of hyperketonemia in early lactation. J Dairy Sci 2022;105(5):4410–20.
30. Croushore WS Jr, Ospina PA, Welch DC, et al. Association between β-hydroxybutyrate concentration at surgery for correction of left-displaced abomasum in dairy cows and removal from the herd after surgery. J Am Vet Med Assoc 2013;243(9): 1329–33.
31. Reynen JL, Kelton DF, LeBlanc SJ, et al. Factors associated with survival in the herd for dairy cows following surgery to correct left displaced abomasum. J Dairy Sci 2015;98(6):3806–13.
32. Duffield T. Subclinical ketosis in lactating dairy cattle. Vet Clin North Am Food Anim Pract 2000;16(2):231–53.
33. Rathbun FM, Pralle RS, Bertics SJ, et al. Relationships between body condition score change, prior mid-lactation phenotypic residual feed intake, and hyperketonemia onset in transition dairy cows. J Dairy Sci 2017;100(5):3685–96. https://doi.org/10.3168/jds.2016-1208.
34. Ruoff J, Borchardt S, Heuwieser W. Short communication: associations between blood glucose concentration, onset of hyperketonemia, and milk production in early lactation dairy cows. J Dairy Sci 2017;100(7):5462–7.
35. Vanholder T, Papen J, Bemers R, et al. Risk factors for subclinical and clinical ketosis and association with production parameters in dairy cows in the Netherlands. J Dairy Sci 2015;98(2):880–8.
36. Chapinal N, Carson ME, LeBlanc SJ, et al. The association of serum metabolites in the transition period with milk production and early-lactation reproductive performance. J Dairy Sci 2012;95(3):1301–9.
37. Loiklung C, Sukon P, Thamrongyoswittayakul C. Global prevalence of subclinical ketosis in dairy cows: a systematic review and meta-analysis. Res Vet Sci 2022; 144:66–76.
38. Compton CW, McDougall S, Young L, et al. Prevalence of subclinical ketosis in mainly pasture-grazed dairy cows in New Zealand in early lactation. N Z Vet J 2014;62(1):30–7.
39. Leal Yepes FA, Mann S, Martens EM, et al. Blood beta-hydroxybutyrate concentrations and early lactation management strategies on pasture-based dairy farms in Colombia. Prev Vet Med 2020;174:104855.

40. McCarthy MM, Mann S, Nydam DV, et al. Short communication: Concentrations of nonesterified fatty acids and beta-hydroxybutyrate in dairy cows are not well correlated during the transition period. J Dairy Sci 2015;98(9):6284–90.
41. McArt JA, Nydam DV, Oetzel GR. Dry period and parturient predictors of early lactation hyperketonemia in dairy cattle. J Dairy Sci 2013;96(1):198–209.
42. Chandler TL, Pralle RS, Dórea JRR, et al. Predicting hyperketonemia by logistic and linear regression using test-day milk and performance variables in early-lactation Holstein and Jersey cows. J Dairy Sci 2018;101(3):2476–91.
43. Gillund P, Reksen O, Gröhn YT, et al. Body condition related to ketosis and reproductive performance in norwegian dairy cows. J Dairy Sci 2001;84(6):1390–6.
44. Pineda A, Cardoso FC. Technical note: Validation of a handheld meter for measuring beta-hydroxybutyrate concentrations in plasma and serum from dairy cows. J Dairy Sci 2015;98(12):8818–24.
45. Leal Yepes FA, Nydam DV, Heuwieser W, et al. Technical note: Evaluation of the diagnostic accuracy of 2 point-of-care beta-hydroxybutyrate devices in stored bovine plasma at room temperature and at 37 degrees C. J Dairy Sci 2018;101(7):6455–61.
46. Iwersen M, Klein-Jobstl D, Pichler M, et al. Comparison of 2 electronic cowside tests to detect subclinical ketosis in dairy cows and the influence of the temperature and type of blood sample on the test results. J Dairy Sci 2013;96(12):7719–30.
47. Iwersen M, Falkenberg U, Voigtsberger R, et al. Evaluation of an electronic cowside test to detect subclinical ketosis in dairy cows. J Dairy Sci 2009;92(6):2618–24.
48. Bach KD, Heuwieser W, McArt JAA. Technical note: Comparison of 4 electronic handheld meters for diagnosing hyperketonemia in dairy cows. J Dairy Sci 2016;99(11):9136–42.
49. Sailer KJ, Pralle RS, Oliveira RC, et al. Technical note: Validation of the BHBCheck blood beta-hydroxybutyrate meter as a diagnostic tool for hyperketonemia in dairy cows. J Dairy Sci 2018;101(2):1524–9.
50. Serrenho RC, Williamson M, Berke O, et al. An investigation of blood, milk, and urine test patterns for the diagnosis of ketosis in dairy cows in early lactation. J Dairy Sci 2022;105(9):7719–27.
51. Duffield TF, Kelton DF, Leslie KE, et al. Use of test day milk fat and milk protein to detect subclinical ketosis in dairy cattle in Ontario. Can Vet J 1997;38(11):713–8.
52. Overton TR, McArt JAA, Nydam DV. A 100-Year Review: Metabolic health indicators and management of dairy cattle. J Dairy Sci 2017;100(12):10398–417.
53. Bach KD, Barbano DM, McArt JAA. Association of mid-infrared-predicted milk and blood constituents with early-lactation disease, removal, and production outcomes in Holstein cows. J Dairy Sci 2019;102(11):10129–39.
54. Caldeira MO, Dan D, Neuheuser AL, et al. Opportunities and limitations of milk mid-infrared spectra-based estimation of acetone and β-hydroxybutyrate for the prediction of metabolic stress and ketosis in dairy cows. J Dairy Res 2020;87(2):196–203.
55. Seely CR, Bach KD, Barbano DM, et al. Effect of hyperketonemia on the diurnal patterns of energy-related blood metabolites in early-lactation dairy cows. J Dairy Sci 2021;104(1):818–25.
56. Mahrt A, Burfeind O, Heuwieser W. Effects of time and sampling location on concentrations of beta-hydroxybutyric acid in dairy cows. J Dairy Sci 2014;97(1):291–8.

57. Suss D, Drillich M, Klein-Jobstl D, et al. Measurement of beta-hydroxybutyrate in capillary blood obtained from an ear to detect hyperketonemia in dairy cows by using an electronic handheld device. J Dairy Sci 2016;99(9):7362–9.
58. Kanz P, Drillich M, Klein-Jobstl D, et al. Suitability of capillary blood obtained by a minimally invasive lancet technique to detect subclinical ketosis in dairy cows by using 3 different electronic hand-held devices. J Dairy Sci 2015;98(9):6108–18.
59. Iwersen M, Thiel A, Suss D, et al. Short communication: repeatability of beta-hydroxybutyrate measurements in capillary blood obtained from the external vulvar skin. J Dairy Sci 2017;100(7):5717–23.
60. Ospina PA, McArt JA, Overton TR, et al. Using nonesterified fatty acids and β-hydroxybutyrate concentrations during the transition period for herd-level monitoring of increased risk of disease and decreased reproductive and milking performance. Vet Clin North Am Food Anim Pract 2013;29(2):387–412.
61. McArt J, Abuelo Á, Mann S. Metabolic disease testing on farms: epidemiological principles. Practice 2020;42(7):405.
62. Gordon JL, Leblanc SJ, Duffield TF. Ketosis treatment in lactating dairy cattle. Vet Clin North Am Food Anim Pract 2013;29(2):433–45.
63. Mann S, Yepes FAL, Behling-Kelly E, et al. The effect of different treatments for early-lactation hyperketonemia on blood beta-hydroxybutyrate, plasma nonesterified fatty acids, glucose, insulin, and glucagon in dairy cattle. J Dairy Sci 2017;100(8):6470–82.
64. Emery RS, Burg N, Brown LD, et al. Detection, occurrence, and prophylactic treatment of borderline ketosis with propylene glycol feeding1. J Dairy Sci 1964;47(10):1074–9.
65. McArt JA, Nydam DV, Ospina PA, et al. A field trial on the effect of propylene glycol on milk yield and resolution of ketosis in fresh cows diagnosed with subclinical ketosis. J Dairy Sci 2011;94(12):6011–20.
66. Nielsen NI, Ingvartsen KL. Propylene glycol for dairy cows: a review of the metabolism of propylene glycol and its effects on physiological parameters, feed intake, milk production and risk of ketosis. Anim Feed Sci Tech 2004;115(2004):191–213.
67. McArt JA, Nydam DV, Oetzel GR. A field trial on the effect of propylene glycol on displaced abomasum, removal from herd, and reproduction in fresh cows diagnosed with subclinical ketosis. J Dairy Sci 2012;95(5):2505–12.
68. Gordon JL, LeBlanc SJ, Kelton DF, et al. Randomized clinical field trial on the effects of butaphosphan-cyanocobalamin and propylene glycol on ketosis resolution and milk production. J Dairy Sci 2017;100(5):3912–21.
69. Capel MB, Bach KD, Mann S, et al. A randomized controlled trial to evaluate propylene glycol alone or in combination with dextrose as a treatment for hyperketonemia in dairy cows. J Dairy Sci 2021;104(2):2185–94.
70. Tatone EH, Duffield TF, Capel MB, et al. A randomized controlled trial of dexamethasone as an adjunctive therapy to propylene glycol for treatment of hyperketonemia in postpartum dairy cattle. J Dairy Sci 2016;99(11):8991–9000.
71. Williamson M, Couto Serrenho R, McBride BW, et al. Reducing milking frequency from twice to once daily as an adjunct treatment for ketosis in lactating dairy cows-A randomized controlled trial. J Dairy Sci 2022;105(2):1402–17.
72. Hubner AM, Canisso IF, Coelho WM Jr, et al. A randomized controlled trial examining the effects of treatment with propylene glycol and injectable cyanocobalamin on naturally occurring disease, milk production, and reproductive outcomes of dairy cows diagnosed with concurrent hyperketonemia and hypoglycemia. J Dairy Sci 2022;105(11):9070–83.

73. Gordon JL, Duffield TF, Herdt TH, et al. Effects of a combination butaphosphan and cyanocobalamin product and insulin on ketosis resolution and milk production. J Dairy Sci 2017;100(4):2954–66.
74. Mann S, McArt J, Abuelo A. Production-related metabolic disorders of cattle: ketosis, milk fever and grass staggers. Practice 2019;41(5):205–19.
75. Pineiro JM, Menichetti BT, Barragan AA, et al. Associations of pre- and postpartum lying time with metabolic, inflammation, and health status of lactating dairy cows. J Dairy Sci 2019;102(4):3348–61.
76. Belaid MA, Rodriguez-Prado M, Lopez-Suarez M, et al. Prepartum behavior changes in dry Holstein cows at risk of postpartum diseases. J Dairy Sci 2021; 104(4):4575–83.
77. Kaufman EI, LeBlanc SJ, McBride BW, et al. Association of rumination time with subclinical ketosis in transition dairy cows. J Dairy Sci 2016;99(7):5604–18.
78. Leal Yepes FA, Mann S, Overton TR, et al. Effect of rumen-protected branched-chain amino acid supplementation on production- and energy-related metabolites during the first 35 days in milk in Holstein dairy cows. J Dairy Sci 2019; 102(6):5657–72. https://doi.org/10.3168/jds.2018-15508.
79. Mammi LME, Guadagnini M, Mechor G, et al. The use of monensin for ketosis prevention in dairy cows during the transition period: a systematic review. Animals 2021;11(7):1988. https://doi.org/10.3390/ani11071988.

Transition Management in Grazing Systems: Pragmatism Before Precision

John Roche, PhD

KEYWORDS

- Magnesium • Dietary cation–anion difference • Body condition score • Pasture

KEY POINTS

- Grazing cows undergo a similar degree of metabolic stress and immune dysregulation as reported in high-yielding housed cows consuming total mixed rations.
- Nutritional requirements are consistent with those presented in National Research Council, 2001, but the ability to manage cow dry matter intake and diet composition is much less; pragmatism in transition management is, therefore, often more important than precision.
- Producers need to manage cows to achieve metabolizable energy intakes of 80% to 100% of requirements;
- The daily diet pre- and post-calving should be fortified with magnesium and trace elements and with calcium early post-calving. Dusting pastures with magnesium oxide pre-grazing is a very effective magnesium supplementation strategy.
- Although the biochemistry is similar in grazing and housed cows, anionic salts are not a pragmatic method of milk-fever control in most grazing systems because dietary potassium is so high in fresh forages and pasture composition variability precludes precise management of dietary cation–anion difference.

BACKGROUND

As in housed systems, the transition period in grazing systems is defined as the 6 to 8 weeks encompassing late pregnancy and early lactation and it involves coordinated changes across multiple tissues and very large changes in the provision of, and requirements for, energy and nutrients.[1,2] Despite the lower milk yields associated with grazing systems relative to housed systems, increases in circulating concentrations of fatty acids and β-hydroxybutyrate (BHB), concentrations of humoral factors associated with immune function and gene expression in leukocytes, and changes in gene expression in metabolically active tissues (eg, liver, adipose tissue) and

School of Biological Sciences, University of Auckland, Private Bag 92019, Auckland 1142, New Zealand
E-mail address: john.roche@mpi.govt.nz
Twitter: down2earth_john (J.R.)

Vet Clin Food Anim 39 (2023) 325–336
https://doi.org/10.1016/j.cvfa.2023.02.005
vetfood.theclinics.com

circulating micro-vesicles all indicate a similar degree of tissue hypertrophy, metabolic stress, and immune dysregulation to those reported in high-yielding housed cows consuming total mixed rations (TMRs).[3–8]

Despite the similarity in physiologic challenges, system-level and nutrition-related differences make management of the grazing transition cow different to what is often recommended for housed cows being offered a TMR. This article provides recommendations for managing the transition dairy cow in a grazing system.

SYSTEM DEFINITION

Grazing systems are not a homogenous entity. They vary from low-input, extensive, tropical grass and legume-based systems, with low-yielding cows, to intensive grazing systems, in which highly digestible forages dominate the annual grazed dry matter (DM) intake (DMI) profile of the cow. Grazing systems may also be hybrid feeding systems, in which high-yielding cows are housed/lotted for large parts of the day, offered most of their nutrient intake from a mixed ration, and grazed pasture is a small part of the milking ration.

In intensive grazing systems, cows graze for 270 to 365 days of the year; pasture growth rates and winter soil conditions in some countries/regions preclude grazing and necessitate the housing of cows (eg, Ireland, United Kingdom, northern United States), whereas housing is not required where rainfall, evapotranspiration, soil conditions, and/or pasture growth favor grazing during winter (eg, New Zealand, Australia, South Africa, mid-Western United States). This article focuses on the intensive grazing system model presented by Roche and coworkers[9] because (1) it is the type of system in which most research into managing grazing transition cows has been undertaken; (2) the recommendations have relevance to more extensive grazing systems; and (3) the most appropriate management of the transition cow in the high-production, mixed ration-based grazing system previously mentioned is arguably better represented by strategies recommended for housed systems.

INTENSIVE GRAZING SYSTEM

Successful, intensive grazing systems revolve around a short calving period, beginning mid-winter, approximately 60 days before pasture growth exceeds herd demand (ie, in mid-winter; **Fig. 1**). Fall-calving systems also exist, especially where milk companies require a flat annual supply curve, but milk production is substantially more expensive and, even with company incentives, these systems are generally less profitable than comparable spring-calving options.[10] Transition cow management is similar in the fall-calving system, although weather-related challenges tend to be greater in the spring-calving system.

The management of intensive grazing systems was reported.[9] Briefly, systems are designed so that cows self-harvest the majority of their lactational feed requirements in situ, with pasture surplus to requirement in spring harvested as silage to be fed, alongside grain and coproduct-based "concentrate" feeds, when pasture supply is less than herd demand (see **Fig. 1**).[9] This latter phase coincides with the transition period in spring-calving seasonal herds.

The pasture growth profile is similar in shape in all intensive grazing systems with peak growth rates and feed quality in spring and growth rates generally declining through summer and autumn to a minimum in winter.[9,11] The total amount grown and the extent of the peaks and troughs in pasture growth rate vary between and within countries; however, conservation policies and supplementary feeding (ie, buffer feeding) strategies vary. As a result, grazing transition cows have varying amounts of

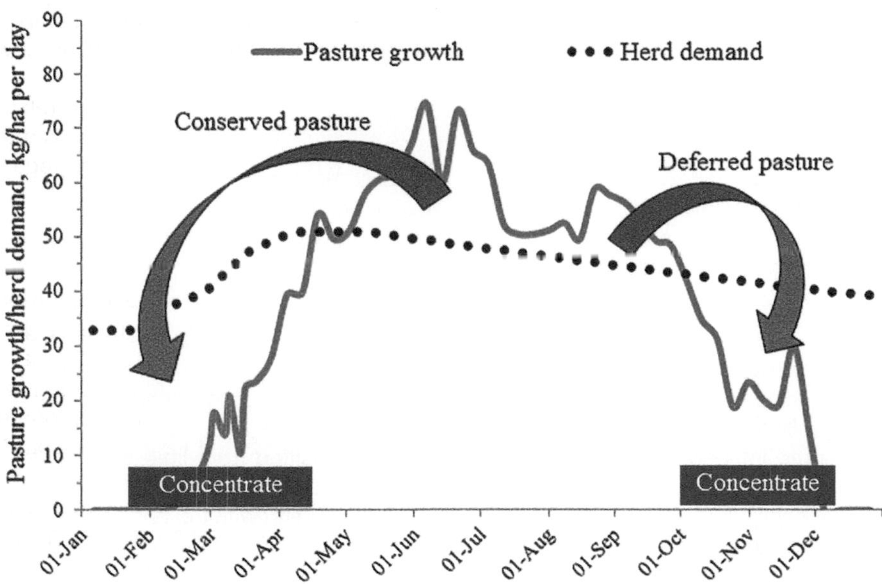

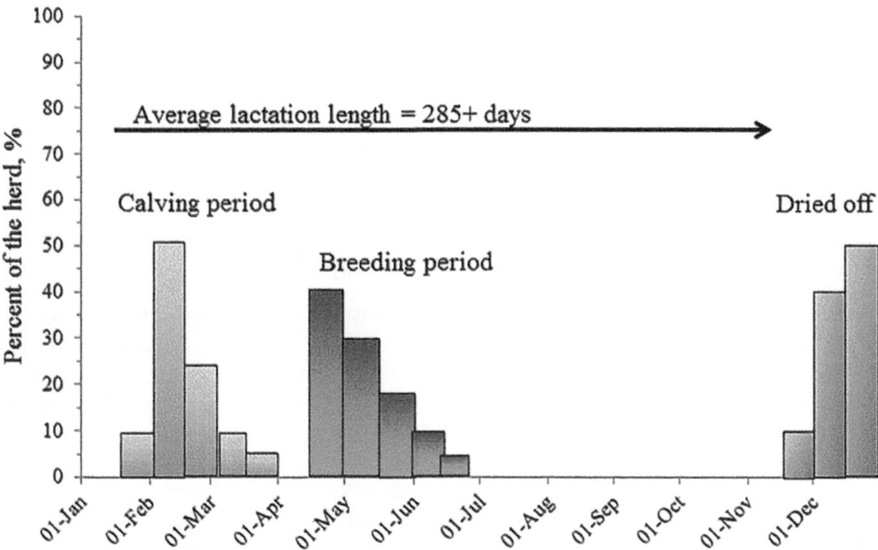

Fig. 1. Temporal pattern of daily pasture supply and herd demand. Pasture surplus to requirements during the first 6 months of the year is conserved as silage, whereas pasture surplus to requirements later in the season is deferred and grazed in situ. In most pasture-based systems, some form of grain- or coproduct-based concentrate is offered to cows in early and late lactation. Planned start of calving is approximately 60 days before pasture growth rate exceeds herd demand. This system requires a very fertile cow.

pasture in the diet pre- and post-calving, and pasture silage and corn silage, in situ-grazed brassica, and beet crops, and concentrate feeds can often be significant components of dry and freshening cow rations.

PROBLEM DEFINITION

Despite the similarity in cow- and tissue-level metabolic and immunologic changes during the transition from pregnancy to lactation in grazing and housed systems, there are system-level and nutrition-related differences that affect the ability of producers in grazing systems to manage the transition cow in a manner as precise as those managing cows in housed systems with TMR. For example:

1. The main feed is fresh and, if not used, is lost[12]; this is an important distinction from TMR-based systems, where forage not used can remain in the silo for later use.
2. The timing of calving increases the risk of weather-associated metabolic diseases (eg, milk fever, hypomagnesemic staggers, ketosis).[13,14]
3. In some intensive grazing systems, cows can transition from little or no grazed pasture before calving to greater than 50% of the diet as grazed pasture immediately post-calving (ie, significant diet transition coinciding with the physiologic transition) and grazed pasture becomes an ever-greater part of the cow's diet during the first 60 days in milk.
4. The producer has limited control over cow DMI, with variable DM yields of pasture in a fixed paddock area and intensive management systems based on area allocation on a daily basis.
5. The nutrient composition of feeds offered and the consistency of these feeds in metabolizable energy (ME) (amount and type), amino acid, and mineral composition vary significantly[11] between and, even, within days, because of individual cow grazing behaviors, variable weather, and the "fresh" and variable quality of pasture as a feed.

These challenges make attempting to "balance" the daily ration futile, with the general approach to nutrition of the transition grazing cow, instead, being pragmatism over precision. Managing the transition cow primarily relates to:

1. ensuring cows reach an adequate body condition score (BCS) before calving
2. managing cow DMI before calving
3. "fortifying" the daily diet with:
   a. Non-fiber carbohydrates (NFC)
   b. trace elements
   c. magnesium pre- and post-calving
   d. anionic salts pre-calving to overcome high levels of potassium
   e. a "starter drench" or calcium supplementation during the fresh/colostrum-producing period and, sometimes, throughout early lactation.

Although requirements for protein increase from pre-calving to peak milk production, post-calving pasture-based diets are, generally, very high in protein and rapid rumen passage rates ensure large quantities of metabolizable protein reach the small intestine.[12] Management strategies to facilitate a successful transition in grazing systems will be further discussed.

BODY CONDITION SCORE

Although not strictly transition cow management, optimizing BCS during the last trimester has been identified as a key factor in successfully transitioning from pregnancy to lactation[15] and therefore is an important point to consider in the management of the grazing transition cow.

Too low a calving BCS reduces milk production and increases the duration of the postpartum anestrous interval, delaying the time to a successful breeding and thereby reducing the efficiency of seasonal calving systems (see Roche and colleagues).[15] This is particularly true in young cows (ie, 2 and 3 year old).[15] Too high a BCS increases the risk of hyperketonemia[16] and associated disorders associated with excessive lipolysis and a lower DMI after calving, including milk fever (clinical hypocalcemia).[13] Roche and colleagues[15] recommended an optimum calving BCS (5-point scale) of 3.0 (adult cows) to 3.25 (young cows) to achieve close to maximum milk production potential while minimizing the DMI-reducing effects of adiposity and the increased risk of hyperketonemia.

A further relevant point regarding grazing systems is that the efficiency with which ME in autumn pasture is used for BCS gain (ie, k_G) is low relative to DM digestibility-comparable feeds. Mandok and coworkers[17] confirmed that even with improved pasture species and varieties, the k_G of autumn pasture is approximately 20% to 30% less than spring pasture, pasture silage derived from spring pasture, maize silage, and concentrate feeds at the same estimated ME content. This means that more feed and more time are required to enable grazing cows to meet their BCS targets.

The speed at which BCS is gained during mid-late gestation does not affect physiologic function in the next lactation,[18] but because of the low k_G of autumn pasture, approximately 300 kg DM of autumn pasture must be consumed above maintenance, lactation, and pregnancy requirements for a 0.5 unit increase in BCS.[17] Because of this, in intensive grazing systems with small inputs of supplementary feeds, low BCS dairy cows need longer non-lactating periods (ie, shorter lactations) before calving to facilitate BCS recovery before the next calving event. This must be factored into the management of mid-gestation grazing cows to optimize the transition from pregnancy to lactation.

Body condition is lost during the post-calving transition phase; the rate of loss occurs at a maximum rate during the first 10-days of lactation,[19] declining for 50 to 70 days, when peak intake of ME is sufficient to meet peak lactation demands. Intake and diet composition during the first 4 to 5 week of lactation has very limited, if any, effects on net BCS change,[15] as the process is primarily under the control of cow genetics,[20,21] with the key management lever being calving BCS.

The management implications of this are multifold. Herd BCS assessment at 200 days post-calving should be used to segregate the herd into BCS categories, and herd management strategies that ensure calving BCS targets are met and not superseded are established (eg, once-daily milking and/or short lactation for low BCS cows, use of supplementary feeds during the non-lactating period). Nutrition of the post-calving transition cow should not be focused on BCS management. Some advisers recommend feeding concentrate feeds to grazing dairy cows during early lactation to increase milk production and minimize BCS loss. Although concentrates will increase milk production, the smallest response to supplements is in early lactation[22–24] and this strategy does not influence BCS loss. The management focus must be on ensuring the cow is at the correct BCS entering the pre-calving phase of the transition period.

MANAGING PRE-CALVING DRY MATTER INTAKE

In most situations, the "drive to eat" increases with energy and nutrient requirements, an evolutionary feature regulated by the central nervous system.[25] The exception to this rule is, putatively, the prepartum dairy cow, whose DMI has been reported to decline during the weeks preceding parturition,[26,27] despite the increased energy requirements for fetal growth and lactogenesis.[1] This decline has been associated with elevated blood BHB concentrations and a greater risk of hepatic steatosis at calving.[27]

The reported decline in DMI, however, is not universal and is not generally of concern in the transition cow in intensive grazing systems. There was no decline in DMI in the weeks preceding calving in dairy cows fed a 50:50 mixture of fresh pasture and pasture hay, irrespective of whether cows were fed to ME requirements or restricted to 80% of requirements[28] and there was no change in feeding activity until the final 3 days pre-calving.[29] The difference in DMI profile between forage- and TMR-fed animals is probably diet-related, with high-estrogen concentrations associated with late pregnancy reported to reduce the consumption of starch but not fermentable fiber.[26,30,31]

Alongside the concern regarding the prepartum decline in DMI, the amount consumed has also been a topic of debate. Since the early twentieth century, researchers have been attentive to the importance of DMI pre-calving. Boutflour[32], for example, postulated the importance of pre-calving nutrient intake, identifying "*the neglect of the preparation of the cow for her lactation period*" as one of the four most important factors limiting milk production. Early studies in grazing transition cows[33] agreed, concluding that cows fed to gain liveweight during the last 4 weeks of pregnancy produced 15% to 21% more milk fat in the subsequent lactation compared with cows fed to lose liveweight. Furthermore, the difference could not be redressed through better feeding in early lactation. These early results, however, may reflect very low feeding levels, poor quality forages, and, potentially, low BCS cows.

More recently, epidemiologic assessments have linked blood markers of energy state pre-calving (as a proxy for DMI) with health post-calving.[34,35] These studies concluded that improved energy state pre-calving was associated with positive outcomes post-calving, confirming results of Bertics and colleagues.[27] The recommendation for producers and their advisers therefore became one of ensuring cow DMI and diet ME density was increased in the weeks preceding calving.

A closer examination, however, reveals inconsistencies[27]; for example, cows in the high pre-calving DMI group had greater plasma circulating fatty acid concentrations and almost double the plasma BHB concentrations at 2 week postpartum compared with cows in the low pre-calving DMI group and there was no effect of pre-partum DMI on liver triacylglycerol (TAG) content at 4 week postpartum. Two decades of research in grazing cows and housed cows consuming a TMR have concluded that cows that are "limit fed" to between 80% and 100% of ME requirements for several weeks before calving enter lactation in a more "metabolically-fit" state and have increased capacity for hepatic gluconeogenesis and β-oxidation, reduced hepatic TAG accumulation, and a reduced risk of milk fever and ketosis.[2,36]

In summary, although epidemiologic studies have pointed to a positive effect of increased DMI prepartum on subsequent health and productivity, experiments to test this hypothesis do not support such an effect, with increasing evidence that a small negative energy balance pre-calving may improve post-calving energy balance, metabolic health indices, immune function, and milk production.

The collective results have implications for how grazing transition dairy cows are managed. As protein intakes are generally in excess of requirements, because of the high-protein content of the predominant forages in grazing systems, ME intake can generally be limited without resulting in an amino acid deficiency. This can be achieved by reducing the allocation of DM each day (ie, a smaller grazing area) or through the inclusion of forages with a lower energy density (eg, silages, hay, straw) in lieu of fresh forage. The system will dictate the most appropriate strategy. For example, if cows are being offered predominantly precision-chopped pasture silage, reducing DMI might increase the risk of displaced abomasum (anecdotal reports); instead, ME intake should be limited by incorporating lower digestibility forages. However, if long-chop silage, baleage, or fresh pasture is the predominant feed, reducing the amount of DM consumed through access restriction is an effective way to best manage the grazing transition cow.

FORTIFYING THE TRANSITION COW DIET

Fresh pasture is a highly digestible feed with a good amino acid profile and reasonable vitamin and mineral composition.[11,12] Inductive reasoning of some requirements relative to diet supply has resulted in recommendations that are poorly supported by evidence. For moderate producing dairy cows, there is limited need to fortify the diet nutritionally, with the factor first limiting production in most scenarios being intake of ME.[12] Nevertheless, diet variability and prevailing weather can impact the cow's ability to consume sufficient quantities of some nutrients, particularly during the transition period. There can be a need, therefore, to fortify the diet with key items.

Nonfiber Carbohydrates

The metabolic requirements for glucose increase exponentially in the weeks preceding calving and into lactation,[1] leading some to recommend the need for including glucogenic precursors (NFC) in the pre-calving diet of grazing cows (for a detailed review of this rationale, see Roche and colleagues).[2] Overton and Waldron[37] reported that some studies observed increased DMI, reduced blood fatty acids and BHB, and increased postpartum milk production in cows supplemented with NFC sources pre-calving, but that most of these studies were confounded by energy intake as well as carbohydrate source. TMR-fed cows[38] and pasture-grazed cows[39] were offered isoenergetic diets that differed in their carbohydrate composition. Smith and colleagues[38] compared 34% and 40% NFC and Roche and colleagues[39] compared 13% and 32% NFC in the prepartum ration. Post-calving milk yield, composition, and BCS change were not affected by pre-calving carbohydrate type in either TMR or pasture-fed cows, refuting the hypothesized benefits of pre-calving dietary NFC inclusion. Higgs and colleagues[40] concluded similarly when they compared fermentable-fiber, starch, and sugar-based supplements in early lactation. In short, there is no basis for a specific recommendation to supplement grazing cows with NFC before calving, as the applied research identified no effect of carbohydrate type- pre- or post-calving when compared in isoenergetic diets.[2]

Trace Elements

Trace elements concentrations vary seasonally (eg, copper) and with weather (eg, iodine) and can be compromised by anti-nutritive factors in some grazed forages (eg, goitrogens). As a result, it is generally recommended that the grazing transition cow is supplemented with copper, cobalt, selenium, iodine, and zinc.[41]

Magnesium Supplementation Pre- and Post-Calving

Pre-calving magnesium intake is, arguably, the single greatest dietary factor influencing the risk of milk fever.[13,42] In an analysis of 30 years of data, milk fever prevalence dropped from greater than 10% to less than 5% following the introduction of pre-calving magnesium supplementation in the late 1970s/early 1980s.[13] Although pasture often has adequate magnesium concentration (0.18%–0.20% DM),[11] it is variable within and between paddocks, is combined with high dietary potassium in fresh forages (>3.3% DM),[11] which reduces ruminal magnesium absorption, and high rainfall events, as are common during the transition period, can reduce DMI and hence daily magnesium intake. As a result, magnesium supplementation is recommended.[43]

Magnesium sulfate and magnesium chloride are more effective than magnesium oxide in maintaining periparturient eucalcemia,[44] but dusting pastures with magnesium oxide pre-grazing is a very pragmatic and effective strategy, allowing cows to consume the magnesium while grazing. Because of the daily need for magnesium and limitations to achieving necessary uptake on a high potassium forage diet in winter, it is recommended that cows receive 0.35% DM and 0.28% DM magnesium in their diet pre- and post-calving.

Anionic Salts Pre-Calving to Overcome High Levels of Potassium

Research undertaken in TMR-feeding systems suggests that potassium is the primary nutritional factor contributing to milk fever through its effect on the dietary cation–anion difference (DCAD).[2,45] Because of this, high potassium forages should be minimized in the weeks before calving.[46] If this contraindication was appropriate for pasture-fed cows, 100% of cows would get milk fever due to the very high potassium content of temperate pastures. In contrast, the incidence of milk fever in pasture-based herds is low[8,47] and New Zealand data indicated no difference in blood calcium around calving when cows were fed pastures varying between 3.3% and 4.2% DM potassium, the natural range in productive temperate pastures during winter–spring.[44] This does not mean that potassium is unimportant. Potassium interferes with the ruminal absorption of magnesium and, as magnesium is important for calcium absorption, thereby increases the risk of milk fever. However, in grazing cows, it seems secondary in importance to magnesium supplementation.

The proportion of potassium, sodium, chlorine, and sulfur in the diet are used to calculate the DCAD, which influences the acidity/alkalinity of blood (blood pH)[48] and, thereby, calcium absorption from the intestine and bone calcium homeostasis.[49,50] The DCAD of pasture is very high, particularly during the transition period (+300–500 meq/kg DM).[51] Blood and urine pH drop when DCAD is less than +150 meq/kg DM,[49,51,52] although this fall is precipitous, as is the risk of milk fever, when DCAD is less than 0 meq/kg DM.[53] Achieving such a low DCAD is not practical when fresh or conserved pasture is a significant part of the transition cow ration.

A "Starter Drench" or Calcium Supplementation During the Fresh/Colostrum-Producing Period and Sometimes Throughout Early Lactation

Calcium supplementation during early lactation increases blood calcium concentrations[44,54] and thereby reduces the risk of hypocalcemia and clinical milk fever. However, this effect seems limited to the first 2-days post-calving[44] in moderate yielding pasture-grazed cows, with increased intestinal absorption and bone resorption initiated with colostrogenesis. In grazing systems, calcium can be provided as part of a "fresh cow" concentrate feed at milking, as a ground limestone or dicalcium phosphate powder applied to fresh pasture or the silage supplement, or as part of a "starter drench" in grazing systems in which supplementary feeds are not provided.

Starter drenches are commercially available products or mixes created by the producer to supplement "fresh cows" during the 4-days immediately post-calving. They vary in constituents, but generally contain calcium and an energy source, such as molasses, propylene glycol or propionate supplements, and, in some cases, sodium monensin as a gluconeogenic stimulant. There are limited research studies investigating the use of "starter drenches" in grazing systems and results are inconsistent.[2] Use in "at risk" cows (eg, older, high BCS cows), if they can be easily identified, could improve health and productivity, but the lack of consistent health or production responses across experiments do not support the routine administration of starter drenches.

CLINICS CARE POINTS

- Approximately 200 days after the start of the seasonal calving period, assess cow BCS and separate thin cows for preferential BCS management.
- Thin cows can be transferred to a herd to be milked once a day or dried off and offered additional feed to ensure appropriate BCS at calving.
- Speed of BCS gain in mid-late gestation does not affect post-calving BCS loss.
- During the 2-3 weeks preceding calving, management should aim to feed cows 80-100% of metabolizable energy requirements.
- If long chop forages are the predominant feed (e.g., fresh pasture, hay, long chop silage), the limit feeding can be maintained by physical feed restriction.
- If diet forages are precision chopped or more than one-third of the diet is concentrate feeds, care to avoid displaced abomasum is required and limit feeding should be achieved through inclusion of low energy-high fiber feeds (e.g., straw, coarse hay).
- Supplement cows with 20-30 g magnesium for 2-3 weeks before and up to 3 months after calving, even when pasture magnesium concentration would appear adequate.
- A trace element supplementation strategy should be developed by the producer and their veterinary adviser to ensure cows before and after calving have adequate copper, cobalt, selenium, iodine, and zinc.
- Supplement cows during the first few days post-calving with up to 100 g calcium.
- Starter drenches may benefit cows at greater risk of metabolic diseases (eg, older, over-conditioned cows), but routine administration is costly and is not supported by the scientific evidence.

SUMMARY

Grazing systems are not homogenous, and pasture quantity and quality vary within and between farms, such that management of the transition cow is focused more on pragmatism than precision. Achieving target BCS before calving is a foundation on which to manage the transition period. Cow metabolism is optimized when cows consume 80% to 100% of their ME requirements; DMI does not decline in cows consuming a primarily forage-based diet until the onset of parturition and type of carbohydrate fed has little or no impact on a successful transition.

A very large amount of anionic salts is required to achieve less than 0 meq/kg DM DCAD if fresh or conserved pasture is an appreciable component of the cow diet before calving. This, and the inability to precisely manage DCAD because of the variability in mineral intake, means that it is not an effective strategy for milk fever prevention in grazing cows. In pre-calving and post-calving, the cow should receive supplementary magnesium and trace elements, with calcium supplementation an important milk fever prevention strategy during the days immediately post-calving.

REFERENCES

1. Bell AW. Regulation of organic nutrient metabolism during transition from late pregnancy to early lactation. J Anim Sci 1995;73:2804–19.

2. Roche JR, Bell AW, Overton TR, et al. Nutritional management of the transition cow in the 21st century – a paradigm shift in thinking. Anim Prod Sci 2013;53: 1000–23.
3. White HM, Donkin SS, Lucy MC, et al. Short communication: Genetic differences between New Zealand and North American dairy cows alter milk production and gluconeogenic enzyme expression. J Dairy Sci 2012;95:455–9.
4. Lucy MC, Verkerk GA, Whyte BE, et al. Somatotropic axis components and nutrient partitioning in genetically diverse dairy cows managed under different feed allowances in a pasture system. J Dairy Sci 2009;92:526–39.
5. Grala TM, Lucy MC, Phyn CVC, et al. Somatotropic axis and concentrate supplementation in grazing dairy cows of genetically diverse origin. J Dairy Sci 2011;94: 303–15.
6. Crookenden MA, Heiser A, Murray A, et al. Parturition in dairy cows temporarily alters the expression of genes in circulating neutrophils. J Dairy Sci 2016;99: 6470–83.
7. Crookenden MA, Walker CG, Peiris H, et al. Short communication: Proteins from circulating exosomes represent metabolic state in transition dairy cows. J Dairy Sci 2016;99:7661–8.
8. Spaans OK, Kuhn-Sherlock B, Hickey A, et al. Temporal profiles describing markers of inflammation and metabolism during the transition period of pasture-based, seasonal-calving dairy cows. J Dairy Sci 2022;105:2669–98.
9. Roche JR, Washburn SP, Berry DP, et al. Seasonal pasture-based dairy production systems. In: Beede D, editor. Large dairy herd management. 3rd edition. Champaign, IL, USA: American Dairy Science Association; 2017. p. 99–114.
10. Spaans OK, Macdonald KA, Neal M, et al. A quantitative case study assessment of biophysical and economic effects from altering season of calving in temperate pasture-based dairy systems. J Dairy Sci 2019;102:11523–35.
11. Roche JR, Turner LR, Lee JM, et al. Weather, herbage quality and milk production in pastoral systems. 2. Temporal patterns and intra-relationships in herbage quality and mineral concentration parameters. Anim Prod Sci 2009;49:200–10.
12. Roche JR. Nutrition management of grazing dairy cattle. In: Webster J, editor. Achieving sustainable production of milk. Volume 3: dairy herd management. Cambridge, UK: Burleigh-Dodds Science Publishing; 2017. p. 251–72.
13. Roche JR, Berry DP. Periparturient climatic, animal, and management factors influencing the incidence of milk fever in grazing systems. J Dairy Sci 2006;89: 2775–83.
14. Hendriks SJ, Phyn CVC, Turner S-A, et al. Effect of weather on activity and lying behaviour in clinically healthy grazing dairy cows during the transition period. Anim Prod Sci 2020;60:148–53.
15. Roche JR, Friggens NC, Kay JK, et al. Berry DP Invited review: Body condition score and its association with dairy cow productivity, health, and welfare. J Dairy Sci 2009;92:5769–801.
16. Gillund P, Reksen O, Grohn YT, et al. Body condition related to ketosis and reproductive performance in Norwegian dairy cows. J Dairy Sci 2001;84:1390–6.
17. Mandok KM, Kay JK, Greenwood SL, et al. Efficiency of use of metabolizable energy for body weight gain in pasture-based, nonlactating dairy cows. J Dairy Sci 2014;97:4639–48.
18. Roche JR, Heiser A, Mitchell MD, et al. Strategies to gain body condition score in pasture-based dairy cows during late lactation and the far-off nonlactating period and their interaction with close-up dry matter intake. J Dairy Sci 2017;99: 1720–38.

19. Roche JR, Berry DP, Lee JM, et al. Describing the body condition score change between successive calvings: A novel strategy generalizable to diverse cohorts. J Dairy Sci 2007;90:4378–96.
20. McNamara JP, Hillers JK. Regulation of bovine adipose tissue metabolism during lactation. 1. Lipid synthesis in response to increased milk production and decreased energy intake. J Dairy Sci 1986;69:3032–41.
21. McNamara JP, Hillers JK. Regulation of bovine adipose tissue metabolism during lactation. 2. Lipolysis response to milk production and energy intake. J Dairy Sci 1986;69:3042–50.
22. Stockdale CR. Levels of pasture substitution when concentrates are fed to grazing dairy cows in northern Victoria. Aust J Exp Agric 2000;40:913–21.
23. Bargo F, Muller LD, Kolver ES, et al. Invited review: Production and digestion of supplemented dairy cows on pasture. J Dairy Sci 2003;86:1–42.
24. Poole C, Donaghy DJ, White RR, et al. Association among pasture-level variables and dairy cow responses to supplements. Anim Prod Sci 2019;60:118–20.
25. Roche JR, Blache D, Kay J, et al. Neuroendocrine and physiological regulation of intake, with particular reference to domesticated ruminant animals. Nutr Res Rev 2008;21:207–34.
26. Coppock CE, Noller CH, Wolfe SA, et al. Effect of forage-concentrate ratio in complete feeds fed ad libitum on feed intake prepartum and the occurrence of abomasal displacement in dairy cows. J Dairy Sci 1972;55:783–9.
27. Bertics SJ, Grummer RR, Cadorniga-Valino C, et al. Effect of prepartum dry matter intake on liver triglyceride concentration and early lactation. J Dairy Sci 1992; 75:1914–22.
28. Roche JR. Short Communication: Dry matter intake precalving in cows offered fresh and conserved pasture. J Dairy Res 2006;73:273–6.
29. Hendriks SJ, Phyn CVC, Turner S-A, et al. Lying behavior and activity during the transition period of clinically healthy grazing dairy cows. J Dairy Sci 2019;102: 7371–84.
30. Forbes JM. Effects of oestradiol-17β on voluntary food intake in ruminants. J Endocrino 1972;52:8–9.
31. Forbes JM. Voluntary food intake and diet selection in farm animals. 2nd edition. Wallingford, UK: CAB International; 2007.
32. Boutflour RB. Limiting factors in the feeding and management of milk cows. In: Report from World's dairy Congress. 1928. p. 15-20.
33. Hutton JB, Parker OF. 1973. The significance of differences in levels of feeding, before and after calving, on milk yield under intensive grazing. N Z J Agric Res 1973;16:95–104.
34. Dyk PB, Emery RS, Liesman JL, et al. Prepartum non-esterified fatty acids in plasma are higher in cows developing periparturient health problems. J Dairy Sci 1995;78(Suppl 1):337.
35. Sheehy MR, Fahey AG, Aungier SPM, et al. A comparison of serum metabolic and production profiles of dairy cows that maintained or lost body condition 15 days before calving. J Dairy Sci 2017;100:536–47.
36. Kay JK, Loor JJ, Heiser A, et al. Managing the grazing dairy cow through the transition period: a review. Anim Prod Sci 2015;55:936–42.
37. Overton TR. Waldron MR Nutritional management of transition dairy cows: strategies to optimize metabolic health. J Dairy Sci 2004;87(E. Suppl):E105–19.
38. Smith KL, Waldron MR, Ruzzi LC, et al. Metabolism of dairy cows as affected by prepartum dietary carbohydrate source and supplementation with chromium throughout the periparturient period. J Dairy Sci 2008;91:2011–20.

39. Roche JR, Kay JK, Phyn CVC, et al. Dietary structural to nonfiber carbohydrate concentration during the transition period in grazing dairy cows. J Dairy Sci 2010;93:3671–83.
40. Higgs RJ, Sheahan AJ, Mandok K, et al. The effect of starch-, fiber-, or sugar-based supplements on nitrogen utilization in grazing dairy cows. J Dairy Sci 2013;96:3857–66.
41. Dairy NZ. Farmfact: Trace elements. 2023. Available at: https://www.dairynz.co.nz/animal/cow-health/trace-elements/. Accessed January 20, 2023.
42. Lean IJ, DeGaris PJ, McNeil DM, et al. Hypocalcemia in dairy cows: meta-analysis and dietary cation anion difference theory revisited. J Dairy Sci 2006;89:669–84.
43. Dairy NZ. Farmfact: Magnesium supplementation. 2023. Available at: https://www.dairynz.co.nz/publications/farmfacts/animal-health-welfare-and-young-stock/farmfact-3-1/. Accessed January 20, 2023.
44. Roche JR, Morton J, Kolver ES. Sulfur and chlorine play a non-acid base role in periparturient calcium homeostasis. J Dairy Sci 2002;85:3444–53.
45. Goff JP, Horst RL. Effects of the addition of potassium or sodium, but not calcium, to prepartum rations on milk fever in dairy cows. J Dairy Sci 1997;80:176–86.
46. National Research Council. Nutrient requirements of dairy cattle. 7th revised edition. Washington, DC: National Academy Press; 2001.
47. McDougall S. Effects of periparturient diseases and conditions on the reproductive performance of New Zealand dairy cows. N Z Vet J 2001;49:60–7.
48. Stewart PA. Modern quantitative acid-base chemistry. Can J Physiol Pharmacol 1983;61:1444–61.
49. Roche JR, Dalley DE, O'Mara FP. Effect of a metabolically created systemic acidosis on calcium homeostasis and the diurnal variation in urine pH in the non-lactating pregnant dairy cow. J Dairy Res 2007;74:34–9.
50. Van Mosel M, Wouterse HS, Van't Klooster AT. Effects of reducing dietary [Na + K]-[Cl+S] on bone in dairy cows at parturition. Res Vet Sci 1994;56:270–6.
51. Roche JR, Dalley D, Moate P, et al. Variations in the dietary cation-anion difference and the acid-base balance of dairy cows on a pasture-based diet in south-eastern Australia. Grass Forage Sci 2000;55:26–36.
52. Roche JR, Dalley D, Moate P, et al. Dietary cation-anion difference and the health and production of pasture-fed dairy cows 2. Nonlactating periparturient cows. J Dairy Sci 2003;86:979–87.
53. Charbonneau E, Pellerin D, Oetzel G. Impact of lowering dietary cation-anion difference in nonlactating dairy cows: a meta-analysis. J Dairy Sci 2006;89:537–48.
54. Roche JR, Dalley D, Moate P, et al. A low dietary cation-anion difference precalving and calcium supplementation postcalving increase plasma calcium but not milk production in a pasture-based system. J Dairy Sci 2003;86:2658–66.

Metabolic Diseases in Beef Cattle

Megan S. Hindman, MS, DVM

KEYWORDS

• Beef cattle • Metabolic diseases • Hypomagnesemia • Acidosis
• Nutritional deficiency

KEY POINTS

- Diagnosis of hypomagnesemia can be determined antemortem via serum samples.
- Physical examination findings, feeding history, and type of feedstuff all can be used to diagnose rumen acidosis.
- Sulfur toxicity can be one of the precursors to polioencephalomalacia.
- Manganese deficiency has been shown to cause chrondrodysplastic calves.
- Protein-energy malnutrition is primarily due to low forage quality being fed during gestation.

INTRODUCTION

Metabolic diseases are typically thought of as dairy cattle problems. Management type and structure come to top of mind when discussing metabolic diseases in cattle and can be one of the predisposing factors as far as how it occurs. In one study, a prevalence of 2% was found for ruminant acidosis in a feedlot; however, there is little prevalence information published with regard to metabolic diseases in beef cattle.[1] Metabolic diseases covered in this article are hypomagnesemia, ruminal acidosis, and all of the common sequelae, polioencephalomalacia, manganese deficiency, and protein-energy malnutrition (PEM). Urinary calculi would also be considered a metabolic disease but is covered in depth in elsewhere in this issue.

HYPOMAGNESEMIA

Magnesium (Mg) is an essential macromineral needed to complete many biochemical processes throughout the body. Deficiencies of Mg, also known as *hypomagnesemic tetany, grass staggers, grass tetany,* or *wheat pasture poisoning,* are caused by a metabolism disorder in ruminants. This disease affects goats, sheep, beef, and dairy

Veterinary Production Animal Medicine Department, Iowa State University, 1712 S Riverside Dr, Ames, IA 50010, USA
E-mail address: mpieters@iastate.edu

Vet Clin Food Anim 39 (2023) 337–353
https://doi.org/10.1016/j.cvfa.2023.02.011

cattle. Magnesium is well absorbed from the small intestine of young calves and lambs.[2,3] As the animal ages, the rumen and reticulum become more developed, becoming the main site for Mg absorption.[4–7] Several ions can alter Mg absorption in the body. The most common ion known to disrupt Mg absorption is potassium (K). Increased oral K intake can significantly reduce Mg absorption from the gastrointestinal tract, suggested by reducing the passive driving force for luminal Mg uptake by changing the gradient across the membrane.[4,8–13] Sodium (Na) also alters Mg absorption by increasing aldosterone production and secretion, increasing K concentrations in the saliva and further into the rumen.[14,15] This has been confirmed in research with sheep that decreased Na, increased ruminal K concentration, and reduced Mg absorption in the forestomaches.[16] Several studies have demonstrated acute increases in ruminal NH_4^+ concentration, such as forages with a higher concentration of crude protein, have decreased Mg absorption.[17–19] In addition, organic acids such as trans-aconitate, which can be found in range grasses such as timothy (*Phleum pratense*), have been suggested to be involved in the pathogenesis of grass tetany.[20–23] This is a proposed pathogenesis due to the three exposed carboxyl groups that are sites for Mg-chelation. [24] Hypomagnesemia can affect calcium (Ca) absorption in two ways. Moderate hypomagnesemia interferes with parathyroid hormone action, reducing the tissues' sensitivity and inhibiting secretion in response to hypocalcemia.[25] In a study on grazing beef calves on pastures at risk for tetany developing, observed clinical signs of cows with tetany were when both Mg and Ca concentrations were below normal.[26]

Pathogenesis/Clinical Signs

Hypomagnesemia is commonly observed in lush pastures high in K and nitrogen and low in Mg and Na but can also be observed with any feedstuffs that contain previously listed ion relationships. Once plasma Mg falls below 0.5 mmol/L (1.1 mg/dL), muscle fasciculations of the face, shoulder, and flank can be observed.[3,13] Hypomagnesemia overtime will lower Mg in the cerebrospinal fluid, causing neurologic signs such as chomping of the jaws, frothy salivation, arched head, paddling of the legs, aggression, marked nystagmus, and eyelids fluttering. The heartbeat can be markedly increased with the heart rate approaching 150 beats per minute and the heart audible without a stethoscope.[3] In addition, the respiratory rate is increased to 60 breaths/min, and rectal temperature can also be increased.[3] Hypomagnesemia also affects Ca status by reducing sensitivity to parathyroid hormone or reducing its secretion in response to hypocalcemia.[25] Therefore, clinical signs can also mimic secondary acute hypocalcemia.

Diagnosis

Diagnosis of hypomagnesemia is based on clinical signs paired with a history of suggestive low Mg-containing feedstuff. The serum is an appropriate antemortem sample to determine Mg status. Serum Mg less than 0.41 to 0.57 mmol/L (<1.0–1.4 mg/dL) indicates hypomagnesemia, and less than 0.21 mmol/L (0.5 mg/dL) indicates imminent tetany.[27] Caution is warranted as additional stress of working cattle suspected of hypomagnesemia can exacerbate the clinical signs of disease, such as convulsions or death. Vitreous humor or cerebrospinal fluid can be used postmortem to diagnose hypomagnesemia. Cerebrospinal fluid less than 0.51 mmol/L (1.25 mg/dL) or vitreous humor concentrations less than 0.24 mmol/L (1.16 mg/dL) is diagnostic of hypomagnesemia.[27] Vitreous humor samples can be obtained by an 18-gauge needle 2 to 4 mL volume up to 48 hours after death at ambient temperature.[28,29]

Treatment/Prevention

Animals exhibiting clinical signs of hypomagnesemia need immediate treatment. This generally requires 1.5 to 2.25 g Mg intravenous (IV) in the adult cow paired with IV calcium.[3] Once administered, cows should not be stimulated to increase for at least 30 minutes after therapy due to the potential initiation of convulsions. Magnesium enemas can be an alternative to IV therapies in a convulsing or aggressive patient. For an adult cow, 60 g of Mg chloride or 60 g of Mg sulfate dissolved in 200 mL of water can be administered into the descending colon.[30] Once administered, it has been demonstrated to increase plasma Mg concentration within 10 minutes.[31,32] Finally, if the esophageal function is present, oral administration of Mg salts can provide a sustained response to plasma Mg concentration. This can be achieved by drenching the cow with a slurry of 100 g Mg oxide mixed with 100 g Ca chloride, 100 g Na phosphate, and 50 g Na chloride.[30] Alternatively, 200 to 400 mL of 50% Mg sulfate solution is more bioavailable for absorption than Mg oxide.[30]

Once a clinical case of hypomagnesemia has been diagnosed in a herd, getting 10 to 15 g of Mg into each pregnant cow and 20 g of Mg into a lactating beef cow can prevent hypomagnesemia tetany from occurring.[33] Owing to palatability concerns, adding Mg oxide to grain, feeding hay, or mixing it with more palatable ingredients, such as molasses, can ensure adequate uptake and decrease feed refusals.

In addition, a forage risk ratio (K mEq./[Ca mEq. + Mg mEq.]) can be calculated using wet chemistry on forages to determine the risk of inducing hypomagnesemia and placing preventative measures in place before forages being fed.[34] A forage risk ratio greater than 2.2 is considered to be indicative of hypomagnesemia risk.

RUMEN ACIDOSIS

Rumen acidosis is the most common metabolic disease in feedlot beef cattle as a result of the typical high-grain diets being fed to finishing cattle. The excessive production of volatile fatty acids (VFA) and potentially lactate exceeds the rumen's ability to maintain a stable pH and precipitate clinical disease conditions. A variety of dietary, management, and environmental factors contribute to rumen acidosis (**Box 1**).

Pathophysiology

Rumen Acidosis can be broken down into two categories: subacute rumen acidosis (SARA) and acute rumen acidosis. SARA is defined as intermittent periods of low pH that are acute and chronic. Clinical acute rumen acidosis occurs when an increase in organic acids accumulates, resulting in a rumen fluid pH of less than 5.2.[36,37]

Box 1
Predisposing factors influencing a decrease in rumen pH

Predisposing factors influencing a decrease in rumen pH.

- Feedstuffs with small particle size (hay 75–125 mm and silage 13–19 mm)[35]
- Highly fermentable feeds and types of processing (ie, whole corn vs steam flake corn)
- Weather changes
- Equipment or personnel errors
- Short adaption period
- Feeding high-concentrate feed long term
- Introduction of concentrate feeds without proper adaption period

The main difference between SARA and acute acidosis, besides the duration of decreased rumen pH, is the mechanism that causes the decline in pH. In acute rumen acidosis, VFAs and lactate influence the rumen pH decline, whereas in SARA, only VFAs are involved.[36,38] **Fig. 1** illustrates the common disease processes and sequelae that occur when a beef feedlot animal undergoes an SARA event.

Clinical Signs

Clinical signs can vary depending on the amount and type of feedstuff ingested. For cattle affected with SARA, clinical signs can be rather nonspecific such as transient anorexia, mild to moderate dehydration, and decreased rumen motility and may or may not have diarrhea.[40,41] Clinical signs for acute acidosis are separated into mild and severe categories. Mild clinical signs of acute acidosis may present as weak ruminal contraction, mild distention of the rumen, and mild signs of colic and may resolve with or without therapy.[42] Cattle with severe clinical signs of acute acidosis may present with dehydration, weakness, recumbency, profuse diarrhea, and death.[42] Temperature may vary depending on the duration of the disease; in early stages, temperatures may be elevated, compared with later progressions, and hypothermia is often observed.[43] Cardiovascular signs for acute acidosis may include increased heart rate, increased respiration rate, delayed jugular filling, prolonged capillary refill times, weak peripheral pulses, and cold distal extremities.[44] In addition, neurologic clinical signs may be observed in acute acidosis, such as obtundation, blindness, head pressing, opisthotonos, and altered gait.[44]

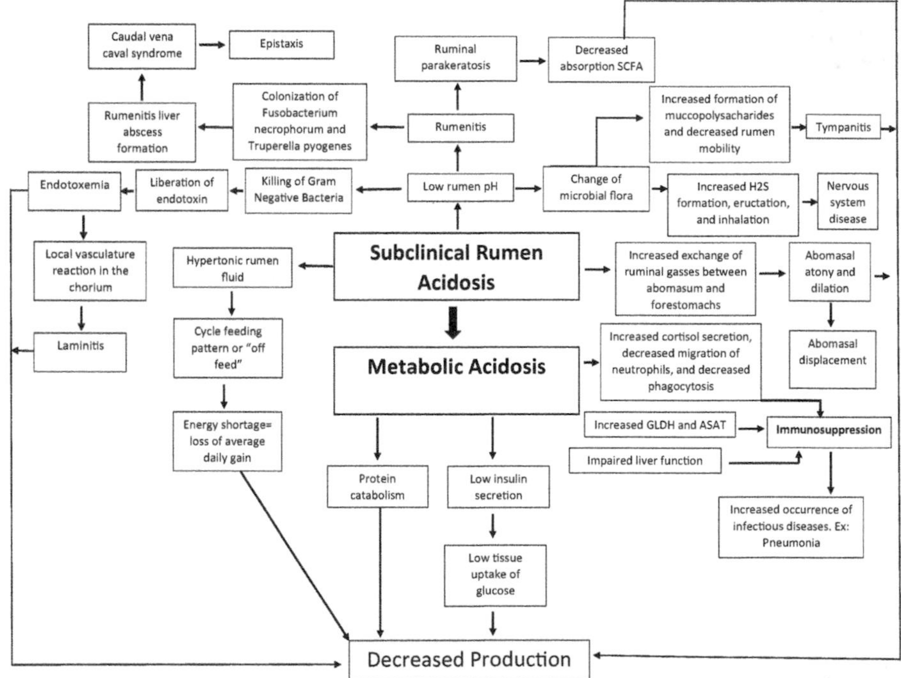

Fig. 1. Pathogenesis that occurs in a subclinical rumen acidosis event and the predisposing disease that can occur after. Figure extrapolated from Enemark and colleagues[39]. (Enemark JM, Jorgensen RJ, Enemark PS. Rumen acidosis with special emphasis on diagnostic aspects of subclinical rumen acidosis: a review. Veterinarija ir zootechnika. 2002 Jan 1;20(42):16-29. https://vetzoo.lsmuni.lt/data/vols/2002/20/pdf/enemark.pdf.)

Diagnosis

Rumen acidosis is initially diagnosed based on the history of feedstuff, feeding behavior, and clinical signs. Although clinical signs can mimic other disease manifestations, analysis of rumen fluid and other ancillary diagnostic tests can solidify an individual animal's initial diagnosis. There are two methods to determine rumen pH: rumenocentesis and oral stomach tube. Several studies have looked at difference between the methods of sample collection and observed differences in pH between the two methods.[45–50] This has been suggested due to the intraruminal location of the stomach tube, saliva contamination, and time of sampling about feeding can alter the ruminal pH reading when collected via stomach tube.[51] Despite the mild inconsistency in location, the author recognizes that completing a rumenocentesis for a herd-level diagnosis is not always feasible.

Additional telltale signs of acidosis in a beef feedlot situation can be:[36]

- Fecal scores with more than 20% loose stool or more than 5% watery
- Ten percent of cattle are lame
- Smeared wet areas lateral to the anus, "windshield wiper butt"
- Increased respiratory rate

Treatment/Prevention

In clinical acute rumen acidosis, aggressive treatment is required. An emergency rumenotomy and removal of the rumen contents should be completed initially before the contents exit into the lower gastrointestinal tract. IV fluids should be administered intraoperatively and continued postoperatively to correct electrolyte imbalances, control metabolic acidosis, and support against hypovolemic shock.[44] In addition, restoration of rumen contents or buffers that have been added may be accomplished by transfaunation post-rumenotomy. In less severe cases, flushing the rumen with warm water and magnesium hydroxide via an orogastric tube combined with IV 5% sodium bicarbonate solution may be enough to counter the acidosis.[42] Immediate harvest may be warranted in severe acute rumen acidosis cases if the animal can ambulate. Animals exhibiting mild clinical disease may recover spontaneously with no specific treatment. Prevention is a treatment strategy for animals affected by SARA.

The prevention of SARA in beef cattle revolves around one factor: management. Adequate acclimation between a roughage diet and a high-concentration diet is one of the main management strategies for preventing SARA. Managing feed bunks ensuring timely delivery of ration, a consistent amount the entire length of the bunk, and timely increase in total ration diets based on observed bunk scores also fall into feed bunk management. An example of a bunk scoring system used in a slick bunk setting for a feedlot can be seen in **Table 1**.[52] Ensuring proper mixing time based

Table 1
South Dakota State University feed bunk scoring system

Score	Description
0	No feed remaining in bunk
0.5	Scattered feed remaining, most of the bunk is exposed
1	Thin uniform layer of feed remaining, about one corn kernel deep
2	25%–50% of feed remaining
3	More than 50% of feed remaining
4	Feed is virtually untouched.

on the type of mixing equipment used has been shown to improve the consistency of a total mixed ration in beef cattle over time and reduce sorting, thus reducing risks for rumen acidosis.[53]

Common Sequelae

Ruminal Tympany. One of the common sequelae that occur after a rumen acidosis incidence is ruminal tympany. During the periods of acidosis, ruminal generation of lactic acid, VFAs, endotoxin, and histamine reduces ruminal contractions via chemoreceptors causing ruminal tympany or bloat to occur.[54] In addition, an increase of VFAs and lactic acid changes the rumen microflora, which can also lead to increased gas production in the rumen, leading to bloat.[37,54] Clinical signs that occur with bloat are mild to moderate distention of the paralumbar fossa. As it progresses, animals may show signs of respiratory distress due to increased intra-abdominal pressure from the expansion of the rumen, pressing on the diaphragm. If not treated, it may result in death. Treatment for bloat is completed by passing an orogastric tube to determine the type of bloat present. If free gas is present, maintain the stomach tube into the rumen until the gas is released and the paralumbar fossa is returned to normal. If froth is found at the end of the tube, placing a surface-active agent such as mineral oil, dioctyl sodium sulfosuccinate, or poloxalene down the tube can reduce the bubbles present in the rumen. Caution must be considered when administering agents as the animal is not in respiratory distress already, or an orogastric tube is placed in the rumen to reduce the risk of aspiration pneumonia of these products. When animals are in severe distress due to bloat, a temporary trocar with a cannula or a rumenostomy can be completed to relieve pressure from the bloat. Humane euthanasia or harvest is an option for cattle with chronic bloats.

Ruminitis. Another common sequela that can occur, particularly in prolonged SARA-affected animals, is ruminitis. Ruminitis is thought to occur by low rumen pH, causing the weakening of cellular adhesion and epithelial cells.[39,55] This results in inflammation of the epithelial cells and hypertrophy of the ruminal epithelium's stratum corneum, creating parakeratosis, which can lower future VFA absorption. Mycotic ruminitis occurs due to the prolonged decrease in ruminal pH, which favors the growth of yeast and fungi that grow in acidic environments.

Liver Abscesses. Previous research has shown a positive association between ruminal lesions associated with acidosis and liver abscesses.[56,57] The decrease in ruminal pH predisposes the animal to an acid-damaged wall which facilitates entry and colonization of *Fusobacterium necrophorum*.[58] Once the rumen wall is colonized, infection leads to ruminal wall abscesses and enters the portal circulation.[58] Bacteria are trapped within the capillary portal system leading to infection and liver abscess formation.[58] Cattle with liver abscesses are asymptomatic and often found during harvest. Tylosin in-feed is labeled to control liver abscesses. Ultimately, prevention is key with feed bunk management practices described above.

Laminitis. Laminitis is an additional sequela to a ruminal acidosis event. The decrease in metabolic pH activates a vasoactive mechanism that increases digital pulse and total blood flow.[59] This releases endotoxins and histamine, which creates vasoconstriction and dilation, leading to unphysiological arteriovenous shunts.[59] Through increased blood pressure, vessel walls become leaky and are damaged, resulting in internal hemorrhaging and edema of the solar corium.[59] This is followed by ischemia and hypoxemia, which increases arteriovenous (AV) shunting and perpetuates the cycle to continue damaging the digit's lower part.[59] Ultimately, the bones shift in position due to the laminar supports being broken down, leaving the claw more prone to damage. Clinical signs of cattle with laminitis are acute lameness, discoloration of the hoof, sole hemorrhages, ulcers, abscesses, misshapen hooves, or double-walled soles.[50,59,60] Diagnosis of laminitis in cattle is based on history, clinical signs, and foot examination to rule out other claw insults. Treatment of laminitis can be, but is not limited to, corrective foot trims and the utilization of anti-inflammatories to reduce pain and inflammation associated with lameness.

Sulfur Toxicity

Sulfur is a macronutrient that can be considered toxic at excessive concentration. The recommended daily dietary intake of sulfur is 0.15% to 0.2% for beef cattle and not to exceed 0.4%.[61] Sulfur is an important factor in essential molecules such as biotin, chondroitin sulfate, cartilage mucopolysaccharides, coenzyme A, fibrinogen, glutathione, heparin, lipoic acid, mucins, and thiamine.[61] It is also needed as a component of methionine, cysteine, cystine, homocysteine, and taurine.[61] Sulfur is also a necessary component for the growth and metabolism of many ruminal bacteria, particularly cellulolytic bacteria.[62] A meta-analysis suggested the incidence of polioencephalomalacia induced by sulfur toxicity in feedlot cattle consuming 0.5% sulfur and 4% neutral detergent fiber from roughage was about 1% from roughly 16,760 cattle on feed.[63] Ruminants tend to be more sensitive to toxic effects of dietary sulfur/sulfate due to efficient microbial conversion to bioactive sulfur species in the rumen. [64] This, paired with the increase frequency of economically beneficial dietary feedstuffs that contains high sulfur concentrations (eg, ethanol distillers grains), can increase the risk of ruminants' toxicity to sulfur.

Pathophysiology

Feedstuff consumed by the animal containing sulfate or amino acids with sulfur is reduced to sulfide in the rumen.[65–67] Incidentally, as pH decreases due to fermentable carbohydrates in the diet, the amount of hydrogen sulfide in the gas cap increases.[68] Research has shown sulfides are turned into hydrogen sulfide gas, which can be inhaled through eructation and pass into system circulation through the pulmonary membranes.[69] Once present in circulation, it inhibits cytochrome C oxidase, essential for cellular respiration, and directly impacts tissues with a high oxygen demand, such as the heart and brain.[70–73] Although it was once thought to be associated with a systemic thiamine deficiency, several studies have shown thiamine concentrations within normal limits in animals with polioencephalomalacia.[65,66,74–76] However, the pathophysiology is unclear as to why sulfide-induced cytotoxicity induces polioencephalomalacia, and more research is needed.[77]

Clinical Signs

Clinical presentation can vary depending on the amount of sulfur consumed. Acute toxicities can include abdominal pain, rumen stasis, fetid diarrhea, dehydration, metabolic acidosis, tachypnea, recumbency, and hydrogen sulfide-smelling breath.[64] As toxicity progresses, it can present as dull mentation, head pressing, circling, blindness, ataxia, and death.

Diagnosis

Diagnosis can be made by gross and histologic lesions of the brain. Gross pathologic lesions include softening and yellowing of the cortex, with fluorescence associated with multifocal to coalescing laminar cortical necrosis by a ultraviolet (UV) light. On histopathology, the evidence of acute necrosis involving the outer cortical laminae shows hypereosinophilia of the neuropil and neurons being shrunken and eosinophilic. Pale staining and vacuolation of the sulci may also be seen.[65]

Treatment/Prevention

A recent literature review of treatment regiments for polioencephalomalacia shows that little clinical data support the varying treatment regiments.[78] The recommended dose of thiamine is administered at 10 to 20 mg/kg every 8 hours intramuscularly but is noted to be empirical.[78,79] IV thiamine can be completed; however, diluting the dose and giving it over a sustained period is recommended to prevent adverse reactions. In addition, using nonsteroidal and steroidal anti-inflammatories has been shown with varying outcomes and sometimes exacerbates clinical signs and pathologies.[78] Other ancillary therapies, such as diuretics, also show varying degrees of outcomes and exacerbate clinical signs.[78] Care needs to be considered when implementing ancillary therapies for polioencephalomalacia to not cause more harm when implementing a treatment strategy. Prevention for polioencephalomalacia can be completed by providing a well-mixed balanced ration.

Manganese Deficiency

Manganese (Mn) is an essential trace element that is required for numerous biochemical processes in the body. Manganese is involved in proper bone development and maintenance, including is required for glycosyltransferases which are involved in synthesizing glycosaminoglycans and glycoproteins of bone and cartilage matrix. [80] Manganese is also essential for incorporating carbohydrates into mucopolysaccharides at the epiphyseal plate through manganese-dependent activation, which transport trisaccharide to link polysaccharide to protein in bone.[81,82] The daily requirement for Mn requirements in mature beef cows is 40 mg/kg.[61] The overall bioavailability from ingested plants is 1% of intestinal absorption in cattle.[80,83–85] **Table 2** illustrates Mn availability in common feedstuff for ruminants in the United States.[86] There are conflicting studies about glyphosate's role in the uptake of Mn from the soil to the plant crops.[87–90] A considerable amount of iron, copper, zinc, sulfur, calcium, and phosphorus in the diet has been shown to interfere with the absorption of Mn, even though the mechanism is unknown.[91]

Pathophysiology and Clinical Signs

Manganese accumulation does not occur in the fetus as other trace minerals do.[82,92] It is normal to see fetal Mn liver concentrations (wet weight basis) at or below the dams.

Table 2
Manganese content (dry matter basis) and availability in various feedstuffs. adapted from APHIS NAHMS Beef Cattle cow/calf 1997[86]

Feedstuff	Availability (%)	Mean ± SE (ppm)
Alfalfa/alfalfa mix	74.90	56.97 + 2.17
Brome	85.00	69.31 ± 6.02
Fescue	97.26	151.84 ± 11.38
Orchard grass	94.12	121.46 ± 12.26
Sudan	83.61	67.54 ± 4.56
Cereal-type forages	84.78	94.98 ± 14.46
Native grasses	86.84	117.25 ± 18.63
Silage/silage mix	74.19	61.313 ± 8.37

Abbreviation: APHIS, Animal and Plant Health Inspection Service; NAHMS, National Animal Health Monitoring System

Manganese deficiency is associated with congenital abnormalities of bone formation of the fetus. However, the pathophysiology is still in question. Several studies have investigated calves born to Mn-deficient dams and have found lower birth weights, disproportionate dwarfism, fetal ataxia, swollen joints, joint laxity, and superior brachygnathism of varying degrees of severity.[91,93–95]

Diagnosis

Manganese deficiency can be diagnosed by samples from the dam, fetus, and feed. For the dam, liver, whole blood, or serum can be collected, with liver and whole blood having higher concentrations of Mn than serum.[87] The fetus's long bones can be evaluated for both histopathology and Mn concentration and fetal liver concentration. Feedstuff can be collected to determine the level of Mn in the ration and determine if the diet is deficient.

Treatment/Prevention

Unfortunately, treatment of the fetus directly is unrewarding and unresponsive. If the fetus is viable, low growth rates are to be expected. Humane euthanasia is an acceptable treatment method. Prevention becomes the strategy for gestating cows. Ensuring proper Mn supplementation in the feed for gestating cows, 20 to 40 mg/kg, with the lower limit possibly leading toward deficiency.[61] In addition, injectable mineral supplementation with Mn has levels returning to normal 8 days after injection and therefore could be considered a short-term solution.[96]

PROTEIN-ENERGY MALNUTRITION

PEM, also known as pregnancy toxemia in beef cows, is when pregnant beef cattle are provided marginal diets causing weight loss, weakness, depression, and inability to rise. The nutrient requirements for a pregnant beef cow are shown in **Table 3**.

Pathophysiology

PEM occurs in cattle with poor quality forage and feedstuff, increased energy demand, and environments below the thermoneutral zone, which results in a negative energy balance. **Table 3** presents energy and protein requirements for a beef cow during gestation. When animals fall into a negative energy balance, the body's glycogen stores are catabolized. Once the glycogen stores have been used, protein and lipid reserves are also catabolized. Using stored energy sources triggers many clinical signs observed in PEM cases.

Clinical Signs

Clinical signs of animals experiencing PEM have a low body condition score, long hair, weakness, inability to rise but still alert, and normal to subnormal temperature.[98] In some cases, diarrhea is often noted, and elevated ketones are present in the blood. Clinical signs appear gradually, often unnoticed until the animal is recumbent and down. [99]

Diagnosis

Diagnosis is made by history and physical examination. Cows will have varying ranges of minor serum abnormalities that may be considered a variation of normal such as low glucose, urea nitrogen, low packed cell volume, and creatinine concentrations. [100–102] Unfortunately, no diagnostic tests provide a confirmatory diagnosis for PEM, only to be used as supportive evidence. Postmortem diagnosis of PEM can be supported

Table 3
Nutrient requirements of beef cows: effects of physiologic state and time

	Month of Gestation									
	1	2	3	4	5	6	7	8	9	10
Net energy for maintenance required (Mcal/d)	15.25	14.01	12.82	11.86	11.04	9.64	10.14	11.04	12.54	14.54
Metabolizable protein required g/d	901	810	719	646	585	466	487	522	582	673

Animal was defined as a Hereford × Angus crossbred cow, approximately 5 years in age and calf at side. Calculations also assume thermoneutral conditions, confinement housing, and dry hair coat.[61,97]

by the loss of fat stores in the pelvic, kidney, and coronary regions.[98,103] Decreased muscle mass will also be present on postmortem examination.

Treatment

Treatment can often be unrewarding, especially for a recumbent animal.[98,104] Gradual protein supplementation can be introduced slowly, such as soybean meal and good-quality legume hay. Force-feeding animals may include softening the feed with water to form a gruel and drenching it orally at approximately 11 kg/d of alfalfa.[98] Parenteral nutrition may also be used to correct electrolyte derangements and increase glucose parameters, in an adult cow a 6.5 L of 50% glucose solution on a continuous drip may be used for metabolized energy supplementation.[98] Propylene glycol can also be used at 33 mL/100 kg of body weight twice a day as a glucose precursor to provide additional energy.[98,105] The induction of parturition may be another viable treatment strategy to lessen the energy demands on the cow. Prognosis is guarded, and humane euthanasia is also a viable treatment option.

Prevention

Prevention of PEM ultimately is understanding and providing the core nutritional requirements of cows at any stage of gestation and lactation. Feeding higher quality and properly stored forages will also help prevent PEM. Environmental management to ensure cattle is comfortable even in cooler weather; the examples of such can be increasing bedding and providing adequate windbreaks. Cows coming into colder weather with low body condition scores can be supplemented separately to ensure adequate nutrition without providing an abundance of supplementation to the rest of the herd. Ultimately, providing sound science-based nutrition and managing the environment is a good investment to producers and not only prevents PEM and can increase reproductive efficiency, performance, calf viability, and fetal programming.

CLINICS CARE POINTS

- Hypomagnesemia prevention should target appropriate dietary supplementation of magnesium using agronomic practices to increase forage magnesium content or with offering a palatable magnesium supplement.
- Beef cattle gestation diets should preferably contain 40 mg/kg dry matter of manganese to ensure sufficient placental transfer and minimize fetal deficiency leading to chondrodystrophic bone lesions.
- Dietary sulfur intake, including what is provided via water, should be less that 0.4% dry matter to minimize potential for ruminal hydrogen sulfide production potentially inducing polioencephalomalacia.
- Rumen adaptation to a high-grain diet, attention to starch sources, bunk management, and dietary particle size are critical factors in addressing ruminal acidosis.
- High neutral detergent fiber (NDF >60%) forages most often are associated with protein-energy malnutrition in pregnant beef cows as estimated NDF intake capacity is approximately 1% of body weight.

DISCLOSURE

The author has nothing to disclose.

REFERENCES

1. Castillo-Lopez E, Wiese BI, Hendrick S, et al. Incidence, prevalence, severity, and risk factors for ruminal acidosis in feedlot steers during backgrounding, diet transition, and finishing. J Anim Sci 2014;92:3053–63.
2. Dillon J, Scott D. Digesta flow and mineral absorption in lambs before and after weaning. J Agric Sci 1979;92:289–97.
3. Hart KA, Goff JP, McFarlane D, et al. Chapter 41 - Endocrine and Metabolic Diseases. In: Smith BP, Van Metre DC, Pusterla N, editors. Large animal internal medicine. Sixth Edition. St. Louis (MO): Mosby; 2020. p. 1352–420.e1312.
4. Tomas F, Potter B. The effect and site of action of potassium upon magnesium absorption in sheep. Aust J Agric Res 1976;27:873–80.
5. Axford RF, Tas MV, Evans RA, et al. The absorption of magnesium from the forestomachs, stomach and small intestine of sheep. Res Vet Sci 1975;19:333–4.
6. Greene LW, Fontenot JP, Webb KE. Site of Magnesium and Other Macromineral Absorption in Steers Fed High Levels of Potassium. J Anim Sci 1983;57:503–10.
7. Care AD, Brown RC, Farrar AR, et al. Magnesium absorption from the digestive tract of sheep. Q J Exp Physiol 1984;69:577–87.
8. Fontenot JP, Wise MB, Webb KE Jr. Interrelationships of potassium, nitrogen, and magnesium in ruminants. Fed Proc 1973;32:1925–8.
9. Greene LW, Webb KE Jr, Fontenot JP. Effect of potassium level on site of absorption of magnesium and other macroelements in sheep. J Anim Sci 1983;56:1214–21.
10. Khorasani GR, Armstrong DG. Effect of sodium and potassium level on the absorption of magnesium and other macrominerals in sheep. Livest Prod Sci 1990;24:223–35.
11. Schonewille JT, Beynen AC, Klooster ATV, et al. Dietary Potassium Bicarbonate and Potassium Citrate Have a Greater Inhibitory Effect than Does Potassium Chloride on Magnesium Absorption in Wethers. J Nutr 1999;129:2043–7.
12. Suttle NF, Field AC. Studies on magnesium in ruminant nutrition. Br J Nutr 1967;21:819–31.
13. Martens H, Monika S. Pathophysiology of Grass Tetany and other Hypomagnesemias: Implications for Clinical Management. Veterinary Clinics of North America. Food Animal Practice 2000;16:339–68.
14. Denton DA. The effect of Na+ depletion on the Na+:K+ ratio of the parotid saliva of the sheep. J Physiol 1956;131:516–25.
15. Morris JG, Gartner RJW. The effect of potassium on the sodium requirements of growing steers with and without α-tocopherol supplementation. Br J Nutr 1975;34:1–14.
16. Martens H, Kubel OW, Gäbel G, et al. Effects of low sodium intake on magnesium metabolism of sheep. J Agric Sci 1987;108:237–43.
17. Head MJ, Rook JAF. Hypomagnesæmia in Dairy Cattle and its Possible Relationship to Ruminal Ammonia Production. Nature 1955;176:262–3.
18. Martens H, Rayssiguier Y. Magnesium metabolism and hypomagnesaemia. In: Ruckebusch Y, Thivend P, editors. Digestive physiology and metabolism in ruminants: proceedings of the 5th International symposium on ruminant physiology, held at Clermont-Ferrand, on 3rd–7th September, 1979. Dordrecht: Springer Netherlands; 1980. p. 447–66.
19. Martens H, Heggemann G, Regier K. Studies on the Effect of K, Na, NH4+, VFA and CO2 on the Net Absorption of Magnesium from the Temporarily Isolated Rumen of Heifers. J Vet Med Ser A 1988;35:73–80.

20. Grunes DL, Stout PR, Brownell JR. Grass tetany of ruminants. Adv Agron 1970; 22:331–74.
21. Stout PR, Brownell J, Burau RG. Occurrences of Trans-Aconitate in Range Forage Species. Agron J 1967;59:21–4.
22. Russell JB, Forsberg N. Production of tricarballylic acid by rumen microorganisms and its potential toxicity in ruminant tissue metabolism. Br J Nutr 1986; 56:153–62.
23. Fontenot JP, Allen VG, Bunce GE, et al. Factors influencing magnesium absorption and metabolism in ruminants. J Anim Sci 1989;67:3445–55.
24. Russell JB, Van Soest PJ. In vitro ruminal fermentation of organic acids common in forage. Appl Environ Microbiol 1984;47:155–9.
25. Goff JP. Calcium and Magnesium Disorders. Veterinary Clinics of North America. Food Animal Practice 2014;30:359–81.
26. Littledike E, Stuedemann J, Wilkinson S, et al. Grass tetany syndrome. Role of magnesium in animal nutrition 1983;173–95.
27. John M. Diagnostic Considerations for Evaluating Nutritional Problems in Cattle. Vet Clin Food Anim Pract 2007;23:527–39.
28. Lincoln SD, Lane VM. Postmortem magnesium concentration in bovine vitreous humor: comparison with antemortem serum magnesium concentration. American journal of veterinary research 1985;46:160–2.
29. Mccoy MA, Hutchinson T, Davison G, et al. Postmortem biochemical markers of experimentally induced hypomagnesaemic tetany in cattle. Vet Rec 2001;148: 268–73.
30. Goff JP. Treatment of Calcium, Phosphorus, and Magnesium Balance Disorders. Vet Clin Food Anim Pract 1999;15:619–39.
31. Bacon JA, Bell MC, Miller JK, et al. Effect of magnesium administration route on plasma minerals in Holstein calves receiving either adequate or insufficient magnesium in their diets. J Dairy Sci 1990;73:470–3.
32. Reynolds CK, Bell MC, Sims MH. Changes in plasma, red blood cell and cerebrospinal fluid mineral concentrations in calves during magnesium depletion followed by repletion with rectally infused magnesium chloride. J Nutr 1984;114: 1334–41.
33. Goff JP. Ruminant hypomagnesemic tetanies. *Current veterinary therapy: food animal practice.* Philadelphia, PA: WB Saunders Co; 1998. p. 215.
34. Kemp A, Hart M. Grass tetany in grazing milking cows. Neth J Agric Sci 1957; 5:4–17.
35. Meyer NF, Bryant TC. Diagnosis and Management of Rumen Acidosis and Bloat in Feedlots. Vet Clin Food Anim Pract 2017;33:481–98.
36. Nagaraja TG, Lechtenberg KF. Acidosis in Feedlot Cattle. Veterinary Clinics of North America. Food Animal Practice 2007;23:333–50.
37. Owens FN, Secrist DS, Hill WJ, et al. Acidosis in cattle: a review. J Anim Sci 1998;76:275–86.
38. Oetzel G, Nordlund K, Garrett E. Effect of ruminal pH and stage of lactation on ruminal lactate concentrations in dairy cows. J Dairy Sci 1999;82:38.
39. Enemark JM, Jorgensen RJ, Enemark PS. Rumen acidosis with special emphasis on diagnostic aspects of subclinical rumen acidosis: a review. Vet Zootech 2002;20(42):16–29.
40. Radostits OM, Gay CC, Hinchcliff KW, et al. Acute carbohydrate engorgement of ruminants (Ruminal lactic acidosis, rumen overload). Vet Med 2007;10: 314–25.

41. Van Metre DC, Tyler JW, Stehman SM. Diagnosis of enteric disease in small ruminants. Vet Clin Food Anim Pract 2000;16:87–115.
42. Chapter 32 - Diseases of the Alimentary Tract. In: Bradford BP, Van Metre DC, Pusterla N, editors. Large animal internal medicine. Sixth Edition. St. Louis (MO): Elsevier; 2020. p. 702–920.e735.
43. Cebra CK, Cebra ML, Garry FB, et al. Forestomach acidosis in six New World camelids. J Am Vet Med Assoc 1996;208:901–4.
44. Snyder E, Credille B. Diagnosis and Treatment of Clinical Rumen Acidosis. Veterinary Clinics of North America. Food Animal Practice 2017;33:451–61.
45. Hollberg W. Vergleichende Untersuchungen von mittels Schambye-Sørensen-Sonde oder durch Punktion des kaudoventralen Pansensacks gewonnenen Pansensaftproben. Dtsch Tierärztliche Wochenschr (DTW) 1984;91:317–20.
46. Höltershinken M, Vlizzo V, Mertens M, et al. Untersuchungen zur Zusammensetzung von über Sonde bzw. Fistel genommenen Pansensaft des Rindes. Dtsch Tierärztl Wochenschr 1992;99:228–30.
47. Duffield T, Plaizier J, Fairfield A, et al. Comparison of techniques for measurement of rumen pH in lactating dairy cows. J Dairy Sci 2004;87:59–66.
48. Enemark JMD, Jørgensen RJ, Kristensen NB. An evaluation of parameters for the detection of subclinical rumen acidosis in dairy herds. Vet Res Commun 2004;28:687–709.
49. Garrett E, Pereira M, Nordlund K, et al. Diagnostic methods for the detection of subacute ruminal acidosis in dairy cows. J Dairy Sci 1999;82:1170–8.
50. Garrett EF, Pereira MN, Nordlund KV, et al. Diagnostic methods for the detection of subacute ruminal acidosis in dairy cows. J Dairy Sci 1999;82(6):1170–8.
51. Jörg MDE. The monitoring, prevention and treatment of sub-acute ruminal acidosis (SARA): A review. Vet J 2008;176:32–43.
52. Pritchard R. Bunk management–Observations from research plains nutrition council spring conference. San Antonio, TX: Texas Agriculture Research and Extension Publication; 1998.
53. Marchesini G, Cortese M, Ughelini N, et al. Effect of total mixed ration processing time on ration consistency and beef cattle performance during the early fattening period. Anim Feed Sci Technol 2020;262:114421.
54. Huber T. Physiological effects of acidosis on feedlot cattle. J Anim Sci 1976;43: 902–9.
55. Krause KM, Oetzel GR. Understanding and preventing subacute ruminal acidosis in dairy herds: A review. Anim Feed Sci Technol 2006;126:215–36.
56. Jensen R. Rumenitis-liver abscess complex in feedlot cattle. The Calif Vet 1960; 13:26.
57. Rezac D, Thomson D, Bartle S, et al. Prevalence, severity, and relationships of lung lesions, liver abnormalities, and rumen health scores measured at slaughter in beef cattle. J Anim Sci 2014;92:2595–602.
58. Amachawadi RG, Nagaraja TG. Pathogenesis of Liver Abscesses in Cattle. Vet Clin Food Anim Pract 2022;38:335–46.
59. Nocek JE. Bovine acidosis: implications on laminitis. J Dairy Sci 1997;80: 1005–28.
60. Philipot J, Pluvinage P, Luquet F. Clinical characterization of a syndrome by ecopathology methods: an example of dairy cow lameness. Veterinary research 1994;25:239–43.
61. National Academies of Sciences Engineering, and Medicine. Nutrient requirements of beef cattle. 8th edition. Washington, DC: National Academy Press; 2016.

62. Spears J, Ely D, Bush L, et al. Sulfur supplement and in vitro digestion of forage cellulose by rumen microorganisms. J Anim Sci 1976;43:513–7.
63. Nichols C, Bremer V, Watson A, et al. The effect of sulfur and use of ruminal available sulfur as a model to predict incidence of polioencephalomalacia in feedlot cattle. Bov Pract 2013;47–53.
64. Jeffery OH. Chapter 35 - Sulfur. In: Ramesh C.G, *Veterinary toxicology.* Third Edition. New York, NY: Academic Press; 2018. p. 483–7.
65. Gould DH, McAllister MM, Savage JC, et al. High sulfide concentrations in rumen fluid associated with nutritionally induced polioencephalomalacia. Am J Vet Res 1991;52:1164–9.
66. Gould DH, Cummings BA, Hamar DW. In vivo indicators of pathologic ruminal sulfide production in steers with diet-induced polioencephalomalacia. J Vet Diagn Invest 1997;9:72–6.
67. Loneragan GH, Gould DH, Callan RJ, et al. Association of excess sulfur intake and an increase in hydrogen sulfide concentrations in the ruminal gas cap of recently weaned beef calves with polioencephalomalacia. J Am Vet Med Assoc 1998;213:1599–604, 1571.
68. Daniel HG. Update on Sulfur-Related Polioencephalomalacia. Veterinary Clinics of North America. Food Animal Practice 2000;16:481–96.
69. Bird P. Sulphur metabolism and excretion studies in ruminants vii. Secretion of sulphur and nitrogen in sheep pancreatic and bile fluids. Aust J Biol Sci 1972; 25:817–34.
70. Smith L, Kruszyna H, Smith RP. The effect of methemoglogin on the inhibition of cytochrome c oxidase by cyanide, sulfide or azide. Biochem Pharmacol 1977; 26:2247–50.
71. Beauchamp R, Bus JS, Popp JA, et al. A critical review of the literature on hydrogen sulfide toxicity. CRC Crit Rev Toxicol 1984;13:25–97.
72. Khan IA, Schuler M, Prior M, et al. Effects of hydrogen sulfide exposure on lung mitochondrial respiratory chain enzymes in rats. Toxicol Appl Pharmacol 1990; 103:482–90.
73. Nicholls P, Kim J-K. Sulphide as an inhibitor and electron donor for the cytochrome c oxidase system. Can J Biochem 1982;60:613–23.
74. Olkowski AA, Christensen DA, Rousseaux CG. Association of sulfate-water and blood thiamine concentration in beef cattle: Field studies. Can J Anim Sci 1991; 71:825–32.
75. Loew F, Bettany J. Apparent thiamin status of cattle and its relationship to polioencephalomalacia. Can J Comp Med 1975;39:291.
76. Hamlen H, Clark E, Janzen E. Polioencephalomalacia in cattle consuming water with elevated sodium sulfate levels: A herd investigation. Can Vet J 1993;34: 153–8.
77. Drewnoski ME, Pogge DJ, Hansen SL. High-sulfur in beef cattle diets: A review. J Anim Sci 2014;92:3763–80.
78. Michael DA. Consideration of evidence for therapeutic interventions in bovine polioencephalomalacia. Vet Clin Food Anim Pract 2015;31:151–61.
79. Loneragan G, Gould D. Polioencephalomalacia (cerebrocortical necrosis). SMITH, BP Large animal internal medicine 2002;3:920–6.
80. Mclaren PJ, Cave JG, Parker EM, et al. Chondrodysplastic Calves in Northeast Victoria. Veterinary Pathology 2007;44:342–54.
81. Graham TW. Trace element deficiencies in cattle. Vet Clin Food Anim Pract 1991;7:153–215.

82. Leach R Jr, Muenster A-M, Wien EM. Studies on the role of manganese in bone formation: II. Effect upon chondroitin sulfate synthesis in chick epiphyseal cartilage. Arch Biochem Biophys 1969;133:22–8.
83. Hidiroglou M. Manganese in ruminant nutrition. Can J Anim Sci 1979;59:217–36.
84. Spears JW. Trace Mineral Bioavailability in Ruminants. J Nutr 2003;133: 1506S–9S.
85. Van Bruwaene R, Gerber G, Kirchmann R, et al. Metabolism of 51Cr, 54Mn, 59Fe and 60Co in lactating dairy cows. Health Phys 1984;46:1069–82.
86. Mortimer RG, Dargatz DA, Corah LR. Forage analyses from cow-calf herds in 23 states In: USDA:APHIS:vs. Fort Collins, CO: Centers for Epidemiology and Animal Health; 1997.
87. Steve E. Evaluating Mineral Status in Ruminant Livestock. Vet Clin Food Anim Pract 2020;36:525–46.
88. Bott S, Tesfamariam T, Candan H, et al. Glyphosate-induced impairment of plant growth and micronutrient status in glyphosate-resistant soybean (Glycine max L.). Plant Soil 2008;312:185–94.
89. Rosolem CA, Andrade GJMD, Lisboa IP, et al. Manganese uptake and redistribution in soybean as affected by glyphosate. Rev Bras Ciência do Solo 2010;34: 1915–22.
90. Nelson N. Manganese response of conventional and glyphosate-resistant soybean in Kansas. Insights: International Plant Nutrition Central Great Plains Reg July 2009;3.
91. Rojas M, Dyer I, Cassatt W. Manganese deficiency in the bovine. J Anim Sci 1965;24:664–7.
92. Aschner JL, Aschner M. Nutritional aspects of manganese homeostasis. Mol Aspect Med 2005;26:353–62.
93. Hansen S, Spears J, Lloyd K, et al. Feeding a low manganese diet to heifers during gestation impairs fetal growth and development. J Dairy Sci 2006;89: 4305–11.
94. Howes A, Dyer I. Diet and supplemental mineral effects on manganese metabolism in newborn calves. J Anim Sci 1971;32:141–5.
95. Ribble CS, Janzen ED, Proulx JG. Congenital joint laxity and dwarfism: A feed-associated congenital anomaly of beef calves in Canada. Can Vet J 1989; 30:331.
96. Pogge DJ, Richter EL, Drewnoski ME, et al. Mineral concentrations of plasma and liver after injection with a trace mineral complex differ among Angus and Simmental cattle. J Anim Sci 2012;90:2692–8.
97. Olson K, Bailey E, Duncan Z, et al. Nutrition and reproduction in the beef cow. 2nd edition. Bovine Reproduction; 2021. p. 372–88.
98. Chapter 33 - Diseases of the Hepatobiliary System. In: Bradford BP, Van Metre DC, Pusterla N, editors. Large animal internal medicine. 6th Edition. St. Louis (MO): Elsevier; 2020. p. 921–55.e926.
99. Moustgaard J. Nutritive influences upon reproduction. J Reprod Med 1971;7: 275–8.
100. Lister E, Fisher L, Jordan W, et al. Influence of shelter, level of feeding, and method of forage conservation on packed cell volume and plasma metabolite levels in pregnant beef cows. Can J Anim Sci 1973;53:81–8.
101. Kunz PL, Blum JW. Relationships between energy balances and blood levels of hormones and metabolites in dairy cows during late pregnancy and early lactation. Zeitschrift für Tierphysiologie Tierernährung und Futtermittelkunde 2009; 54:239–48.

102. Lee AJ, Twardock AR, Bubar RH, et al. Blood metabolic profiles: Their use and relation to nutritional status of dairy cows. J Dairy Sci 1978;61:1652–70.
103. Thompson RG. Emaciation in calves fed artificial diets. Can Vet J 1967;8:242–3.
104. Blood D. Diseases caused by nutritional deficiencies. Veterinary Medicine: a Textbook of the Diseases of Cattle Sheep, Pigs and Horses. In: Lea &. Philadelphia PA: Febiger; 1979.
105. Oetzel GR. Protein-energy malnutrition in ruminants. Vet Clin Food Anim Pract 1988;4(2):317–29.

Urinary Calculi of Small Ruminants

Meredyth Jones Cook, DVM, MS, DACVIM

KEYWORDS

• Urolithiasis • Sheep • Goats • Nutrition

KEY POINTS

- Obstructive urolithiasis in small ruminants is a multifactorial disease affecting intact and castrated males.
- Due to the cost and associated prognosis associated with the various treatment methods for urolithiasis, the focus should be on dietary and other preventative strategies for controlling this disease.
- Intravenous fluids, anxiolytics, antimicrobials, and anti-inflammatories are frequently used in combination with surgical techniques, such as tube cystostomy, perineal urethrostomy, urinary bladder marsupialization, and others in order to resolve urinary obstruction.

INTRODUCTION

Obstructive urolithiasis is a multifactorial condition of male ruminants causing significant economic losses and compromising animal welfare. Although significant strides have been made through decades of research on nutrition, body water balance, urine pH, and other factors, cases continue to be presented to veterinary practitioners. Urolithiasis remains an exciting area for research, as evidenced by continued publication of studies evaluating risk factors, preventative strategies, and new and improved treatment modalities. Although the published data and techniques presented in this article will focus on small ruminants, much of what we know about urolithiasis regarding treatment and prevention is common across all ruminants.

Risk Factors

Whether treatment of obstructive urolithiasis is successful or not, affected animals suffer substantial pain, and there is often significant financial and emotional loss for the animal owner. For this reason, the prevention of stone formation and obstruction should be an important part of any small ruminant herd health plan. Designing effective prevention plans requires a solid understanding of the currently known risk factors,

Oklahoma State University and Large Animal Consulting & Education, 2115 W. Farm Road, Stillwater, OK 74078, USA
E-mail address: meredyth.jones@okstate.edu

Vet Clin Food Anim 39 (2023) 355–370
https://doi.org/10.1016/j.cvfa.2023.02.006

which include anatomic factors, urine pH, dietary composition, water intake, and genetic factors.

Anatomic Factors

Although the anatomic design of the male ruminant urinary tract does not predispose to stone formation, it does contribute to obstruction. As urine passes through the urethra, it encounters the 2 curves of the proximal and distal sigmoid flexures of the penis and the vermiform appendage (urethral process) at the distal tip of the penis. The urethra narrows at both the distal sigmoid flexure, due to the insertion of the retractor penis muscles, and the vermiform appendage. These are the most common sites of obstruction in male small ruminants.

Urine pH

The alkaline pH of ruminant urine is a risk factor for urolith formation. The alkaline urine pH of herbivores is largely influenced by the potassium content of forages. High potassium increases the dietary cation anion difference (DCAD) of the diet, resulting in a progression toward increased alkalinity of the blood and urine. Phosphatic and calcium carbonate uroliths are known to precipitate in alkaline urine. Struvite crystallization occurs at a pH range of 7.2 to 8.4, with dissolution occurring at a pH of less than 6.5.[1] Apatite stones form at a urine pH of 6.5 to 7.5.[2] Urine pH may have little or no effect on silicate and calcium oxalate uroliths.

Water Intake

Simplified, uroliths are structurally an organic matrix of cells or proteins on which inorganic minerals crystallize. There are 3 main theories of how stones form; however, essentially urolithiasis represents supersaturation of urine by these organic and inorganic components.[3]

Water deprivation and negative water balance contribute to this supersaturation and precipitation of crystalloids. Further, improved water intake should result in more frequent urination and removal of stone components from the urinary tract. Highlighting the importance of frequent urination, in sheep, the urolith risk factors of increased urine pH, increased urine concentration, and increased urine calcium concentration, occurred 1 hour after the initiation of feeding a calculogenic diet.[4] A reduction in urine output has been noted when sheep were changed from an alfalfa hay diet to a concentrate pellet,[5] and a reduction in water intake is proposed for grain feeding over roughage feeding.

Dietary Composition

Anatomic factors and water intake are general risk factors that likely apply to all stone types. However, in order to converse about dietary risk factors and prevention of urolithiasis, the target stone type must be known. Reported stone types in small ruminants include phosphatic (including struvite, magnesium ammonium phosphate, calcium phosphate/apatite), calcium carbonate, calcium oxalate, and silicate. Phosphatic and calcium carbonate both form in alkaline urine, which is normal in ruminants consuming typical diets.

Historically, phosphatic stones have been associated with grain feeding, whereas calcium carbonate uroliths develop with legume feeding.[6–9] However, one small study of 49 cases of obstructive urolithiasis in sheep and goats that directly evaluated diet and stone type did not confirm this,[10] and the author has observed numerous exceptions. Silicate uroliths are diet-dependent and geography-dependent, with these forming in the western United States and Canada in animals grazing siliceous soils.

Phosphatic Uroliths

Phosphatic uroliths include struvite (magnesium ammonium phosphate), amorphous magnesium calcium phosphate and apatite (calcium phosphate), making the control of phosphorus and magnesium levels in the diet important. Although 2 of these stone types include calcium, the focus has generally been on controlling phosphorus levels in the diet over limiting calcium. Because these macrominerals compete for absorption, calcium has been used to reduce the impact of phosphorus. In some scenarios where by-product feeds are used, elevated phosphorus levels may contribute to urolithiasis regardless of its ratio to calcium.

Obviously, this is not a perfect plan and may account for some of the inconsistency seen in stone type versus diet. In addition to grains providing high dietary phosphorus, animal-fed diets that require little mastication, such as grains or pellets, decrease salivary excretion of phosphorus and increase urinary excretion.[11] In the case of magnesium, it has been shown to be more efficiently absorbed in animals fed higher concentrate rations.[12]

Calcium Carbonate Uroliths

Elevated calcium in diets is likely a risk factor for the development of calcium carbonate urolithiasis. It is the perception of the author and other clinicians that the rate of calcium carbonate urolithiasis has increased over time. This may be due to a number of factors but one theory is that the addition of calcium to diets to decrease phosphorus absorption without tight control over the ratio may actually predispose to calcium carbonate urolithiasis. Another control measure for phosphatic urolithiasis is adding anionic salts to diets to acidify the urine through systemic acidosis. Systemic acidosis increases calcium excretion in urine. It is possible that these control measures for phosphatic urolithiasis may be predisposing animals to calcium carbonate urolithiasis although it must be emphasized that this disease is multifactorial with other possible explanations.

Organic nidus

Although the focus of conversation regarding stone formation is often the inorganic mineral formations, it is worth noting that stones generally contain an organic nidus, which becomes layered with inorganic components. In sheep, this matrix has been shown to include nitrogen, various sugars, amino acids, erythrocytes, leukocytes, and epithelial cells.[13] Suture, tissue debris, blood clots, or bacteria may also comprise this nidus.[3] Urinary tract excretion of excess dietary protein[9,13] and metaplasia of the uroepithelium from vitamin A deficiency[13] therefore provides matrix materials. Infection of the urinary tract may also provide components but infection is not considered an important contributing factor to urolithiasis in ruminants.

Genetic Factors

Breed predispositions have been postulated for urolithiasis risk; Pygmy and Nigerian Dwarf are overrepresented,[14,15] whereas other anecdotal reports indicate the diseased population is representative of the hospital population, such as in areas where Boer goats are common. A genetic predisposition to be a "stone former" has been suggested or confirmed in humans,[16] dogs,[17] and cats.[18] This has been discussed but not well documented in small ruminants. Across 2 studies of experimentally induced calcium carbonate urolithiasis where animals received an artificial, intracystic nidus and an alfalfa-based diet, the same 2 goats (out of 8 in study 1; out of 6 in study 2) produced significantly more stone mass than the remaining goats.[19]

Age

Obstructive urolithiasis may occur in any age animal. When age and stone composition are evaluated together, phosphatic urolithiasis is not significantly associated with age,[10] whereas calcium carbonate urolithiasis is significantly associated with increasing age.[10,15] The odds of obstruction with calcium carbonate uroliths were 0.07 (95% CI [0.02, 0.32], P = .001) for animals 5 to 36 months of age compared with animals 4 months old and younger.[10]

Table 1 Preventative measures based on risk factors for obstructive urolithiasis in small ruminants. Due to the multifactorial nature of this disease, consensus on preventative measures across studies is rare. The recommendations in this chart are general guidelines based on current knowledge.

Treatment

Evaluation and initial steps

Many animals who present with obstructive urolithiasis will require surgical intervention at some point in their disease in order to survive. There are initial steps; however, that may resolve the obstruction temporarily or permanently, along with medical care for support. A suggested workflow to patient assessment and medical and surgical decision-making is presented.

It is prudent to consider that any ill male small ruminant is a candidate for urinary obstruction. Important history questions include dietary history, age at castration, intended use, any recent illnesses, and when last observed to urinate normally.

A thorough physical examination should be performed, and findings may include stones, crystals, or blood clots on preputial hairs, pulsation of the pelvic urethra, peri-preputial swelling, and pain on palpation of the distal penis. Behavioral observations may include straining, bruxism, flank watching, sawhorse stance, or simply a quiet, depressed animal.

If available, transabdominal ultrasound is valuable for visualization of the urinary bladder to determine diameter or detect rupture and evaluate the kidneys for hydronephrosis. The mean urinary bladder diameter in obstructed small ruminants was 9.7 $\pm$ 2.9 cm.[31] Poor clinical condition, obesity, previous castration, and uroperitoneum are associated with an increased risk of nonsurvival.[31] In multivariable analysis, severely increased creatinine (>5.9 mg/dL), abnormal packed cell volume (high or low), and increased creatine kinase activity were significantly associated with nonsurvival.[31] Another important consideration is loss of use. Breeding animals with ruptured urethra will no longer be able to breed due to penile adhesions.

If the index of suspicion is high for urinary obstruction, the vermiform appendage should be examined. This may be performed with sedation with or without lumbosacral epidural. In prepubescent animals or early castrates, exteriorization of the penis is challenging due to preputial adhesions. The author uses butorphanol 0.05 mg/kg (or morphine 0.1 mg/kg), midazolam 0.2 mg/kg, and ketamine 1 to 2 mg/kg, combined intravenously for sedation in these cases. Xylazine or other alpha 2 agonists should be avoided due to their effect of increasing urine volume, which could rupture an intact urinary tract.[32] A lumbosacral epidural can also be useful for this procedure by aseptically administering 2% lidocaine at 1 mL/7 kg. The patient may be placed in a sitting position or laterally recumbent with the hind limbs extended cranially and the free portion of the penis is passed through the preputial orifice where it is grasped by an assistant. Preputial adhesions, if present, will need to be broken down, which may require the use of hemostats or Allis tissue forceps (**Fig. 1**).

Table 1
. Summary of major risk factors for urolithiasis in ruminants and specific strategies to address each

Risk Factor		Suggested Preventative Strategies	Comments	Reference
Anatomic factors		Delay castration	May increase urethral diameter. This is controversial and not all studies agree across small ruminant species. The general belief is that, if intact males can be managed to allow delayed castration past 4–6 mo, it should be done	20–22
		Amputate vermiform	Some references state that no effect on fertility is expected from amputation but there are no primary studies evaluating this	Bani Ismail et al,[23] 2007 & Boundy [24] 1998
Urine pH		Balance DCAD to 0 mEq/kg of feed using chloride salts	Reduces urinary pH to <6.5 in goats to prevent crystallization of phosphatic components	12,25,26
		Titrating individual urine pH to <6.5 ammonium chloride and pulse dosing 3 d on, 4 d off	Customizes urine acidification to individual animal and helps reduce renal tolerance to salts	Sprake et al,[27] 2012
		Monitor urine pH 5–7 h after feeding and salt administration	Target urine pH is <6.5	Jones [26] 2009
		D, L-methionine 200 mg/kg PO daily	Reduces urine pH	Grissett [28] 2012
Water intake		Make clean, palatable, and temperature appropriate water readily available	Increased water intake and urine excretion may increase the removal of organic and inorganic urolith components	Swingle [5] 1962 & Crookshank [11] 1965
		Limit grain and pelleted feed, increase forage and grazing	Forage and grazing requires additional water for mastication and digestion; meal feeding grains and pellets shunts water to rumen and releases antidiuretic hormone	Gaebel [12] 1987
Dietary composition	Phosphatic uroliths	Reduce dietary grain	Magnesium and phosphorus highly available from grain	Hoar [29] 1970 & Hoar [30] 1970
		Increase dietary fiber	Increases salivary excretion of phosphorus	Jones [19] 2018
		Balance Ca:P to 2–3:1		

(continued on next page)

Table 1
(continued)

Risk Factor	Suggested Preventative Strategies	Comments	Reference
		Competition for absorption between calcium and phosphorus reduces phosphorus availability	
Calcium carbonate uroliths	Limit legume feeding	High calcium in alfalfa encourages calcium carbonate urolith formation	
	Balance Ca:P to 2:1	This ratio limits availability of phosphorus through competitive absorption without a calcium level that selects for calcium-containing stones	
	Monitor for over acidification with anionic salts	Metabolic acidosis increases calcium excretion into the urine	
Organic nidus	Palatable water	Increased water intake an urine excretion may increase the removal of organic and inorganic urolith components	
	Adequate trace mineral access and intake; routine screening	Helps maintain mineral balance and vitamin A levels for mucosal health	Packett [13] 1965
Genetic factors	Consider breed and familial history	Large-scale studies will be needed to track the incidence of obstructive urolithiasis in families but individual susceptibility has been strongly suggested in goats and other species	14,15,19
Age	Consider age-related risk by stone type	Animals of increasing age may be at increased risk of calcium carbonate formation	Jones [10] 2017

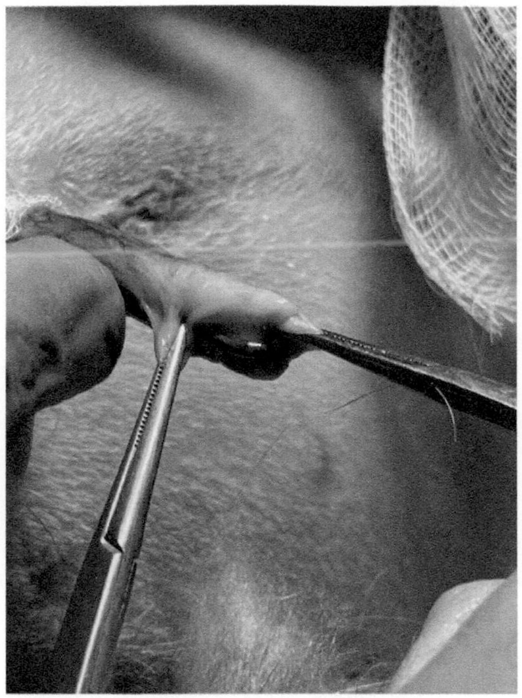

Fig. 1. Penis and prepuce of an early castrate 5-year-old Boer wether. The prepuce is still tightly adhered to the penis and those adhesions must be broken to allow full extension of the penis.

The vermiform appendage is observed for stone material. **Fig. 2**A and B demonstrate the typical appearance of calcium carbonate and phosphatic uroliths. It is common for a one or more stones to be present (**Fig. 3**). Whether or not stones are present, the appendage should be amputated at the tip of the penis at an angle with a sharp instrument to ensure a large, ovoid opening and minimal trauma to the tissue, which could encourage stricture (**Fig. 4**). This may result in emptying of the urinary bladder. If it does not, retrograde catheterization should be attempted.

Male artiodactyls have a urethral diverticulum present at the level of the urethral arch, which prevents retrograde catheterization of the urinary bladder in the absence of specialized catheters.[33] However, passing a catheter to that level can help identify the location of an obstruction or help clear an obstruction. Using a tomcat or 3.5-fr polypropylene urinary catheter, 2 to 3 mL of 2% lidocaine is instilled in the urethra with the distal end occluded. This provides both pain relief and may help reduce urethrospasm. The long polypropylene catheter is passed in a retrograde manner to detect any obstruction, which may feel gritty or hard. At this point, saline is flushed gently to see if the stone will dislodge. This should not be an aggressive hydropulsion because of the possibility of the saline passing the stone into the bladder, increasing volume and pressure. If the stone is not easily dislodged, flushing is stopped.

If the obstruction is resolved by either vermiform amputation or by hydropulsion, it is appropriate to initiate medical management with caution to the owner that reobstruction is likely due to additional stones in the urinary bladder. If the obstruction is not resolved, the client must make a decision to proceed with further medical or surgical management.

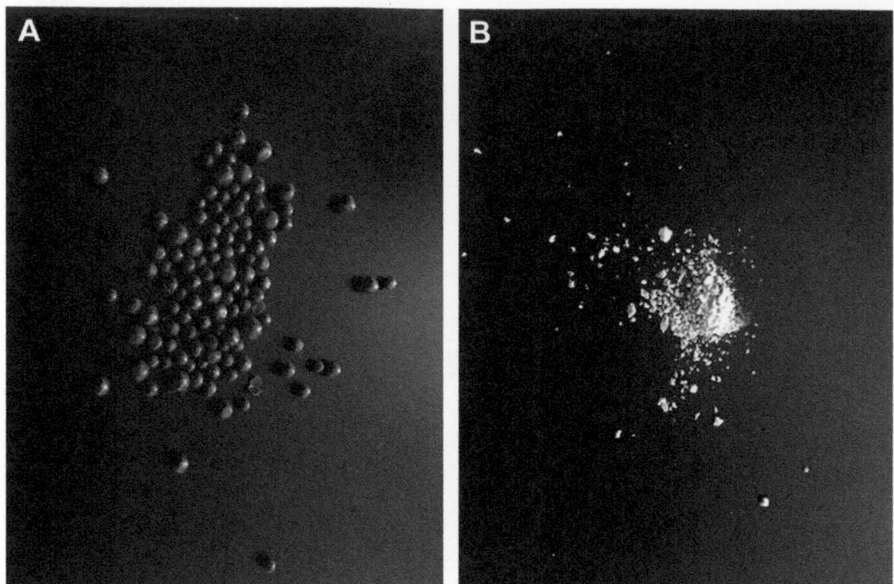

Fig. 2. (*A and B*): Typical appearance of calcium carbonate uroliths (gold beads) versus phosphatic uroliths (sand).

In cases where calcium carbonate stones are suspect, radiography is particularly valuable early in the workup. These stones are radiopaque and easily seen in the urinary bladder and urethra.[34] Knowing the number and locations of calcium carbonate uroliths can be useful in determining treatment options and prognosis. Calcium carbonate uroliths are stable and highly resistant to dissolution in acidic solutions or acidic urine. Urinary acidification with or without surgery would be unlikely to be successful in relieving the obstruction in cases with multiple calcium carbonate stones in the urethra. Although phosphatic uroliths are radiopaque,[10] they often do not show up on radiographs due to the technique necessary to penetrate the small ruminant abdomen. Negative radiographs should not be interpreted to indicate that no uroliths are present.

Medical management

Medical management includes therapies to relax the urethra, relieve pain, acidify the urine, support systemic circulation, and address other abnormalities as indicated. Medications used with the intent to relax the urethra include acepromazine (0.05 mg/kg, subcutaneously, q 4 hours) and midazolam (0.2 mg/kg, subcutaneously, q 4 hours) or diazepam (0.1 mg/kg, slow intravenously, q 4 hours). Morphine (0.05–0.1 mg/kg, subcutaneously, q 4–6 hours) and flunixin meglumine (1 mg/kg, intravenously) or meloxicam (2 mg/kg, orally, initial dose) may be considered for pain management. nonsteroidal antiinflammatory drugs (NSAIDs) should be used with great caution in animals with urinary obstruction, so one may choose to delay until the obstruction is relieved and fluid therapy is initiated.

Ammonium chloride (100–200 mg/kg, orally, initial dose) is administered for urine acidification. If clients are reticent to pursue surgery, animals under this protocol may be placed in a dry stall without bedding and observed for urination from the urethra for a few hours to overnight. For animals to be left overnight with a distended urinary bladder, needle decompression is indicated to reduce the risk of rupture.

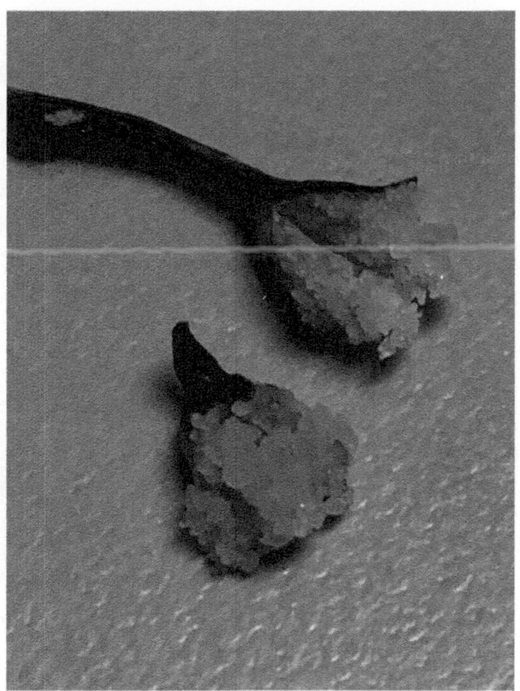

Fig. 3. Opened vermiform appendage from a urinary obstructed small ruminant. The lumen is obstructed by phosphatic-type crystals.

When medical management, vermiform amputation, and time have failed, a noninvasive intervention is the Walpole's cystocentesis.[35] In this procedure, under ultrasound guidance, urine is withdrawn from the urinary bladder and replaced with 50 mL Walpole's solution. After 2 minutes, urine is withdrawn and the pH tested. This procedure is repeated until the urine pH reaches 4 to 5. The initial report of this

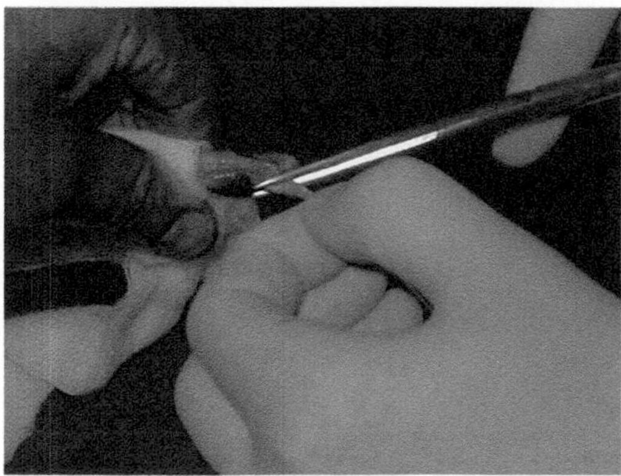

Fig. 4. Amputation of the vermiform appendage in a goat. An assistant maintains penile extension using gauze. The vermiform appendage is amputated using sharp scissors or scalpel at a slight angle to create an oblong, larger orifice.

procedure showed 80% (20/25 animals) short-term success. A subsequent data set obtained by the author (MJC) at the same institution indicated a 38% success rate, or 7/19 animals (Jones and colleagues, unpublished, 2016). Walpole's cystocentesis should only be considered in cases for which surgery is not an option for the owner and euthanasia is the only other option. Leakage of Walpole's solution into the abdomen at surgery or via a bladder perforation may be fatal and leakage from an undetected urethral rupture results in massive tissue damage and pain.

Surgical Management

Surgical intervention for urolithiasis is indicated in most cases for resolution. Several procedures have been described over time and continue to be modified by surgeons working to decrease common side effects, reduce treatment costs, and optimize outcomes.

Tube Cystostomy and Modifications

The objective of tube cystostomy is to divert urine away from the urethra out through the body wall in order to allow the urethra to heal and the obstructing uroliths to be expelled or dissolved. The traditional tube cystostomy is an open-abdomen procedure. The abdomen is entered through an 8-cm parapreputial incision midway between the preputial orifice and scrotum. The urinary bladder is identified and stay sutures placed and a cystostomy performed for the removal of uroliths and attempted normograde flushing of the urethra. A Foley catheter is placed through an additional incision in the body wall and into the urinary bladder. The cuff is inflated using saline and secured in place with a pursestring suture in the urinary bladder. In cases of urinary bladder rupture, the defect is repaired, and then the catheter is placed.[36] The urinary bladder is pulled to the body wall by the balloon and a Chinese finger trap suture pattern is used in the skin to secure the external portion of the tube to the body wall. A Heimlich valve or closed urinary system is used to prevent aspiration of air and contaminants into the urinary bladder. Medical management is instituted during hospitalization. The urine is diverted for at least 4 to 5 days, at which time a hemostat is used to occlude the tube and the patient is observed for urination from the urethra. This is repeated daily until urination occurs, which occurs in a mean of 11.5 days.[36] Once a strong urine stream from the urethra is achieved for at least a day, the holding suture is removed, the balloon deflated, and the tube pulled.

Success rates for surgical tube cystostomy in small ruminants have been reported to be 48%,[37] 52%,[31] 76%,[14] and 83% to 86%.[36,38,39] The most common complication rates reported in these studies include displacement of the tube and recurrence of the obstruction. This procedure requires general anesthesia, a long surgical time, and a long hospitalization making it financially prohibitive for some owners. For this reason, efforts to modify this procedure were undertaken to make it more economical. These include ultrasound-guided percutaneous methods of placing the tube into the urinary bladder using a variety of suprapubic catheters.[37,40,41] These have been described for use for preoperative stabilization or as an adjunct to medical management without full tube cystostomy. In one study of goats using a straight suprapubic catheter, 10/10 failed due to tube displacement, persistent obstruction, reoccurrence, and urethral rupture.38 Use of a percutaneous catheter with a memory curve to facilitate retention has been described.[41] Although obstruction or migration of the catheter and accidental gastrointestinal puncture may occur, these complications are relatively rare (12/43 goats), making this a good option to use in conjunction with medical management or until surgery is performed.[41]

Perineal Urethrostomy and Modifications

Perineal urethrostomy also diverts urine away from the obstructed portion of the urethra but permanently compromises the urethra and is therefore not suitable for breeding animals. In most situations, perineal urethrostomy is considered a short-term solution to obstruction due to the high rate of stricture that can occur postoperatively, resulting in reobstruction.[42]

To address the complication of strictures, a modified proximal perineal urethrostomy (MPPU) technique has been described for use in goats with persistent or recurrent obstruction. This approach involves an extensive dissection around the proximal penile body such that the ventral 180° of the penile body is completely free of its pelvic attachments. Further, careful mucocutaneous apposition is created for the urethral stoma. The goal is reduced tension on the stoma, which may play a role in stricture formation.[43] The most common complications were hemorrhage (1 out of 11 goats required blood transfusion), errant urine stream, and recurrent urolithiasis but urethrostomy sites remained patent in 9 out of 11 goats for more than a year postoperatively.[43]

In a retrospective including both traditional and MPPU, hemorrhage was the most common complication of MPPU while the most common complications of traditional perineal urethrostomy were related to reobstruction (stricture, stone) and urine scald.[42]

Urinary bladder marsupialization is a method of urine diversion where a stoma is created between the urinary bladder and body wall. A parapreputial celiotomy incision is created lateral to the prepuce and a cystostomy performed to remove debris. A second, smaller (approximately 4 cm) parapreputial incision is created on the contralateral side lateral to the prepuce where the urinary bladder is repositioned and tacked at 4 points. The seromuscular layer of the urinary bladder is sutured circumferentially to the abdominal fascia with interrupting sutures. The cystostomy margins are then sutured circumferentially to the skin with simple interrupted sutures. Absorbable, 2 to 0 or 3 to 0 suture material is used for these 2 layers and the contralateral celiotomy is closed in routine fashion.[44] Complications of urinary bladder marsupialization include urinary bladder mucosal prolapse, incontinence, partial dehiscence, occluding serum formation, cystitis, urine scald, and stricture of the marsupialization site.[37,44,45] It is reported that goats may urinate normally through the urethra after stoma stricture,[44] and some animals are able to develop urinary continence.[45] Other described surgical approaches to small ruminant urolithiasis include vesicopreputial anastomosis,[46] minimally invasive surgical tube cystostomy,[47] and laser lithotripsy.[48]

Preventative Management

Planning for the prevention of urolithiasis should be a topic included in any herd health or nutritional consultation where male small ruminants are involved. Due to the cost, prognoses, and potential complications associated with each of the treatment modalities listed, a proactive, multifaceted approach to prevention is necessary. This is not a simple disease with a simple solution.

The risk factors outlined earlier in this article serve as a guide to address specific risks on a given farm. What type of animals are in the group? What is their expected use? What is their current or planned diet? Understanding the goals and expectations of the client can facilitate the construction of a plan that helps clients attain their goals while minimizing disease. Further, this information can help predict the stone type most likely to appear in this herd or flock so that strategies specific to that stone type can be used.

There are some general recommendations that we can make that can be expected to limit stone formation, regardless of stone type. Delaying castration past 4 to 6 months can result in an increase in urethral diameter, increasing the capacity to pass formed stones.[20–22] Delayed castration must be carefully considered especially in miniature breeds because they are precocious breeders who may breed their female peers at an early age. Sex separation is recommended. Amputation of the vermiform appendage is challenging in prepubescent animals but removes the most common site of urolith obstruction due to its small diameter at the terminal urethra. The effect of this on fertility of breeding animals has not been evaluated,[23,24] and the procedure is not commonly performed as a preventative measure.

Dilution of urine and frequent urination helps rid the urinary bladder of both organic and inorganic components of uroliths, regardless of stone type. Making sure that clean, palatable, temperature-appropriate water sources are readily available at all times in all seasons can facilitate this dilution and regular urination. Water balance is also influenced by feed type. Foraging and grazing requires additional water for mastication and digestion, while meal feeding grains and pelleted feeds shunt water to the rumen. This results in the release of antidiuretic hormone, reducing urine output and dilution. For these and other reasons, limiting grains and pellets and increasing forage and grazing time are good practices toward preventing urolithiasis.[5,11]

The organic nidus may include cellular, protein, sugar, and other components. Providing protein at a level necessary for the stage of life and production but not in excess helps limit excess protein in the urine. Palatable trace minerals that include adequate Vitamin A prevent metaplasia and cellular sloughing of the uroepithelium that can serve as a nidus.[13]

We can take our recommendations beyond the general to the specific by identifying the specific stone types associated with certain groups of animals. A basic generalization is that younger, grain-fed animals tend to develop phosphatic type stones, whereas young adults, miniature breeds, and those consuming alfalfa or other legumes tend to develop calcium carbonate stones.[10] Other stone types, such as silicate, form in animals in sandy western soils in the United States and Canada but we know very little about preventing these other than to limit the access of males to these grazing areas.

For animals with anticipated risk for phosphatic urolithiasis, urine pH and mineral balance are important factors to address. A goal for controlling phosphatic urolithiasis is to, at least periodically, reduce the urine pH less than 6.5, the target pH for dissolution.[1,2] This can be done in a variety of ways, including reducing the DCAD of the total diet to 0 mg/kg using chloride salts.' D, L-Methionine at a dosage of 200 mg/kg orally daily has been shown to effectively reduce urine pH.[28] A strategy that addresses concerns about individual susceptibility to urinary acidifiers and renal adaptation to acidification is to titrate an ammonium chloride dose in the individual animal to a urine pH of less than 6.5 and then pulse dose 3 days on, 4 days off.[27] It is clear that DCAD balancing is a more appropriate approach to herd-level control, whereas titration and pulse dosing are more appropriate for individual animals, although pulse dosing can be used with DCAD balanced diets. Regardless of the acidification method used, urine pH should be regularly monitored in meal-fed animals 5 to 7 hours after receiving an acidifier to confirm that the target pH is being achieved.[26] Balancing magnesium, phosphorus, and calcium is important in the control of struvite and other phosphatic stones. In general, the goal is to keep magnesium and phosphorus low, while using calcium to offset absorption of phosphorus. We know that magnesium and phosphorus are highly available when obtained through grains,[12] whereas forages increase salivary excretion of phosphorus, resulting in our consistent recommendation of reducing grains and increasing forage intake. Calcium competes for absorption with phosphorus, leading to the recommendation that the Ca:P ratio of diets to prevent phosphatic stones be 2 to 3:1.[29,30] This ratio must be closely monitored and not exceeded because it may predispose to calcium-containing uroliths.

For animals at risk for calcium carbonate urolithiasis, the dietary Ca:P ratio should be limited to 2:1 in order to keep phosphorus absorption at bay while not allowing calcium to be available in excess. Exclusion of legumes, particularly alfalfa, is generally recommended for these at risk animals.[19] Although calcium carbonate forms in alkaline urine, it is not readily dissolved by urine pH reduction. Acidifying urine pH may be limited to helping to prevent formation but may be a 2-edged sword due to the effect of acidification on renal calcium excretion. Calcium availability in the urine is increased in metabolic acidosis because it is induced by the chloride salts. For this reason, the use of chloride salts should be limited to the dose, which reduces urine pH to 6.5 without over acidification. This highlights the need to be specific regarding target stone type when addressing preventative measures. The use of acidifying measures to prevent phosphatic stones may actually increase the formation of calcium-containing stones.

Although it has not been confirmed in large, controlled studies, it has been strongly suggested that there is individual susceptibility to urolithiasis (stone formers), and there are instances where urolithiasis of the same stone type has been repeated in families.[14,15,19]

Prevention of urolithiasis will likely never be able to be distilled to a simple, formulaic plan; however, preventative measures addressed here can significantly reduce incidence of the disease. Decades of research and data generated regarding urolithiasis can leave us frustrated when breakthrough cases occur. However, in most cases of obstructive urolithiasis, at least one breach of these recommendations can be readily identified. We must be vigilant in educating livestock producers about proper nutrition, husbandry, and other risk factors, as well as help them understand the physiologic basis for these recommendations to encourage a commitment to multimodal prevention over the long term.

CLINICS CARE POINTS

- Obstructive urolithiasis should be screened for in any ill male small ruminant presenting for veterinary care.
- It is imperative that the urolith type be identified, or initially presumed based on appearance and risk factors, in order to make recommendations regarding disease prevention.
- Conversations with livestock owners regarding prevention of urolithiasis should address anatomic factors, urine pH, water intake, dietary composition, and genetic factors.
- A thorough diagnostic evaluation, which determines the extent of urinary bladder and urethral damage, the location of the obstruction(s), and systemic stability of the animal facilitates selection of treatments and the estimation of prognosis.
- The most common causes of failure of medical and surgical treatments across all types is failure to resolve the obstruction and recurrence of the obstruction.

DISCLOSURE

The author has no financial conflict of interest to disclose.

REFERENCES

1. Jacobs D, Heimbach D, Hesse A. Chemolysis of struvite stones by acidification of artificial urine. Scand J Urol Nephrol 2001;35:345–9.
2. Elliot JS, Quaide WL, Sharp RF, et al. Mineralogical studies of urine: The relationship of apatite, brushite and struvite to urinary pH. J Urol 1958;80(4):267–71.
3. Osborne CA, Polzin DJ, Abdullahi SU, et al. Struvite urolithiasis in animals and man: Formation, detection and dissolution. Adv Vet Sci Comp Med 1985;29:1–45.
4. Trueman NA, Stacy BD. Ovine urolithiasis: Some mineralogic and physiologic observations. Invest Urol 1969;7(2):185–91.
5. Swingle KF, Cornelius CE. Ruminant urolithiasis V. Excretion of certain urinary biocolloid fractions by sheep on alfalfa and grain rations. Am J Vet Res 1962;23:972–6.
6. Romanowski RD. Biochemistry of urolith formation. J Am Vet Med Assoc 1965;147(12):1324–6.
7. Cornelius CE, Moulton JE, McGowan B. Ruminant urolithiasis: I. Preliminary observations in experimental ovine calculosis. Am J Vet Res 1959;20:863–71.
8. Cornelius CE. Studies on ovine urinary biocolloids and phosphatic calculosis. Ann New York Acad Sci 1963;104:638–57.
9. Packett LV, Lineberger RO, Jackson HD. Mineral studies in ovine phosphatic urolithiasis. Am J Clin Nutr 1971;24(10):1716–21.
10. Jones ML, Gibbons PM, Roussel AJ, et al. Mineral composition of uroliths obtained from sheep and goats with obstructive urolithiasis. J Vet Intern Med 2017;31:1202–8.
11. Crookshank HR, Packett LV Jr, Kunkel HO. Ovine urinary calculi and pelleted rations. J Anim Sci 1965;24:638–42.
12. Gaebel G, Martens H, Suendermann M, et al. The effect of diet, intraruminal pH and osmolarity on sodium, chloride and magnesium absorption from the temporarily isolated and washed reticulo-rumen of sheep. Q J Exp Pays 1987;72:501–11.
13. Packett LV, Coburn SP. Urine proteins in nutritionally induced ovine urolithiasis. Am J Vet Res 1965;26(10):112–9.
14. Ewoldt JM, Anderson DE, Miesner MD, et al. Short- and long-term outcome and factors predicting survival after surgical tube cystostomy for treatment of obstructive urolithiasis in small ruminants. Vet Surg 2006;35(5):417–22.
15. Nwakorie EE, Osborne CA, Lulich JP. Risk factors for calcium carbonate urolithiasis in goats. J Am Vet Med Assoc 2015;247:293–9.
16. Griffin DG. A review of the heritability of idiopathic nephrolithiasis. J Clin Pathol 2004;57:793–6.
17. Harnevik L, Hoppe A, Soderkvist P. SLC7A9 cDNA cloning and mutational analysis of SLC3A1 and SLC7A9 in canine cystinuria. Mamm Genome 2006;17:769–76.
18. Thumchai R, Lulich J, Osborne CA, et al. Epizootiologic evaluation of urolithiasis in cats: 3,498 cases (1982-1992). J Am Vet Med Assoc 1996;208:547–51.
19. Jones ML, Dominguez BJ, Deveau MA. An experimental model for calcium carbonate urolithiasis in goats. J Vet Intern Med 2018;32:1268–73.
20. Marsh H, Safford JW. Effect of deferred castration on urethral development in calves. J Am Vet Med Assoc 1957;'30:342–6.
21. Kumar R, Kumar A, Singh H, et al. Effect of castration on urethra and accessory sex glands in goats. Indian Vet J 1982;59:304–8.

22. Bani Ismail ZA, Al-Zghoul MF, Al-Majali AM, et al. Effects of castration on penile and urethral development in Agassi lambs. Bulg J Vet Med 2007;10(1):29–34.
23. Smith MC. Urinary system. In: Smith MC, Sherman DM, editors. Goat medicine. Philadelphia: Lea & Febiger; 1994. p. 388–9.
24. Boundy T. Routine ram examination. In: Melling M, Alder M, editors. *Sheep and goat practice* 2. Philadelphia: WB Saunders Co; 1998. p. 1–18.
25. Stratton-Phelps M, House JK. Effect of a commercial anion dietary supplement on acid-base balance, urine volume, and urinary ion excretion in male goats fed oat or grass hay diets. Am J Vet Res 2004;65(10):1391–7.
26. Jones ML, Streeter RN, Goad CL. Dietary cation anion difference for the control of risk factors for urolithiasis in goats. Am J Vet Res 2009;70(1):149–55.
27. Sprake P, Roussel AJ, Stewart R, Bissett WT. The effect of ammonium chloride treatment as a long-term preventative approach for urolithiasis in goats and a comparison of continuous and pulse dosing regimes. J Vet Intern Med 2012; 26:760.
28. Grissett G, Fleming S, Neizman K. Evaluation of orally supplemented D, L-methionine as a urine acidifier for small ruminants. J Vet Intern Med 2012;26:760.
29. Hoar DW, Emerick RJ, Embry LB. Potassium, phosphorus and calcium interrelationships influencing feedlot performance and phosphatic urolithiasis in lambs. J Anim Sci 1970;30(4):597–600.
30. Hoar DW, Emerick RJ, Embry LB. Influence of calcium source, phosphorus level and acid-base-forming effects of the diet on feedlot performance and urinary calculi formation in lambs. J Anim Sci 1970;31(1):118–25.
31. Reidi AK, Nathues C, Knubben-Schweizer G, et al. Variables of initial examination and clinical management associated with survival in small ruminants with obstructive urolithiasis. J Vet Intern Med 2018;32:2105–14.
32. Thurmon JC, Nelson DR, Hartsfield SM, et al. Effects of xylazine hydrochloride on urine in cattle. Aus Vet J 1978;54:178–80.
33. Reppert EJ, Streeter RN, Simpson KM, et al. Retrograde catheterization of the urinary bladder in healthy male goats by use of angiographic catheters. Am J Vet Res 2016;77(11):1295–9.
34. Kinsley MA, Semevolos S, Parker JE, et al. Use of plain radiography in the diagnosis, surgical management, and postoperative treatment of obstructive urolithiasis in 25 goats and 2 sheep. Vet Surg 2013;42:663–8.
35. Janke JJ, Osterstock JB, Washburn KE, et al. Use of Walpole's solution for treatment of goats with urolithiasis: 25 cases (2001-2006). J Am Vet Med Assoc 2009; 234(2):249–52.
36. Rakestraw PC, Fubini SL, Gilbert RO, et al. Tube cystostomy for treatment of obstructive urolithiasis in small ruminants. Vet Surg 1995;24:498–505.
37. Fortier LA, Gregg AJ, Erb HN, et al. Caprine obstructive urolithiasis; requirement for 2nd surgical intervention and mortality after percutaneous tube cystostomy, surgical tube cystostomy, or urinary bladder marsupialization. Vet Surg 2004; 33(6):661–7.
38. Jacobs CC, Fecteau ME. Urethrotomy in combination with or after temporary tube cystostomy for treatment of obstructive urolithiasis in male goats. Vet Surg 2019; 48(3):315–20.
39. Gamsjager L, Chigerwe. Risk factors for, frequency, and type of complications after temporary tube cystostomy in goats, sheep, and pigs. Vet Surg 2021;50: 283–93.

40. Streeter RN, Washburn KE, McCauley CT. Percutaneous tube cystostomy and vesicular irrigation for treatment of obstructive urolithiasis in a goat. J Am Vet Med Assoc 2002;221(4):546–9.
41. Chigerwe M, Heller MC, Balcomb CC, et al. Use of a percutaneous trans abdominal catheter for management of obstructive urolithiasis in goats, sheep, and pot-bellied pigs: 69 cases (2000-2014). J Am Vet Med Assoc 2016;248(11):1287–90.
42. Oman RE, Reppert EJ, Streeter RN, et al. Outcome and complications in goats treated by perineal urethrostomy for obstructive urolithiasis: 25 cases (2010-2017). J Vet Intern Med 2019;33:292–6.
43. Tobias KM, van Amstel SR. Modified proximal perineal urethrostomy technique for treatment of urethral stricture in goats. Vet Surg 2013;42:455–62.
44. May KA, Moll HD, Wallace LM, et al. Urinary bladder marsupialization for treatment of obstructive urolithiasis in male goats. Vet Surg 1998;27:583–8.
45. May KA, Moll HD, Duncan RB, et al. Experimental evaluation of urinary bladder marsupialization in male goats. Vet Surg 2002;31:251–8.
46. Cypher EE, van Amstel SR, Videla R, et al. Vesicopreputial anastomosis for the treatment of obstructive urolithiasis in goats. Vet Surg 2017;46:281–8.
47. Fazili MR, Malik HU, Bhattacharyaa HK, et al. Minimally invasive surgical tube cystostomy for treating obstructive urolithiasis in small ruminants with an intact urinary bladder. Vet Rec 2010;166(17):528–32.
48. Halland SK, House JK, George LW. Urethroscopy and laser lithotripsy for the diagnosis and treatment of obstructive urolithiasis in goats and pot-bellied pigs. J Am Vet Med Assoc 2002;220:1831–4.

Hepatic Lipidosis in Ruminants

Josef J. Gross

KEYWORDS

- Hepatic lipidosis • Fatty liver • Fat cow syndrome • Pathophysiology • Liver
- Dairy cow

KEY POINTS

- The start of lactation is accompanied by distinct metabolic and endocrine adaptations to meet the increased energetic demands for lactation.
- Hepatic lipidosis develops when the capacities for oxidation and export of fatty acids are overwhelmed.
- Hepatic lipidosis has an active role in the development and manifestation of other metabolic and infectious diseases.

INTRODUCTION

Hepatic lipidosis (HL), fatty liver or fat cow syndrome, occurs primarily during the first few weeks of lactation in dairy cows but may already be pronounced shortly before or at parturition.[1–3] Because of the prevailing energy deficiency at the onset of lactation imposed by a lack of feed intake at concomitantly elevated requirements, adipose tissue is mobilized and concentrations of nonesterified fatty acids (NEFA) increase in blood. Once the hepatic uptake exceeds the capacity for export and oxidation, lipids accumulate in the form of triacylglycerides (TAG). Consequently, various functions and activities of the liver are reduced or impaired.[1,4] Particularly due to the considerable increases in milk production over the last years, factors contributing to the extent of lipomobilization during the negative energy balance further aggravate the expression of HL, resulting in high incidence rates. Although numerous clinical research was completed in the past 4 decades, HL still represents a major metabolic disease in dairy cows, associated with decreased animal health, milk yield, and welfare. Costs for fatty liver derive from increased veterinary costs and losses of reproductive and lactational performance. Furthermore, HL is associated with an increased culling rate and a reduction of lifetime performance.

Coinciding with other health disorders such as ketosis, a differential diagnosis of HL is only possible to a limited extent. On the other hand, early lactation dairy cows

Veterinary Physiology, University of Bern, Bremgartenstrasse 109a, 3012 Bern, Switzerland
E-mail address: josef.gross@unibe.ch

Vet Clin Food Anim 39 (2023) 371–383
https://doi.org/10.1016/j.cvfa.2023.02.007 vetfood.theclinics.com
0749-0720/23/

suffering from metritis, ketosis, or lameness have a great likelihood to express HL as well. So far, deviations of different diagnostic biomarkers characteristic for other health disorders are also associated with the presence of fatty liver. On the other hand, the question arises if fatty liver is causative or supportive for the development of secondary health disorders.

Numerous excellent review papers exist that address the cause of HL and ways of its treatment and prevention.[2,5–7] Treatment and prevention shall therefore not be the scope here. The aim of this review paper is to elucidate the role of HL hepatic lipidosis as a disease component of ruminant metabolic disease conditions. Besides the cause of HL, the focus is set on mechanisms and pathophysiological pathways related to an impaired hepatic function due to increased TAG accumulation, which cause further metabolic diseases.

INCIDENCE AND CLINICAL RELEVANCE

The clinical relevance of HL emanates primarily from the reduction in milk yield, increased incidence of metabolic diseases, lowered fertility, loss of animal welfare, and costs for veterinary treatments. Although categorization of HL according to the lipid concentration in hepatic tissue varies between scientific reports, the relatively broad gradation into normal, mild, moderate, and severe fatty liver allows an estimation of the animal's general health status and risk for developing concomitant metabolic diseases.[2,8] Whereas cows with a normal or mild fatty liver are often clinically unapparent, determined odds ratios to express further health disorders are several fold higher in cows with a greater extent of hepatic fat infiltration.

Earlier studies by Jorritsma and colleagues assumed that between 50% and 60% of all cows show increased hepatic lipid concentrations during early lactation.[9,10] Estimations for the prevalence of HL during the first month after parturition assigned up to 10% of dairy cows having severe hepatic infiltration and up to 40% having moderate fatty liver.[2] In more than 80% of downer cows during the early postpartum period, moderate and severe, respectively, hepatic fat infiltration was observed.[11] In addition, the clinical relevance of HL can indirectly be quantified by incidence rates of closely associated metabolic disorders such as ketosis.

Reports on prevalence rates for subclinical ketosis range from 3% to 42% in the first 2 to 3 months of lactation,[12–15] whereas prevalence of clinical ketosis ranges at lower levels from 2% to 15%.[16,17] At a herd level, subclinical ketosis may affect up to 40% of cows in a herd although the incidence can be as high as 80%.[18,19] Herds with more than a 15% to 20% prevalence of excessively elevated concentrations of NEFA and β-hydroxybutyrate (BHB) in early lactation have higher rates of subsequent health disorder.[18,20] A review by van der Kolk and colleagues indicated that cows first testing subclinical ketosis positive from 3 to 5 days postpartum were 6.1 times more likely to develop a displaced abomasum than cows first testing subclinical ketosis positive at later lactational stages.[19] Moreover, cows first testing subclinical ketosis positive from 3 to 7 days postpartum were 4.5 times more likely to be removed from the herd. Cows with ketosis often show a reduced performance in terms of milk yield and fertility.[20,21] Furthermore, ketosis triggers the susceptibility toward further production diseases such as retained placenta, fatty liver, displaced abomasum, metritis, and lameness.[13,22,23] Besides the impairment of animal welfare, significant economic losses occur due to costs for reduced milk yield and veterinary treatments.[24,25] Costs for fatty liver in the United States' dairy cow population almost 20 years ago were estimated to be more than $60 million.[2] With increasing milk yields in dairy cows, nowadays even more cows can be assumed to have HL.

CAUSE OF HEPATIC LIPIDOSIS

Milk production of dairy cows has increased globally over the past few decades.[26] During the last 40 to 50 years, average milk production per cow more than doubled in many countries. Concomitantly, a considerable number of dairy cows are affected by health disorders that are primarily associated with the high-performance level and associated failures of metabolic and immunologic adaptation. However, the selection toward higher milk yield continues worldwide.[27,28] Therefore, a further increase of prevalence and incidence rates of ketosis can be expected, as the risk toward developing health disorders increases with increasing milk production.

In contrast to the rapidly increasing nutrient and energy demands for milk production, the concomitant feed intake increases slowly after parturition,[29] whereas toward the end of lactation and during the dry period a risk of overconditioning exists. Consequently, cows face a considerable energy deficiency during the first weeks of lactation until feed intake can meet the energy requirements for maintenance and lactation.[4,30] Furthermore, the onset of lactation in dairy cows is characterized by a high priority in directing nutrients to the mammary gland.[31–33] To compensate for the temporary negative energy balance (NEB), cows mobilize body reserves (predominantly adipose tissue) until the peak of lactation is reached, in order to replenish and accumulate corresponding reserves again later. Thus, the prevailing NEB triggering lipolysis exposes high-producing cows to metabolic stress already at the time of calving.[32,34] Consequently, predisposition to metabolic and infectious diseases is initiated at the very beginning of lactation. Additional factors such as inadequate feeding and overconditioning during the dry period may further aggravate metabolic adaptation and favor hypocalcemia, endometritis, and so forth.[35,36]

The beginning of lactation requires considerable metabolic adaptations to meet increased energy demands for milk production of dairy cows.[30,32,37] Dairy cows experience an abrupt change from anabolic to catabolic metabolism when passing through a period of NEB from late gestation to early lactation.[18,29,38] During the transition period, cows are highly susceptible to developing metabolic and related diseases such as ketosis, liver lipidosis, retained placenta, mastitis, displaced abomasum, laminitis, or reproduction problems.[39–41] An affected cow may enter a vicious circle, as postpartum disorders are interrelated and one metabolic disorder may predispose the cow to other disorders.

Glucose is a key nutrient and limiting source for lactation, and the capacity of gluconeogenesis and dietary intake of glucogenic precursors remain low during early lactation.[42] Considering the essentiality of glucose for other organs and tissues (eg, immune system, reproductive tissues, and so forth), it is not surprising that the health disorders are associated with the period of low circulating glucose concentrations in early lactation.[42,43] Lipids therefore become an alternative metabolic fuel. To address increased fatty acid needs as an energy source and for milk fat synthesis, body lipid stores are mobilized (lipomobilization) via lipolysis. Mobilized NEFA enter the liver, where they are normally metabolized in the presence of oxaloacetate after being activated by binding to acetyl-coenzyme A (acetyl-CoA), thereby releasing energy (**Fig. 1**). Fatty acids that are not completely oxidized are reesterified to TAG, bound to apolipoprotein, and released into the bloodstream as very low-density lipoprotein (VLDL). However, the ability of the liver to export triglycerides is limited. Consequently, fatty liver can develop.[2,3,6]

Although the metabolic load is known to be highest after parturition, metabolic adaptations with respect to lactation already start before calving. Despite no obvious additional need for energy shortly before parturition, insulin and insulinlike growth

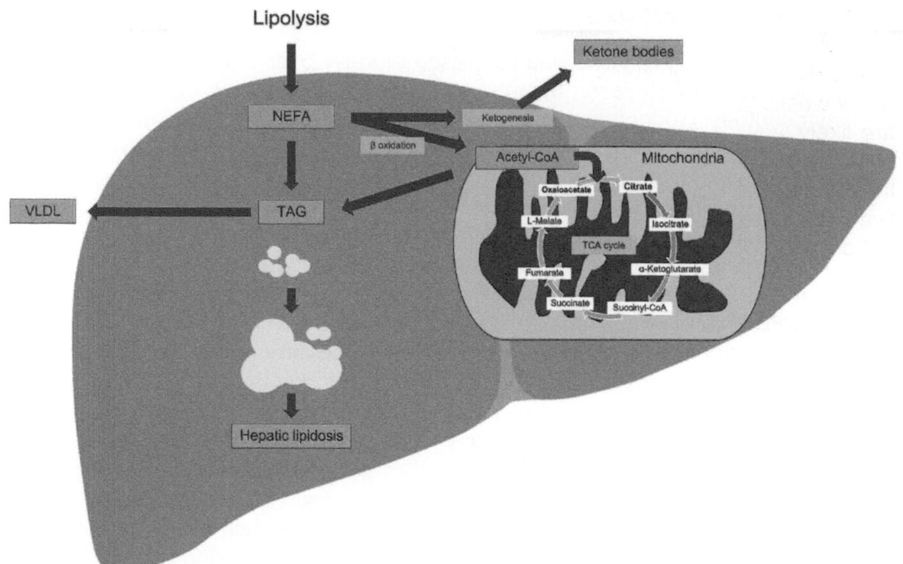

Fig. 1. Metabolism of mobilized fatty acids in the tricarboxylic acid (TCA) cycle and development of hepatic lipidosis.

factor-1 (IGF-1) concentrations already start to decline, and elevated release of growth hormone (GH) and mobilization of adipose tissue commence.[44] The drop of circulating thyroid hormones, leptin, adiponectin, insulin, and IGF-1 shortly before parturition enables the initiation of lipolysis while concomitantly inhibiting lipogenesis.[32,45,46]

Along with enhanced sensitivity to catecholamines, low insulin concentration is one of the main triggers to activate hormone-sensitive lipases in adipose tissue and hence fat mobilization.[47] Low circulating insulin is involved in the uncoupling of the somatotropic axis in the liver via downregulation of the hepatic GH receptor.[44,48] Consequently plasma GH levels increase, whereas plasma IGF-1 concentrations remain low.[49,50] A direct effect of GH is the stimulation of lipolysis from adipose tissue supported by enhanced sensitivity to beta-adrenergic effects of catecholamines.[33]

Glucose originates predominantly from hepatic gluconeogenesis in ruminants. Hepatic gluconeogenesis depends on overall tricarboxylic acid (TCA) cycle activity, especially on the availability of oxaloacetate and substrates, such as propionate, lactate, amino acids, and glycerol (see **Fig. 1**). Upregulation of gluconeogenesis postpartum relies on oxaloacetate reserves, thereby reducing oxaloacetate availability in hepatocyte mitochondria. Consequently, oxidation of fatty acids via the TCA cycle is limited, and an alternative metabolic pathway (besides storage of triglycerides in the liver) is activated through enhanced synthesis of ketone bodies from acetyl-CoA in the liver (see **Fig. 1**). Low insulin concentrations additionally promote ketogenesis.[51]

Cows face a metabolic dilemma by the competition for oxaloacetate either depleted for gluconeogenesis or required to maintain the TCA cycle for oxidation of fatty acids (see **Fig. 1**).[52,53] Cows with a greater milk yield are likely to have a prolonged and more severe NEB. Consequently, high-yielding cows are forced to mobilize more adipose tissue. However, if the TCA cycle becomes overloaded (eg, by capacious drainage of oxaloacetate for gluconeogenesis), the acetyl-CoA is shunted off to produce ketone bodies (acetoacetic acid, acetone, and BHB) in order to prevent cessation of the TCA cycle and accumulation of acetyl-CoA (see **Fig. 1**).[54,55] Consequently, fatty acids that are not oxidized are converted to ketone bodies or reesterified to triglycerides within the liver.[1,2] A mild to severe fatty liver may develop already within a very narrow time after calving, although NEFA concentrations and metabolic load reach highest values a few weeks later.[3] The concomitant low cholesterol concentrations in early lactation are likely limiting the hepatic triglyceride export despite an upregulation of hepatic cholesterol biosynthesis.[56] Forcing NEB with adipose tissue mobilization at a later lactational stage, however, did not result in a considerable lipid accumulation in the liver, as cholesterol concentrations were elevated supporting hepatic triglyceride export as VLDL.[3,57]

HEPATIC LIPIDOSIS AS DISEASE COMPONENT

Pathophysiology and Histologic Changes Associated with Hepatic Lipidosis

To a certain extent, deposition of TAG in hepatocytes is a physiologic response to compensate for the excessive NEFA influx besides ketogenesis. In general, accumulation of TAG is the result of increased NEFA arriving at the liver, elevated local synthesis, decreased oxidation, and limited hepatic export of fatty acids.[53,58] Besides hepatic physical swelling and enlargement, a gross color change toward a yellowish appearance indicates considerable fatty infiltration.[59] Excessive TAG accumulation alters histologic structures of the liver. Bobe and colleagues collated histologic findings in cows diagnosed with fatty liver, which include, depending on the severity and degree of hepatic TAG accumulation; fatty cysts in liver parenchyma; an increased hepatocyte volume; mitochondrial damage; compression and decreased volume of nuclei; rough endoplasmic reticulum, sinusoids, and other organelles; and decreased number of organelles.[2] For diagnostic purposes, increased concentrations of liver enzymes and bile constituents were detected in plasma of dairy cows with severe fatty liver (for details, see review by Bobe and colleagues[2]).

Therefore, it is not surprising that hepatic lipidosis coincides with other health disorders (eg, ketosis, lameness, fertility problems). In part, reasons for fatty liver development are identical with those responsible for concomitant other health disorders (ie, negative energy balance, excessive lipomobilization). However, impaired liver function due to HL can also act as trigger of production diseases. Although associations of HL with production diseases are well known, the following sections specifically elucidate the aspect of HL as disease component in terms of its role for the development of other health disorders. Hepatic lipidosis is, however, not only an acute issue in early lactating dairy animals facing a transient energy deficiency but has long-lasting impacts on physiologic adaptation. Milk production, health status, and reproductive performance of dairy cows can be decreased for weeks after concentrations of liver TAG returned to baseline concentrations.[60,61]

Hepatic Lipidosis and Metabolic Status

Pathologic changes associated with HL affect concentrations of metabolites and minerals in plasma.[2] Because of their individual toxicity at high concentrations and further metabolic effects, elevated concentrations of ammonia, NEFA, and ketone bodies may decrease the physiologic functions of other organs. Elevated concentrations of NEFA have the ability to increase lipogenesis and ketogenesis in hepatocytes.[62] Moreover, increased concentrations of ketone bodies decrease β-oxidation, gluconeogenesis, and TCA activity in hepatocytes.[2] Consequently, metabolic stress is further aggravated in cows with HL. A proteome analysis in feed-deprived dairy cows found downregulation of proteins associated with fatty acid oxidation, glycolysis, electron transfer, protein degradation, antigen processing, and cytoskeletal rearrangement, whereas different enzymes and proteins involved in the urea cycle, fatty acid and cholesterol transport, and calcium signaling were upregulated.[63] Recent research revealed that biomarkers identified by metabolomics may distinguish HL from other peripartal disorders.[64] Similarly, concentrations of serum hepatokines such as angiopoietin-like protein 4 and fibroblast growth factor 21 (FGF21) were greater in cows with HL and clinical ketosis compared with healthy animals.[65]

Increased plasma concentrations of bile constituents (bilirubin, bile acids, and cholic acid) indicate a reduced bile flow in cows with fatty liver.[2] Elevated concentrations of bile are toxic and increase hepatic production of free radicals, which can cause inflammation and tissue damage.[66] Alvarez and colleagues observed that high concentrations of bile damage bovine pancreatic duct epithelial cells.[67]

Hepatic lipidosis is accompanied by decreased concentrations of lipoproteins (free cholesterol, cholesteryl ester, and phospholipids), citrate, and glycogen.[2,68] Low concentration of hepatic glycogen imply an increased risk for metabolic disorders.[69] In addition, different concentrations and activities of components and enzymes related to cholesterol and lipoprotein metabolism (eg, apoprotein B-100, protein kinase C, LDL and VLDL)[68,70] and mitochondrial carnitine palmitoyl transferase involved in β-oxidation and ketogenesis[71] are decreased in liver.[2] Likewise, plasma concentrations of lipoproteins and enzymes involved in hepatic lipid export and transport are also decreased in HL. Consequently, the already limited and additionally decreased capacity for TAG export trigger the lipid accumulation in the liver. Related to the impairment of lipoprotein synthesis, fatty liver results in a reduced formation of cholesteryl esters, which are important precursors for the steroid hormone synthesis.[68] Thus, an impact on reproductive performance can be expected (see later section).

Besides metabolic changes, HL is associated with altered hormonal sensitivity of adipose tissue and pancreas.[2,72,73] At the same time, clearance rates of insulin,[74] endotoxins,[61] and other compounds[75] in hepatocytes are decreased. Based on the decreased clearance of hormones by hepatocytes infiltrated with lipids,[74] Bobe and colleagues[2] assumed that synthesis and secretion of hepatic IGF-1, adrenal glucocorticoids, pancreatic glucagon and insulin, and thyroid hormones is decreased. Reduced concentrations of these respective hormones in plasma are characteristic during the catabolic stage in early lactating dairy cows, which supports lipolysis and the prioritized nutrient direction toward the mammary gland.[30,42]

Hepatic Lipidosis and Immunologic Status

Hepatic lipidosis is closely related to the incidence of other metabolic and infectious diseases such as ketosis, metritis, and mastitis,[2,76] although infectious diseases occur even without the presence of fatty liver.[39] During the peripartal period, immune function and response are suppressed at concomitantly elevated concentrations of proinflammatory cytokines such as tumor necrosis factor-alpha.[61,77] A direct effect of HL on the immune competence can be assumed due to the decreased clearance of endotoxins[61] and increased levels of acute phase proteins such as haptoglobin and serum amyloid A.[68] In combination with the aforementioned HL-related alterations of metabolites, hormones, and factors interacting with the immune system, a direct effect of the degree of hepatic lipid infiltration on the immune responsiveness cannot be denied.[68,78]

Excessive lipolysis and elevated ketogenesis result in increased concentrations of NEFA and BHB in plasma that are known to actively impair immune competence.[77]

Increased circulating concentrations of endotoxins and elevated inflammatory markers are likely to negatively affect claw health, resulting in increased lameness during the coinciding period of HL.[79]

Hepatic Lipidosis and Reproductive Function

The onset of postpartal ovarian activity was reported to start later in cows with a more severe NEB and greater concentrations of plasma BHB.[80] In addition, decreased concentrations of IGF-I, insulin, and lipoproteins[5] and elevated concentrations of NEFA and urea can impair normal ovarian function.[2,81,82] As follicular development commences with the negative energy balance, lower pregnancy rates in cows with HL can be explained by decreased numbers of oocytes that survive during early follicular development.[8]

Another explanation for the delayed start of ovarian activity can be assigned to the decreased and delayed synthesis of steroidogenic hormones (ie, progesterone and luteinizing hormone) in cows with HL. Therefore, it is not surprising that cows with HL have a decreased reproductive performance.[61,83] Under the immune suppressive conditions around parturition, increased incidence, length, and severity of endometritis were observed that cause a delayed uterine involution.[84,85]

PREVENTION OF HEPATIC LIPIDOSIS

Approaches for prevention of HL are similar to those of preventing ketosis and aim at (1) reducing NEFA concentrations in blood by lowering lipolysis, (2) improving oxidation of NEFA, and/or (3) increasing hepatic TAG export.[86] Numerous nutritional and management strategies have been studied in the past. In brief, increasing energy density of diets (eg, supplementary fat and starch) had little effects on hepatic TAG content.[2,86] Although niacin has antilipolytic properties, niacin or nicotinic acid failed in more recent studies to prevent ketosis and HL.[2] However, the administration of monensin and glucose precursors (eg, propylene glycol, propionate salts) seem promising alternatives to mitigate HL.[2,86] Rumen-protected choline and methionine serve as precursors of VLDL constituents and were shown to decrease hepatic TAG accumulation.[87] However, results on choline are discussed controversially.[88] Although choline supplementation may reduce hepatic TAG content[89] and improve oxidative stress and liver function markers,[87] the beneficial effects of the associated increase of dry matter intake are likely to be masked by a concomitant increase of milk yield.[88]

Management strategies may be the most effective way to prevent HL. Overconditioning during the dry period is one of the most potent risk factor for ketosis.[90] Cows that have been overfed during dry period have a lower dry matter intake after calving and mobilize endogenous fat reserves more rapidly during the first weeks of lactation. In these animals, increased lipomobilization provides more fatty acids than can be oxidized, which further triggers ketogenesis and hepatic TAG accumulation. Besides maintenance of a normal body condition, preventive measures for other peripartal health disorders (eg, hypocalcemia, displacement of the abomasum, lameness, and so forth) that are accompanied by reduced feed intake should be promoted. Another promising approach is the reduction of dry period length. Although milk yield in the next lactation period is lower, the metabolic load and therefore the risk to develop ketosis and HL are significantly lower when the dry period was omitted or reduced.[91–93] In a similar manner, lactation periods can be extended before dry-off to mitigate potential failures in body condition score (BCS) adjustments.[94,95]

CONCLUSIONS

Especially in early lactating dairy cows, hepatic lipidosis remains a major issue for animal health and welfare. Besides economic losses due to reduced lactational and reproductive performance, close associations with concomitantly occurring infectious and metabolic health disorders, in particular ketosis, exist. Excessive lipolysis and limited capacities for hepatic oxidation of fatty acids and TAG export are the primary causes for the development of both hepatic lipidosis and ketosis. Despite the similarities in cause, hepatic lipidosis is a direct and indirect disease component of other ruminant metabolic diseases. Particularly, the impaired hepatic function due to increased TAG accumulation (eg, decreased gluconeogenesis, synthesis of lipoproteins, steroid hormones, clearance of endotoxins) at a concomitantly inflammatory status actively supports the development of further metabolic diseases.

SUMMARY

Hepatic lipidosis occurs primarily during the first weeks of lactation in dairy cows as a result of excessive lipolysis beyond the concomitant capacity for beta-oxidation and hepatic export of triglycerides. Besides economic losses due to reduced lactational and reproductive performance, close associations with concomitantly occurring infectious and metabolic health disorders, in particular ketosis, exist. The infiltration of fat in hepatocytes manifests in an altered histologic structure and is accompanied by changes in their function. Hence, hepatic lipidosis is not only the consequence of the postpartal negative energy balance but also a disease component actively involved in the cause of further health disorders. In this paper, the pathophysiological pathways leading to the hepatic triglyceride accumulation, disturbances of metabolic status, impairment of immunocompetence, and reproductive performance are elucidated. Changes of concentrations of metabolites, endocrine factors, and other compounds in serum are able to alter metabolic adaptation and the responsiveness of the immune system. Furthermore, a reduced clearance of various compounds partly increases their toxicity, negatively affects synthesis of hormones, and tissue responsiveness.

CLINICS CARE POINTS

- Prevention and treatment of hepatic lipidosis indirectly follows that for ketosis (glucogenic precursors, glucocorticoids, insulin, niacin, and so forth).
- Treatment success depends on the severity of hepatic fat infiltration.
- Preventive measures in dairy cow management to avoid excessive metabolic imbalances reduce the degree of hepatic lipidosis (no overconditioned cows, high feed intake after parturition).

DISCLOSURE

The author declares no conflict of interest.

REFERENCES

1. Grummer RR. Etiology of lipid-related metabolic disorders in periparturient dairy cows. J Dairy Sci 1993;76(12):3882–96.
2. Bobe G, Young JW, Beitz DC. Invited review: pathology, etiology, prevention, and treatment of fatty liver in dairy cows. J Dairy Sci 2004;87(10):3105–24.
3. Gross JJ, Schwarz FJ, Eder K, et al. Liver fat content and lipid metabolism in dairy cows during early lactation and during a mid-lactation feed restriction. J Dairy Sci 2013;96(8):5008–17.

4. Drackley JK, ADSA Foundation Scholar Award. Biology of dairy cows during the transition period: the final frontier? J Dairy Sci 1999;82(11):2259–73.
5. Herdt TH. Relationship of fat metabolism to health and performance in dairy cattle. Bovine Pract. 1991;26:92–5.
6. Herdt TH. Ruminant adaptation to negative energy balance. Influences on the etiology of ketosis and fatty liver. Vet Clin North Am Food Anim Pract 2000; 16(2):215.
7. Pinedo P, Melendez P. Liver Disorders Associated with Metabolic Imbalances in Dairy Cows. Vet Clin North Am Food Anim Pract 2022;38(3):433–46.
8. Wensing T, Kruip T, Geelen MJH, et al. Postpartum fatty liver in high-producing dairy cows in practice and in animal studies. The connection with health, production and reproduction problems. Comp Haematol Int 1997;7:167–71.
9. Jorritsma R, Jorritsma H, Schukken YH, et al. Relationships between fatty liver and fertility and some periparturient diseases in commercial Dutch dairy herds. Theriogenology 2000;54(7):1065–74.
10. Jorritsma R, Jorritsma H, Schukken YH, et al. Prevalence and indicators of postpartum fatty infiltration of the liver in nine commercial dairy herds in the Netherlands. Livest Prod Sci 2001;68:53–60.
11. Kalaitzakis E, Panousis N, Roubies N, et al. Clinicopathological evaluation of downer dairy cows with fatty liver. Can Vet J 2010;51(6):615–22.
12. Dohoo IR. The effects of calving to first service interval on reproductive performance in normal cows and cows with postpartal disease. Can Vet J 1983; 24(11):343–6.
13. McArt JAA, Nydam DV, Oetzel GR. Epidemiology of subclinical ketosis in early lactation dairy cattle. J Dairy Sci 2012;95(9):5056–66.
14. Suthar VS, Canelas-Raposo J, Deniz A, et al. Prevalence of subclinical ketosis and relationships with postpartum diseases in European dairy cows. J Dairy Sci 2013;96(5):2925–38.
15. Brunner N, Groeger S, Canelas Raposo J, et al. Prevalence of subclinical ketosis and production diseases in dairy cows in Central and South America, Africa, Asia, Australia, New Zealand, and Eastern Europe. Transl Anim Sci 2018;3(1): 84–92.
16. Baird GD. Primary ketosis in the high-producing dairy cow: clinical and subclinical disorders, treatment, prevention, and outlook. J Dairy Sci 1982;65(1):1–10.
17. Duffield T. Subclinical ketosis in lactating dairy cattle. Vet Clin North Am Food Anim Pract 2000;16(2):231.
18. McArt JA, Nydam DV, Oetzel GR, et al. Elevated non-esterified fatty acids and β-hydroxybutyrate and their association with transition dairy cow performance. Vet J 2013;198(3):560–70.
19. van der Kolk JH, Gross JJ, Gerber V, et al. Disturbed bovine mitochondrial lipid metabolism: a review. Vet Q 2017;37(1):262–73.
20. Raboisson D, Mounié M, Maigné E. Diseases, reproductive performance, and changes in milk production associated with subclinical ketosis in dairy cows: a meta-analysis and review. J Dairy Sci 2014;97(12):7547–63.
21. Walsh RB, Walton JS, Kelton DF, et al. The effect of subclinical ketosis in early lactation on reproductive performance of postpartum dairy cows. J Dairy Sci 2007;90(6):2788–96.
22. Duffield TF, Lissemore KD, McBride BW, et al. Impact of hyperketonemia in early lactation dairy cows on health and production. J Dairy Sci 2009;92(2):571–80.
23. Ospina PA, Nydam DV, Stokol T, et al. Evaluation of nonesterified fatty acids and beta-hydroxybutyrate in transition dairy cattle in the northeastern United States:

Critical thresholds for prediction of clinical diseases. J Dairy Sci 2010;93(2): 546–54.
24. McArt JA, Nydam DV, Overton MW. Hyperketonemia in early lactation dairy cattle: a deterministic estimate of component and total cost per case. J Dairy Sci 2015; 98(3):2043–54.
25. Cainzos JM, Andreu-Vazquez C, Guadagnini M, et al. A systematic review of the cost of ketosis in dairy cattle. J Dairy Sci 2022;105(7):6175–95.
26. FAOSTAT. Statistics Division. Food and Agriculture Organization of the United Nations. Available at: https://www.fao.org/faostat/en/#data. Accessed November 30, 2022.
27. Capper JL, Cady RA, Bauman DE. The environmental impact of dairy production: 1944 compared with 2007. J Anim Sci 2009;87(6):2160–7.
28. von Keyserlingk MA, Martin NP, Kebreab E, et al. Invited review: Sustainability of the US dairy industry. J Dairy Sci 2013;96(9):5405–25.
29. Gross J, van Dorland HA, Bruckmaier RM, et al. Performance and metabolic profile of dairy cows during a lactational and deliberately induced negative energy balance with subsequent realimentation. J Dairy Sci 2011;94(4):1820–30.
30. Gross JJ, Bruckmaier RM. Invited review: Metabolic challenges and adaptation during different functional stages of the mammary gland in dairy cows: Perspectives for sustainable milk production. J Dairy Sci 2019;102(4):2828–43.
31. Bauman DE, Currie WB. Partitioning of nutrients during pregnancy and lactation: a review of mechanisms involving homeostasis and homeorhesis. J Dairy Sci 1980;63(9):1514–29.
32. Bell AW. Regulation of organic nutrient metabolism during transition from late pregnancy to early lactation. J Anim Sci 1995;73(9):2804–19.
33. Bruckmaier RM, Gross JJ. Lactational challenges in transition dairy cows. Anim Prod Sci 2017;57:1471–81.
34. LeBlanc S. Monitoring metabolic health of dairy cattle in the transition period. J Reprod Dev 2010;56(Suppl):S29–35.
35. Douglas GN, Overton TR, Bateman HG 2nd, et al. Prepartal plane of nutrition, regardless of dietary energy source, affects periparturient metabolism and dry matter intake in Holstein cows. J Dairy Sci 2006;89(6):2141–57.
36. Roche JR, Friggens NC, Kay JK, et al. Invited review: Body condition score and its association with dairy cow productivity, health, and welfare. J Dairy Sci 2009; 92(12):5769–801.
37. Rukkwamsuk T, Kruip TA, Wensing T. Relationship between overfeeding and overconditioning in the dry period and the problems of high producing dairy cows during the postparturient period. Vet Q 1999;21(3):71–7.
38. Herdt TH, Stevens JB, Olson WG, et al. Blood concentrations of beta hydroxybutyrate in clinically normal Holstein-Friesian herds and in those with a high prevalence of clinical ketosis. Am J Vet Res 1981;42(3):503–6.
39. Goff JP, Horst RL. Physiological changes at parturition and their relationship to metabolic disorders. J Dairy Sci 1997;80(7):1260–8.
40. Ingvartsen KL, Dewhurst RJ, Friggens NC. On the relationship between lactational performance and health: Is it yield or metabolic imbalance that cause production diseases in dairy cattle? A position paper. Livest Prod Sci 2003;83: 277–308.
41. Ingvartsen KL, Moyes KM. Factors contributing to immunosuppression in the dairy cow during the periparturient period. Jpn J Vet Res 2015;63(Suppl 1): S15–24.

42. Gross JJ. Limiting factors for milk production in dairy cows: perspectives from physiology and nutrition. J Anim Sci 2022;100(3):skac044.
43. Wankhade PR, Manimaran A, Kumaresan A, et al. Metabolic and immunological changes in transition dairy cows: A review. Vet World 2017;10(11):1367–77.
44. Rhoads RP, Kim JW, Leury BJ, et al. Insulin increases the abundance of the growth hormone receptor in liver and adipose tissue of periparturient dairy cows. J Nutr 2004;134(5):1020–7.
45. Block SS, Butler WR, Ehrhardt RA, et al. Decreased concentration of plasma leptin in periparturient dairy cows is caused by negative energy balance. J Endocrinol 2001;171(2):339–48.
46. Kuhla B, Metges CC, Hammon HM. Endogenous and dietary lipids influencing feed intake and energy metabolism of periparturient dairy cows. Domest Anim Endocrinol 2016;56(Suppl):S2–10.
47. Locher LF, Meyer N, Weber EM, et al. Hormone-sensitive lipase protein expression and extent of phosphorylation in subcutaneous and retroperitoneal adipose tissues in the periparturient dairy cow. J Dairy Sci 2011;94(9):4514–23.
48. Kobayashi Y, Boyd CK, Bracken CJ, et al. Reduced growth hormone receptor (GHR) messenger ribonucleic acid in liver of periparturient cattle is caused by a specific down-regulation of GHR 1A that is associated with decreased insulin-like growth factor I. Endocrinology 1999;140(9):3947–54.
49. Gross J, van Dorland HA, Schwarz FJ, et al. Endocrine changes and liver mRNA abundance of somatotropic axis and insulin system constituents during negative energy balance at different stages of lactation in dairy cows. J Dairy Sci 2011;94(7):3484–94.
50. Kessler EC, Gross JJ, Bruckmaier RM. Different adaptation of IGF-I and its IGFBPs in dairy cows during a negative energy balance in early lactation and a negative energy balance induced by feed restriction in mid lactation. Vet Med Czech 2013;58:459–67.
51. Soeters MR, Sauerwein HP, Faas L, et al. Effects of insulin on ketogenesis following fasting in lean and obese men. Obesity 2009;17:1326–31.
52. Aschenbach JR, Kristensen NB, Donkin SS, et al. Gluconeogenesis in dairy cows: the secret of making sweet milk from sour dough. IUBMB Life 2010;62(12):869–77.
53. White HM. The Role of TCA Cycle Anaplerosis in Ketosis and Fatty Liver in Periparturient Dairy Cows. Animals (Basel) 2015;5(3):793–802.
54. Sato H, Matsumoto M, Hanasaka S. Relations between plasma acetate, 3-hydroxybutyrate, FFA, glucose levels and energy nutrition in lactating dairy cows. J Vet Med Sci 1999;61(5):447–51.
55. Sugden MC, Bulmer K, Holness MJ. Fuel-sensing mechanisms integrating lipid and carbohydrate utilization. Biochem Soc Trans 2001;29(Pt 2):272–8.
56. Kessler EC, Gross JJ, Bruckmaier RM, et al. Cholesterol metabolism, transport, and hepatic regulation in dairy cows during transition and early lactation. J Dairy Sci 2014;97(9):5481–90.
57. Gross JJ, Kessler EC, Albrecht C, et al. Response of the cholesterol metabolism to a negative energy balance in dairy cows depends on the lactational stage. PLoS One 2015;10(6):e0121956.
58. Hoyumpa AM Jr, Greene HL, Dunn GD, et al. Fatty liver: biochemical and clinical considerations. Am J Dig Dis 1975;20:1142–70.
59. Morrow DA, Hillman D, Dade AW, et al. Clinical investigation of a dairy herd with the fat cow syndrome. J Am Vet Med Assoc 1979;174(2):161–7.

60. Veenhuizen JJ, Drackley JK, Richard MJ, et al. Metabolic changes in blood and liver during development and early treatment of experimental fatty liver and ketosis in cows. J Dairy Sci 1991;74(12):4238–53.
61. Breukink HJ, Wensing T. Pathophysiology of the liver in high yielding dairy cows and its consequences for health and production. Isr J Vet Med 1997;52:66–72.
62. Cadórniga-Valiño C, Grummer RR, Armentano LE, et al. Effects of fatty acids and hormones on fatty acid metabolism and gluconeogenesis in bovine hepatocytes. J Dairy Sci 1997;80(4):646–56.
63. Kuhla B, Albrecht D, Kuhla S, et al. Proteome analysis of fatty liver in feed-deprived dairy cows reveals interaction of fuel sensing, calcium, fatty acid, and glycogen metabolism. Physiol Genomics 2009;37(2):88–98.
64. Imhasly S, Naegeli H, Baumann S, et al. Metabolomic biomarkers correlating with hepatic lipidosis in dairy cows. BMC Vet Res 2014;10:122.
65. Wang J, Zhu X, She G, et al. Serum hepatokines in dairy cows: periparturient variation and changes in energy-related metabolic disorders. BMC Vet Res 2018;14(1):236.
66. Ljubuncic P, Tanne Z, Bomzon A. Ursodeoxycholic acid suppresses extent of lipid peroxidation in diseased liver in experimental cholestatic liver disease. Dig Dis Sci 2000;45(10):1921–8.
67. Alvarez C, Nelms C, D'Addio V, et al. The pancreatic duct epithelium in vitro: bile acid injury and the effect of epidermal growth factor. Surgery 1997;122(2):476–84.
68. Katoh N. Relevance of apolipoproteins in the development of fatty liver and fatty liver-related peripartum diseases in dairy cows. J Vet Med Sci 2002;64(4):293–307.
69. Drackley JK, Richard MJ, Beitz DC, et al. Metabolic changes in dairy cows with ketonemia in response to feed restriction and dietary 1,3-butanediol. J Dairy Sci 1992;75(6):1622–34.
70. Gruffat D, Durand D, Graulet B, et al. Regulation of VLDL synthesis and secretion in the liver. Reprod Nutr Dev 1996;36(4):375–89.
71. Mizutani H, Sako T, Toyoda Y, et al. Preliminary studies on hepatic carnitine palmitoyltransferase in dairy cattle with or without fatty liver. Vet Res Commun 1999;23(8):475–80.
72. Rukkwamsuk T, Wensing T, Geelen MJ. Effect of overfeeding during the dry period on regulation of adipose tissue metabolism in dairy cows during the periparturient period. J Dairy Sci 1998;81(11):2904–11.
73. Rukkwamsuk T, Wensing T, Geelen MJ. Effect of overfeeding during the dry period on the rate of esterification in adipose tissue of dairy cows during the periparturient period. J Dairy Sci 1999;82(6):1164–9.
74. Strang BD, Bertics SJ, Grummer RR, et al. Relationship of triglyceride accumulation to insulin clearance and hormonal responsiveness in bovine hepatocytes. J Dairy Sci 1998;81(3):740–7.
75. West HJ. Effect on liver function of acetonaemia and the fat cow syndrome in cattle. Res Vet Sci 1990;48(2):221–7.
76. Hill AW, Reid IM, Collins RA. Influence of liver fat on experimental Escherichia coli mastitis in periparturient cows. Vet Rec 1985;117(21):549–51.
77. Suriyasathaporn W, Heuer C, Noordhuizen-Stassen EN, et al. Hyperketonemia and the impairment of udder defense: a review. Vet Res 2000;31(4):397–412.
78. Shi J, Gilbert GE, Kokubo Y, et al. Role of the liver in regulating numbers of circulating neutrophils. Blood 2001;98(4):1226–30.

79. Abuelo A, Gandy JC, Neuder L, et al. Short communication: Markers of oxidant status and inflammation relative to the development of claw lesions associated with lameness in early lactation cows. J Dairy Sci 2016;99(7):5640–8.
80. Gross JJ, Kawashima C, Dohme-Meier F, et al. Postpartal resumption of ovarian activity in dairy cows: Implications for herbage-based feeding systems in Switzerland. Schweiz Arch Tierheilkd 2020;162(11):667–74.
81. Comin A, Gerin D, Cappa A, et al. The effect of an acute energy deficit on the hormone profile of dominant follicles in dairy cows. Theriogenology 2002;58(5): 899–910.
82. Jorritsma R, Wensing T, Kruip TA, et al. Metabolic changes in early lactation and impaired reproductive performance in dairy cows. Vet Res 2003;34(1):11–26.
83. Geelen MJ, Wensing T. Studies on hepatic lipidosis and coinciding health and fertility problems of high-producing dairy cows using the "Utrecht fatty liver model of dairy cows". A review. Vet Q. 2006;28(3):90–104.
84. Heinonen K, Gröhn Y, Lindberg LA, et al. The effect of mild fat infiltration in the liver on the fertility of Finnish Ayrshire cows. Acta Vet Scand 1987;28(2):151–5.
85. Sheldon IM, Noakes DE, Rycroft AN, et al. Influence of uterine bacterial contamination after parturition on ovarian dominant follicle selection and follicle growth and function in cattle. Reproduction 2002;123(6):837–45.
86. Grummer RR. Nutritional and management strategies for the prevention of fatty liver in dairy cattle. Vet J 2008;176:10–20.
87. Coleman DN, Alharthi A, Lopreiato V, et al. Choline supply during negative nutrient balance alters hepatic cystathionine β-synthase, intermediates of the methionine cycle and transsulfuration pathway, and liver function in Holstein cows. J Dairy Sci 2019;102:8319–31.
88. Humer E, Bruggeman G, Zebeli Q. A Meta-Analysis on the Impact of the Supplementation of Rumen-Protected Choline on the Metabolic Health and Performance of Dairy Cattle. Animals (Basel) 2019;9:566.
89. Cooke RF, Silva Del Río N, Caraviello DZ, et al. Supplemental choline for prevention and alleviation of fatty liver in dairy cattle. J Dairy Sci 2007;90:2413–8.
90. Gerloff BJ. Dry cow management for the prevention of ketosis and fatty liver in dairy cows. Vet Clin North Am Food Anim Pract 2000;16:283–92.
91. Chen J, Gross JJ, van Dorland HA, et al. Effects of dry period length and dietary energy source on metabolic status and hepatic gene expression of dairy cows in early lactation. J Dairy Sci 2015;98:1033–45.
92. Chen J, Remmelink GJ, Gross JJ, et al. Effects of dry period length and dietary energy source on milk yield, energy balance, and metabolic status of dairy cows over 2 consecutive years: Effects in the second year. J Dairy Sci 2016;99: 4826–38.
93. Kok A, Chen J, Kemp B, et al. Review: Dry period length in dairy cows and consequences for metabolism and welfare and customised management strategies. Animal 2019;13(S1):s42–51.
94. Sehested J, Gaillard C, Lehmann JO, et al. Review: extended lactation in dairy cattle. Animal 2019;13(S1):s65–74.
95. van Knegsel ATM, Burgers EEA, Ma J, et al. Extending lactation length: consequences for cow, calf, and farmer. J Anim Sci 2022;100:skac220.